An Odd Kind of Fame

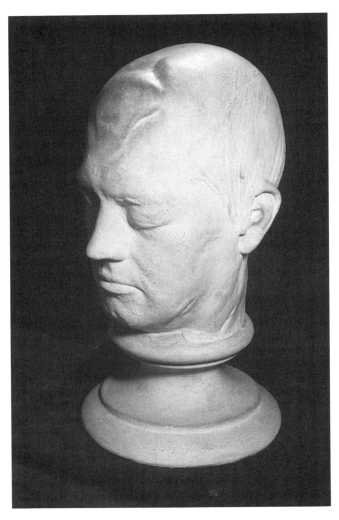

Life mask of Phineas Gage, probably made for Henry Jacob Bigelow in late 1849 From the late Dr. H. M. Constantian of Worcester, Massachusetts, and reproduced by courtesy of the Warren Anatomical Museum, Harvard University.

An Odd Kind of Fame

Stories of Phineas Gage

Malcolm Macmillan

A Bradford Book
The MIT Press
Cambridge, Massachusetts
London, England

This book was set in Sabon by Asco Typesetters, Hong Kong.
Printed and bound in the United States of America.

Library of Congress Cataloging-in-Publication Data

Macmillan, Malcolm, 1929–
  An odd kind of fame : stories of Phineas Gage / Malcolm Macmillan.
    p.   cm.
  "A Bradford book."
  Includes bibliographical references and index.
  ISBN 0-262-13363-6 (alk. paper)
  1. Gage, Phineas—Health. 2. Brain damage—Patients—United States—
Biography. 3. Split brain—History. 4. Psychosurgery—History. 5. Brain—
Localization of functions—History. I. Title.
RC387.5.G34 M33   2000
617.4'81044'092—dc21
[B]   99-056640

Contents

Preface

An Odd Kind of Fame would not have been possible without the help of a very large number of people over a very large number of years. Most of these I have acknowledged at the appropriate part of the text, but I owe very special thanks to India Tresselt of Moretown, New Hampshire. My being in Melbourne meant that she had to be a long-distance research assistant, and she became the most extraordinary one for whom I could have wished. Mara Blosfelds, now of Perth, but then living in Boston, Massachusetts, worked equally competently at completing much of the newspaper reading and record locating. Meanwhile, back in Australia, Dr. Elizabeth Bednall, Ms. Ruth Francis, and Mr. Geoff Griffin did sterling work in locating medical literature for me, mostly via the *Index Catalogue of the Surgeon-General's Library*. I have to thank Mrs. Marian Marquand, genealogist of San Francisco, for establishing the true date of Gage's death and her attempts to trace Gage descendants; the late Dr. Harold Constantian of the Worcester District Medical Society of Massachusetts for leads to the story of Dr. Edward Higginson Williams; Dr. Carol Rifelj of Middlebury College, Vermont, for providing me with my first stock of maps, gazetteers, and other basic information about Vermont and New Hampshire; Dr. Elfriede Ihsen of Melbourne for making a working translation of the key parts of Burckhardt's monograph-sized paper describing his attempts to treat insanity by operating on the brain; and Ken Nahigian of San Francisco.

I am especially indebted to Richard J. Wolfe, then in charge of rare books and manuscripts at the Francis A. Countway Library, Harvard University. He introduced me to Dr. Ken Tyler, through whom I was to meet Dr. Rick Tyler, and he told me about Fred Barker's work and gave me Fred's address. Among other things, Dick directed me or my helpers to J. B. S. Jackson's account of his visit in August 1849 to Lebanon to see Phineas, to the records of the Boston Society for Medical Improvement, and to the letters of David Ferrier about Gage to Henry Pickering Bowditch. Most of what I know about John Martyn Harlow has come from Linda McSweeny, Kathleen O'Doherty, Paul Uek and Tom Smith of the Woburn Public Library, Woburn, Massachusetts. Mara and I both benefited considerably from the very expert assistance of Joyce Ann Tracy, Joanne Chaison, and Tom Knoles of the American Antiquarian Society, Worcester, Massachusetts, and through the kindness of John B. Hench of the Society, I was able to make the best use of my short time at the library by being able to stay in the Society's Daniels-Goddard House, conveniently situated across the road from it. For finding much important information about John Martyn Harlow, Phineas Gage, or Edward Higginson Williams I have to thank Lee Kugler and Lauren Rosen of Boston; Paul Carnahan and his staff at the Vermont State Library in Montpelier, Vermont; David Cramer and Barbara Krieger at Dartmouth College, Hanover, New Hampshire; William Copeley at the New Hampshire State Historical Society in Concord; and Nancy Bacon at the Norman Williams Public Library, Woodstock, Vermont. At all four of these libraries I was also able to make my own searches of their holdings. Liz Marrs and Elizabeth Broad of the Deakin University Library and Brenda Tunbridge of the Biomedical Library, Monash University, helped enormously with references and bibliographic details. Eric Linderman of the College of Physicians of Philadelphia and J. O'Hara of the Massachusetts Medical Society found some especially important details about Harlow. The many other archivists, librarians, and libraries who helped in particularly important ways include Carole Hughes, University of Vermont, Burlington, Vermont; Eva Murphy, Fingold Library, State House, Boston, Massachusetts; David Gunner and Paul Aaron, Warren Anatomical Museum, Harvard University; Julian Holland, Macleay Museum, University of Sydney, Sydney; Samuel Davis and Dan Flanagan, Thomas Jefferson University; Ruth Ann Kierniemen, Green Mountain College, Pultney, Vermont; Dorothy Whitcomb, University of Wisconsin, Madison; Nancy J. Halli, Historical Society of Pennsylvania; Jeff Korman, Enoch Pratt Free Library, Baltimore, Maryland; and the staff of the New England Historic and Genealogical Society Library, Boston; the Massachusetts Historical Society, Boston; the Barcroft Library, University of California, Berkeley; the Green and Lane Libraries, Stanford University; and the Library of the University of Massachusetts, Amherst.

Because the anniversary of Phineas Gage's accident was commemorated during the final phases of writing, I was fortunate enough to meet many people from Cavendish and nearby who were working to make the commemoration the success it undoubtedly became. Despite their heavy work schedules, they found time to help me clarify a host of minor details, and I hope they recognize their contributions in *An Odd Kind of Fame*. They are Denise Natale, Stacia Spaulding, and Tom Sabo of the commemoration committee, and Linda Welch and Bob Drake. In my attempt to document various aspects of the stories about Phineas Gage's pre- and postaccident life, a number of historical and genealogical societies, many of them quite small, provided me with very large amounts of assistance. These include the historical societies of Cavendish, Vermont (Carmine Guica, Sandra Stearns, and Stacia Spaulding), Rutland, Vermont (Jim Davidson, Dawn Hance), New York (Jan Anderson), Lebanon, New Hampshire (Robert Leavitt), and Enfield, New Hampshire (Marjorie Carr, Frances Childs); the Connecticut State Historical Society, Hartford, Connecticut (Judith Ellen Johnson); the Andover Historical Society, Andover, Massachusetts; and the Manchester Historical Society, Manchester, New Hampshire.

I was helped considerably by the railroad historian Jerry Fox of Essex Junction, Vermont, and the works of canal and railway construction historians Peter Way and Walter Licht in arriving at an understanding of the complexities of the background of canal and railroad construction. The very special debt I owe to the many historians of popular entertainments, museums, and circuses in the United States in the nineteenth century is acknowledged in Appendix H. Even though they were unsuccessful, I am grateful to Fabian Aboitiz and Juan S. Gomez-Jeria of the Universidad de Chile, Santiago, for trying so hard to find traces of the time Phineas Gage worked in Chile. Portia Vescio was similarly unsuccessful in finding any record of Phineas in relation to the Boston police.

Halstead, N. Gray, Carew and English, San Francisco, were instrumental in letting me see N. Gray and Co.'s *Funeral Record 1850 to 1862*. Michael Svanevik introduced me to the history of San Francisco's netherworld and joined in the unsuccessful search for records of Gage's exhumation, as did Serafin Mora, General Manager of Cypress Lawn Cemetery, who also took me to the Pioneer Memorial that marks the place where most of Gage now rests. D. Peter Petrakis, also of Cypress Lawn, later assisted me in tracing the burials of other members of the Gage and Shattuck families.

When I was still a member of the Department of Psychology at Monash University, Professor Ross Day of that department provided encouragement as well as ensuring that material and technical support was always available. Leslie Anderson, Cathy Cook, and Cheryl Roberts, Technical Officers, Vladimir Kohout, Photographer, and Judy Sack and Rosemary Williams, Illustrators, all of that department, gave absolutely unstintingly to the project. One phase of the work was supported by a Monash Special Research Grant of $1,300, and another by a grant of $4,400 from the Australian Research Grants Committee. I owe special thanks to my colleagues Dr. Harry Whitaker, who arranged for me to spend time in his department at Northern Michigan University in Marquette, Dr. John Kihlstrom for inviting me to the University of Arizona at Tucson and to Yale where, at the latter, I was able to search for archival material, and Emeritus Professor Frederick Crews, University of California at Berkeley, and Betty Crews, who between them extended hospitality and arranged important introductions for me. I am particularly indebted to my good friend and colleague Nicholas J. Wade, Professor of Visual Psychology at The University, Dundee, for astute advice, for the rare material he obtained for me and, together with Christine Wade, for providing me with hospitality and a base from which to search in Edinburgh and Aberdeen.

I doubt that I would have been able to bring *An Odd Kind of Fame* to a close without the considerable help of my very great friend Dr. Edith Bavin of the Department of Psychology at La Trobe University in Melbourne. She bore the greater burden of our Gage-hunting trips to the United Kingdom and the United States, including driving in the United States, and her capable assistance, her insights, and her careful attention to detail helped solve many of the problems that arose in the course of the work.

I owe special thanks to four people at MIT Press: to Amy Pierce and Michael Rutter for encouraging me to publish with them, to Melissa Vaughn for steering me painlessly—almost—through the production stages, and to Michael Harrup who, as copy editor, provided expert guidance and interesting exchanges over the peculiarities of American as compared with Australian English.

I am extremely grateful to the School of Psychology at Deakin University for giving me the opportunity of completing this work by appointing me to an Adjunct-Professorship after I was retired from active association with Monash University.

Malcolm Macmillan
Box Hill and Burwood, January 1999

Acknowledgments

For generously allowing the use of material contained in some of my previously published papers I thank the following:

Brain and Cognition for A wonderful journey through skull and brains: The travels of Mr. Gage's tamping iron, 1986, 5: 67–107; Inhibition and the control of behaviour: From Gall to Freud via Phineas Gage and the frontal lobes, 1992, 19: 72–104; and The concept of inhibition in some nineteenth century theories of thinking, 1996, 30: 4–19 (© Academic Press);

Journal of the History of the Neurosciences for Experimental and clinical studies of localisation before Flourens, 1994, 4: 139–154; Phineas Gage's contribution to brain surgery, 1996, 5: 56–77; and Restoring Phineas Gage: A 150th. retrospective (2000), 9: 42–62. (© Swets and Zeitlinger);

Lawrence Erlbaum and Associates for Phineas Gage: A case for all reasons, in C. Code, C.-W. Wallesch, A.-R. Lecours, and Y. Joanette, eds., *Classic Cases in Neuropsychology* (pp. 243–262), 1996, London: Erlbaum (© Lawrence Erlbaum and Associates).

1

Introduction

In investigating the reports on diseases and injuries of the brain I am constantly being amazed at the inexactitude and distortion to which they are subjected by men who have some pet theory to support.

—David Ferrier writing to Henry Pickering Bowditch about Gage, 12 October 1877

An Odd Kind of Fame is about a human curiosity: an otherwise unremarkable railway construction worker named Phineas Gage whose quite remarkable injury to his brain in an accident 150 years ago turned him into a major curiosity of medicine, a status that he enjoys, if it can be so put, to this day. Because his behavior changed so dramatically after the injury, his case is also judged to be the first and possibly most important to reveal something of the relation between the brain and complex personality characteristics. Yet in searching for the facts about him, it soon became obvious that little could be said about the changes the injury produced in his behavior, and even less about the parts of his brain that were injured.

My search for the facts about Phineas Gage began about 1983 in a very minor way. I merely required an account of him to include as part of a set of historically based lectures introducing students to various problems in psychology. Each lecture was structured around some issue that had been important in the history of the science and that was currently relevant. Although the emphasis was on the conceptual aspects of the study of the topic, as far as was possible I used original descriptions of the investigations, and as much original pictorial material as I could conveniently find. But for the topic of the localization of brain function, in which I wanted to use Phineas Gage's case, finding material on him proved very difficult. From student days I had some appreciation of the importance ascribed to the case and expected there would be a reasonably extensive literature on it. This turned out not to be true. There were many mentions of him, but few papers solely or mainly about him. There were also plenty of pictures of him (or rather his life mask), his skull, and his tamping iron, but only the reports of John Martyn Harlow from 1848, Henry Jacob Bigelow from 1850, and J. B. S. Jackson from 1870 were available in Australian libraries (and the first of these has now disappeared). On a short study leave in San Francisco that same year, I found the same difficulty in locating holdings of these papers, more in finding holdings of Harlow's crucial follow-up report of 1868, and even more in finding newspaper accounts of his accident and eventual death. Nevertheless, about a year after beginning my search, the first version of *An Odd Kind of Fame* came into existence in the form of a paper read on 16 March 1984 to the Staff Colloquium of the Department of Psychology at Monash University. Dr. Lauren Harris, a proper neuropsychologist, to whom I sent a copy for an opinion, was sufficiently interested to pass it on to Dr. Harry Whitaker, editor of *Brain and Cognition*, in which journal it appeared in 1986. Dr. Whitaker's appreciation, together with the response to the paper itself, encouraged me to develop the work into this book.

The problems I found in investigating Phineas Gage were, I now realize, because I was the victim of what might be termed professional overestimation: because Phineas Gage was said to be important in psychology, everyone would have been interested in him; because his survival was so remarkable, someone must have made a major study of him. Neither was the case. He had made no newspaper headlines—not only because they had hardly been invented in 1848—because the story of his accident, survival, and eventual death had, for the most part, gone unnoticed.

Partly because so little is known about Phineas Gage, and partly because of the grossness of the errors in what is said about him, I have tried in *An Odd Kind of Fame* to describe accurately what we do know, and have done so chronologically. This reflects my belief that it is only when the facts about Gage's case are properly understood in the context of their times that the interpretations of him can be assessed and the significance of his case itself fully appreciated.

The Structure of the Book

Although the chapters comprising *An Odd Kind of Fame* fall into four groups, the book itself is not so divided. Chapters 2 through 6, which constitute the first group, cover Phineas Gage's background and work, his accident, its consequences, and his subsequent history. Chapter 2 begins with a short discussion of the accident that befell Phineas in September 1848, outline his family and personal background, situate his work as a railroad construction foreman in the work and employment practices of the time, and describe the events immediately following his injury. Chapter 3 is devoted to an analysis of contemporary newspaper and medical reports of the accident and its consequences. Appearing between late 1848 and Gage's recovery the following year, both kinds of report show an increasing fascination with the bizarre nature of the case. The medical treatment that Gage received from Dr. John Martyn Harlow is set out in chapter 4 and evaluated against the treatment of similar cases. How his case was gradually adopted as a standard against which others were judged is also traced. From the beginning there was disagreement about the passage of the tamping iron through Gage's skull and which parts of his brain had been damaged; chapter 5 is therefore devoted to the problems of assessing the damage to his skull and brain. I show that modern attempts to resolve the disagreements have not, despite their in-genuity, been successful. The related topic of assessing the psychological damage is taken up in chapter 6. I show that we do not have enough detail about what Gage was like before or after the accident to say much more than that the psychological damage it inflicted was undoubtedly considerable. An extensive search of places that Gage visited or in which he lived and worked failed to find substantially more information than Harlow reported in 1848 and 1868. The lack of reasonably detailed knowledge about which parts of Phineas's brain were injured and about how his mental processes were changed means that we cannot draw other than the most general conclusions about brain-behavior relations from his case.

None of the material in chapters 2–6 is particularly technical or (I hope) difficult to understand. The second set of chapters may be a bit more formidable for the nonspecialist reader. This second section, con-sisting of chapters 7, 8, and 9, sets out Phineas Gage's place in the history of how functions came to be localized in the brain. That story is as complicated as the topic itself and is almost as complex as the forward and backward movements that tend, usually, to result in scientific prog-ress. I have tried to write as simply as I know how, and although I hope that the non–brain surgeon reader will be able to follow developments, the three chapters can be skimmed without too much disruption of con-tinuity, especially if the following synopsis of chapters 7, 8, and 9 is digested thoroughly. The background to localization is set out in chapter 7 with a discussion of the interdependence of knowledge of brain structures, technical methods of brain dissection, and the ways mental functions were conceptualized up to about 1800. Chapter 8 deals with the way Gall localized functions in the brain in the system that became known as phrenology, and with the physiological controversies his doctrine generated. A quite independent development that eventually localized reflex functions in the spinal cord is then contrasted with Gall's position. Simple connections between sensation and movement seen in the spinal reflex were eventually believed to exist in the brain, and a sensory-motor physiology with its accompanying psychology became possible.

Now whereas Gall's system had at least in principle offered an explanation for the effects of Gage's brain damage, nothing in these early sensory-motor conceptualizations could. The brain might be thought of as being a reflex mechanism, but no reflexes had actually been localized in it. Similarly, although new learning could be modeled in terms of the formation of new sensory-motor connections, this new physiology provided only a speculative mechanism for a will that inhibited all but one of a set of associations that led to action. Because Gage's behavior could not be incorporated within that framework, many of the framework's adherents had to disregard or even deny there had been changes in him, especially if they were unwilling to adopt Gall's explanatory system.

Chapter 9 traces two contemporaneous and related but more or less independent developments. One centers on the observations and concepts that led to the two Drs. Dax and Broca localizing a language function in the left lobe of the brain. In the battle over their theses, Gage was judged the most important contrary evidence. The other development came from the way Hughlings Jackson's analysis of epileptic seizures seemed to point to processes for movement being localized in the brain. Jackson's hypothesis was confirmed by experiments, mainly those of David Ferrier, in which the exposed brain of the dog and the monkey were stimulated directly. Ferrier found that although stimulation of the frontal lobes produced no responses, removing parts of the lobes surgically produced behavioral changes he thought resembled those seen in cases like Gage's. Basing his work on the sensory-motor physiology of the day, Ferrier proposed a hypothetical inhibitory-motor mechanism for explaining the effects of the operation, and eventually extended it to Gage. His application was crucial in rescuing Gage from obscurity, even though it forced the changes into a version of sensory-motor psychology that remained inadequate to explain them.

The little known contribution of Phineas Gage to brain surgery is brought out in chapter 10, the first of a group of three chapters exploring various applications of knowledge derived from his case. Following Ferrier, Gage's symptoms were sometimes thought of as showing a loss of inhibition, but more often they were simply classed as "mental changes." In a brief but important period in the development of brain surgery, one that had ended by the beginning of the twentieth century, early brain surgeons drew on both notions indiscriminately. In the 1930s, those who pioneered the psychosurgical procedures of lobotomy or leucotomy revived the peculiarities of their reasoning. My examination in chapter 11 of the oft-remarked connection of Gage with psychosurgery finds it to be very minor, if not entirely mythical. Chapter 12 deals with another application of the concept of inhibition in the nineteenth theory: its application to the theory of thinking formulated by Alexander Bain and David Ferrier. Variants of the theory are found in theories of "insanity" and hypnosis, and possibly in a theory of thinking put forward by Sigmund Freud. My analysis shows that almost all these applications share the defect of forcing the mechanism of inhibition to explain too much.

What we should make of how the knowledge of Gage has been transmitted forms the subject matter of chapters 13, 14, and 15. The first of these chapters analyzes some of the ways in which the Gage case is represented, and misrepresented, in popular, semifictional, and fictional works. The same distortions evident in this literature are also found in the scientific works examined in chapter 14. Many characteristics are attributed to Gage that are neither reported by Harlow nor documented elsewhere. Where the scientific misrepresentations do not come from partial or careless readings of Harlow's 1868 paper, they often attribute characteristics to Gage that were first reported in other patients, particularly those who underwent frontal lobe surgery in the 1930s. Similar attributions emerge in what purports to be Gage's subsequent history. Much of this turns out to be fable, based sometimes on careless readings of Harlow, but most frequently on not reading him at all. Correcting the errors and distortions in the representations of chapter 14 amounts to restoring our picture of Phineas Gage. On my view, that task necessarily involves trying to obtain a clearer picture of John Martyn Harlow. That search is the subject matter of chapter 15. What Harlow tells us is almost all that we know about Phineas Gage, but he gives us only a small amount of information about the changes in Gage's behavior after his accident, and what he tells us about the damage to his brain is really a best estimate. I do not believe that modern attempts to improve on this estimate have resolved the indeterminacy. But without returning to the reality presented and represented by Harlow, we will not free ourselves of the fables with which the case of Phineas Gage has already provided us. Nor will we escape new ones currently being fabricated.

Construction and Fabrication

When I began the work that became *An Odd Kind of Fame*, I intended merely to determine the bearing that Gage's injury had on our knowledge of the functions of the brain, especially its frontal lobes. Although it turned out that I soon had to include considerations of the relevance Gage's case was thought to have for a number of other topics, including phrenology, aphasia, the development of the will, the diagnosis and removal of frontal brain tumors, and psychosurgery, coping with that expansion was not difficult. What then emerged as the most interesting thing about Gage's case was the very different constructions that had been put on it at different times. None were at all arbitrary; they made very good sense from the conceptual standpoints of the different con- tributors to the (mainly) nineteenth-century debate on the localization of brain function. At one time I even thought that the positions taken in that debate were thrown into such relief by the various constructions put on Gage that the main point of tracing the history of the case might be to illuminate the debate itself.

If I now see things slightly differently, it is because of the difficulty of understanding what is meant by "construction." Are Gage, his injury, and subsequent history just a discursive "domain" brought into being or created by the words of those who have spoken and written about him? The history of the Gage case throws the problems surrounding this kind of thinking into very sharp relief. Are the different discourses or con- structions equivalently different ways of talking about Gage, or are they different ways of representing the same reality? More generally, which is primary: the word or the thing for which the word stands? If it is the former, there is no point in asking which construction is the best, but if the latter, it is appropriate to consider whether some construc- tions are more truthful than others.

The essentially self-evident point I want to make is that when we speak or write about *something*, we are speaking or writing about some *thing*, and whatever that thing is, it exists independently of our thinking, writing, and speaking about it. Consequently, we do not build or construct the thing itself, only an idea *of it*. Construction may well be of a "domain," but it is a domain fabricated from a material reality, and we make it in order to represent those aspects of the reality in which we are interested. The value of a given construction is indexed by the closeness with which it approximates that reality.

Fabrication (which I find a good synonym for much of what passes as construction) is always a concrete, sensuous, human activity carried out at a particular time, in a particular place, by particular men and women acting in particular social ways. It is never a passive, soulless, and non-human enterprise. Historically we know that human activity of this kind sometimes results in more or less true constructions and, at other times, in more or less false ones. For example, we now have no difficulty in recognizing that Galileo's "construction" of a solar system that placed our sun at its center is a reasonably true reflection of reality. Most of us also now think it makes sense to ask about the accuracy of Galileo's representation. I cannot imagine even the most dedicated modern constructionist arguing that to ask that question is meaningless.

For the constructivist argument to prevail, one would have to concede that Galileo's thesis contains no more nor less truth than earlier views like the Ptolemaic, which placed our earth at the centre. Ptolemy's was simply a different discursive domain, a different way of talking. Note that on this view, we cannot say "a different way of talking *about* it" because there is no "it" existing independently of the discourse that can be talked "about." To those who reject this thesis, may I suggest the following thought experiment (even though it is slightly flawed). Let them imagine they are members of a team of astronauts trained for the first manned space flight to Mars. As they walk out to the launching pad, they find not the one rocket they had been led to believe would be there, but two. Here they are asked to make a choice: in which capsule do they want to travel? Will their flight be the one planned and directed by Galileo, or can they be talked into being propelled toward Mars by Ptolemy? Which flight path, the one planned and directed according to Galileo's discourse or the one from the Ptolemaic domain, is more likely to get them to their destination? Where is the problem in admitting the role that historical, social, and personal factors play in determining how we think and talk about the solar system or other aspect of reality, and distinguishing between the relative truth or relative falsity of the ideas we construct of it?

With Gage, the established facts are so limited that it is relatively easy to establish what has been manufactured from them. However, if different constructions are compared with one another and we detect a difference between them, we can make little of this discrepancy without reference to the facts. For example, what purpose is served by our mere knowing that one author says Gage was unable to hold a regular job and another that he was not interested in working? Again, consider the significance of our knowing that nothing is recorded in the original corpus of facts about Gage's temper being short, or his lacking emotional responsiveness, or his being a drunkard. Constructions that attribute such characteristics to him are rather more than another discourse or just a way of talking about him: they are simply untrue.

Note that the original description of Gage is not required to represent the truth about him. It is the basis against which we can judge which of the different constructions approximates that limited body of facts more truthfully than others. After making that judgment, we may then consider the contribution the human qualities of the different investigators— their technical skills, their historically conditioned understandings, and their more personal biases and prejudices—make to a particular construction. Siting that contribution where the constructivists place it reverses an important order: words become more important than things.

More generally, we can think of the contemporary descriptions of Gage's behavior and the damage to his skull and brain as loosely analogous to that external reality from which our other and generally more important constructions derive. Allowing that analogy also makes it possible to judge how closely a given construction reflects the truth about him. There's the rub. In Gage's case we know the corpus of facts; in the more general case we don't. Does that mean we can never know? The answer is, "Yes and no." We give a much less qualified "yes" to Galileo when comparing him with Ptolemy than we do to the "no" if we compare him with Einstein. The dual answer results from the systems proposed by all three being approximations to the real state of affairs. Scientific practice—a concrete, sensuous, human activity—leads us to improve our approximations but in most instances never to match them exactly with reality. The real problem is that of the transition from theoretical idea to truth: when do we say that our approximation is close enough to the reality it represents for us to say it is true? Of course, we do make this more general decision. No one would now say that our observation that the sun's rising and setting marks stages in its journey around the earth is *only* a way of speaking. We have long since decided that Galileo's thesis is more than "hypothesis" or "theory" and that he was right to mutter under his breath, if he uttered the words at all, "But it still moves." The decision to move from "theory" to "reality" is one we make in the absence of formal rules. To say that certain representations of Gage are more accurate or truthful than others poses much less of a problem. Defending this materialist constructionist thesis against post-modernist fabrications forms a small, implicit part of *An Odd Kind of Fame*.

2

Background to Fame

Nearly 150 years ago Phineas Gage became famous as the survivor of one of the most remarkable, if not *the* most remarkable, injuries to the brain in medical history. Yet he himself was so ordinary that we do not know for certain when he was born, an uncertainty that we perhaps share with his mother. Nor did we know, until 140 years after his accident, the correct date of his death. We know hardly anything about what he was like before or after being injured, and very little about what he did during the time he survived the accident. Our knowledge of what damage was done to his brain is similarly uncertain: we have his skull and the instrument of his injury, but we do not know and cannot know which parts of his brain were injured. Nor, except in a very gross way, do we know what effect the damage had upon him. Phineas Gage is famous despite our ignorance of these things. His fame is of the kind that is, and in his case literally so, thrust upon otherwise ordinary people. The nature and origins of that fame form the subject matter of this book.

The Case of Phineas Gage

How Phineas Gage's brain was injured is vividly captured in what is apparently the first account of his accident, one written, it seems, within twenty-four hours of the event and published in the Ludlow (Vermont) *Free Soil Union*. Reprinted a few days later in the *Boston Post*, the report was there surrounded by others of more ordinary injury and death (see figure 2.1).[1]

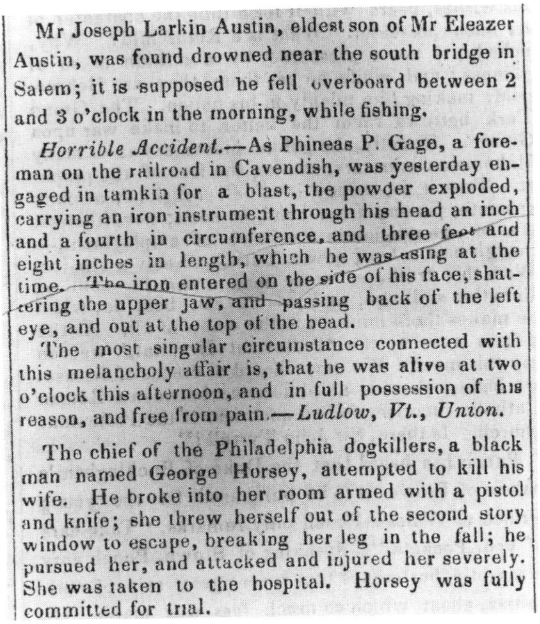

Mr Joseph Larkin Austin, eldest son of Mr Eleazer Austin, was found drowned near the south bridge in Salem; it is supposed he fell overboard between 2 and 3 o'clock in the morning, while fishing.

Horrible Accident.—As Phineas P. Gage, a foreman on the railroad in Cavendish, was yesterday engaged in tamkin for a blast, the powder exploded, carrying an iron instrument through his head an inch and a fourth in circumference, and three feet and eight inches in length, which he was using at the time. The iron entered on the side of his face, shattering the upper jaw, and passing back of the left eye, and out at the top of the head.

The most singular circumstance connected with this melancholy affair is, that he was alive at two o'clock this afternoon, and in full possession of his reason, and free from pain.—*Ludlow, Vt., Union.*

The chief of the Philadelphia dogkillers, a black man named George Horsey, attempted to kill his wife. He broke into her room armed with a pistol and knife; she threw herself out of the second story window to escape, breaking her leg in the fall; he pursued her, and attacked and injured her severely. She was taken to the hospital. Horsey was fully committed for trial.

Figure 2.1
The first report of Phineas Gage's accident. From the *Boston Post* reprinting on 21 September 1848, of the original in the *Free Soil Union* (Ludlow, Vermont). Courtesy of the American Antiquarian Society.

The damage that an iron instrument of the size given by the *Free Soil Union* could do to Gage's brain is almost unimaginable. But in fact, the iron was bigger; the report should have said it was "an inch and a fourth in diameter." Nevertheless Gage survived. Undoubtedly this was due to a number of factors, but the most important among them was the treatment he received from a relatively inexperienced local physician, John Martyn Harlow. Graduated four and a half years earlier, Harlow had been practicing in Cavendish since only January of 1845. Nevertheless, as we shall see from the two reports that Harlow published on the case in 1848 and 1868, his examination of the wound and assessment of the damage was so thorough, his immediate treatment so skillful, and his postaccident care so imaginatively flexible that Gage was well enough to return to his home in Lebanon, New Hampshire, only twelve weeks after the almost total destruction of most of his left frontal lobe.

Phineas Gage was injured at 4:30 P.M. on Wednesday, 13 September, 1848, during the construction of the Rutland and Burlington Railroad

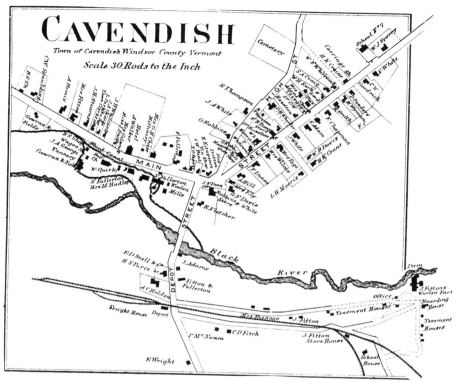

Figure 2.2
Cavendish, c. 1869
From Beers 1869.

immediately south of Duttonsville, then the principal village in the township of Cavendish in Vermont, and soon to be renamed Cavendish after it (figure 2.2). After some months of recuperation, Gage felt well enough to return to this work, but when he asked his contractors they would not give him his position back. The damage to his brain had changed him too profoundly. In 1868 Harlow said that from having been "the most efficient and capable foreman" employed by the contractors, one who was "a shrewd, smart business man," and very energetic and persistent in executing all his plans, Gage now frequently changed what he proposed doing, and was, among other things, fitful, capricious, impatient of advice, obstinate, and lacking in deference to his fellows. The change was so marked that he was, his friends said, "No longer Gage."[2]

The change was also lasting. Gage seems never again to have held a job where he exercised the level of responsibility he had once had as a foreman. According to Harlow, Gage traveled around New England, exhibiting himself and his iron, and for a time did the same at Barnum's Museum. He then worked for eighteen months in a livery stable and stagecoaching business until, four years after the accident, he left for Chile, where he worked for some seven years caring for horses and driving coaches. Ill-health eventually forced him to return to the United States, specifically to San Francisco where, after he regained his health, he was employed as a farm laborer. Not long after resuming work, Gage had an epileptic seizure, and soon had more of increasing frequency and severity. Finally the seizures killed him. Despite the massive damage to his brain that his tamping iron had caused, Gage had lived on for eleven and a half years.

Phineas Gage's fame is primarily that of a medical curiosity, few instances of people surviving similar injuries having been reported subsequently. Even today, on examining Gage's skull and iron, it seems impossible that he should have survived. But his fame is wider. His injury and personality change contributed fundamentally, although not immediately, to our understanding of the functions localized in the brain, particularly in its frontal areas. We will see that the significance of the personality charge was neither known nor appreciated until about thirty years after it was manifested, and that, even today, it is impossible to be very specific about what the Gage case tells us about those functions. Despite this limitation, LeUnes' 1974 survey of nineteenth-century papers referred to in twentieth-century textbooks of psychology found the second most frequently cited such work to be Harlow's paper reporting Gage's final status. As the twentieth century was drawing toward its close, 150 years after the accident his case continued to be mentioned in about 60 percent of introductory psychology textbooks.

The Farming Background

We are limited in what we can learn from Gage's case partly because we have little documented information about him prior to the accident, including his upbringing, education, and occupation. It seems very likely that he was an eighth-generation American of Puritan origin, a descendant of the John Gage who C. V. Gage says:

first appears in Massachusetts as one of the signers of the covenant of the First Church in Boston headed by Governor Winthrop 27th. August, 1630 and from his position in the list it is inferred that he came in Winthrop's Fleet and like the Governor, came from County Suffolk.

The *Genealogy* of Stearns, Whitcher, and Parker is more definite: John "was of Stoneham in Suffolk" and "came to America with John, the son of Governor Winthrop and landed in Salem June 12, 1630." W. M. Gage, C. V. Gage, and Stearns, Whitcher, and Parker agree that this John Gage moved from Boston to Ipswich, Massachusetts, in 1633, where the first three generations of his descendants remained.

With the fourth-generation Solomon Gage, the family seems to have moved to New Hampshire. Solomon's son, the first Phineas in the family, was born in Concord, New Hampshire, in 1772 and became the grandfather of the Phineas Gage with whom we are concerned. According to Child's *Gazetteer*, this first Phineas Gage moved to Enfield, New Hampshire, from Concord "at the age of twenty five years," where he appears in the Enfield census 1800–1840, inclusive, and the Enfield tax lists 1798–1842, inclusive.[3]

Our primary information about the family's occupation also comes from Child's *Gazetteer*. Child describes Phineas's grandfather as "one of the early settlers" of Enfield and implies that he was a farmer by saying that his son Calvin "located as a farmer on the old place, but finally removed to a farm about a mile and a half from the homestead." The occupation given in the record of the second marriage of Phineas's younger brother, Roswell Rockwell, in the New Hampshire Vital Records Office is also "farmer." Through the kindness of the late Mrs. Frances Childs of Canaan, I have been able to see the site of "the old place" on Potato Road, Enfield, as well as the site of Roswell's farm in Grafton. They are also about a mile and a half apart, but neither farmhouse now exists. "The old place," sold to John R. Dresser in 1861, was destroyed by fire in 1967, and all that remains of what was probably brother Roswell's farm are the substantial stones forming the cellar hole, in which the horses were once stabled during the severe winter months.

Roberts's compilation of Enfield records establishes that grandfather Phineas Gage married Phebe (or Phoebe) Eaton of Candia, New Hampshire, at Enfield on 19 February 1797, and that Jesse Eaton Gage, the first of their twelve children, was born at Enfield on 1 April 1798. According to the Town Records of Lebanon in the New Hampshire State Archives in Concord, Jesse, who fathered our Phineas, married Hannah

Trussell Swetland of East Lebanon, New Hampshire, on 27 April 1823. This date is confirmed by records created by the Plummer-Wills families, now in the care of Robert Leavitt, and by C. V. Gage and Roberts. Our Phineas Gage was the first of their five children, the others being Lura G., Roswell Rockwell, Dexter Prichard, and Phebe Jane.

We know most of the dates and places of birth of Phineas's brothers and sisters, but we cannot document his own with anything like the same degree of certainty. Although Harlow (1868, note of 24 September 1848) gave Gage's "native place" as "in New Hampshire" and appears to have been referring to Lebanon, we cannot be certain that he was born there. Neither he nor his birth is noted as such in the Plummer-Wills records for Lebanon, and there is no entry for him in Roberts's compilation of the vital records of Enfield, the town where some of his brothers and sisters, and most of his uncles and aunts, were born. The only definite date given by anyone for his birth is the 9 July 1823, and that appears without a source in C. V. Gage's genealogy. If he was born on that date, Phineas would have been twenty-five years and two months old at the time of his accident, an age which matches the "twenty five years" given by Harlow and Bigelow, and one not inconsistent with that recorded at his death.[4]

Phineas Gage was undeniably of farming stock and may have grown up in East Lebanon, possibly on the farm of his mother's family. However, because "Enfield" is given as the birthplace of the next two children in the family (Lura G. and Roswell Rockwell), it seems to me to be more likely that he grew up on his grandfather's farm there or on his uncle's in nearby Grafton. Although described by Harlow (1868) as "untrained in the schools," and even though no school records from the adjacent towns of Lebanon, Enfield, or Grafton seem to have survived, we can at least assume that Phineas had attended school and was literate. The figures from the U.S. Censuses of 1840 and 1850 for Grafton County (which included the towns of Enfield, Grafton, and Lebanon) show surprisingly high levels of school attendance: in 1840, the population over five and under twenty years of age was 14,830, and, from what their families reported, there were 14,047 children attending universities or academies and primary or secondary schools. The corresponding figures for 1850 give a total attendance of 13,749 of the 14,417 population within the same age range. Literacy levels were consequently high. Further, taking the numbers of "adults" in the population to be those over twenty years of age, the census data yield direct literacy rates for white adults of 99.1 percent and 99 percent for 1840 and 1850, respectively. However, because the information on which these rates were based was obtained in 1840 by simply asking the head of the household for the total number of illiterates in the family, and in 1850 by asking the same question about each family member, the true literacy rates should probably be set somewhat lower.[5]

Had Phineas been brought up on his grandfather's farm, the nearest of the Enfield schools to the Potato Road farmhouse was actually so distant from it that it would have been more convenient for him to attend Grafton District Number 11 Grafton Pond School, almost next door to what seems to have become his brother Roswell's farm, then possibly farmed by his uncle Calvin. If so, it would have provided only a limited education. Like almost all of the schools in the Grafton District, it and its teachers were regularly criticized by the Superintending Committee. From the beginning the population was too sparse to support the school there and what was said about it in 1875 is harshly revealing:

the schoolhouse is totally unfit for school purposes being a mere shelter devoid of comfort or attractions. Blackboards are wanting. Ventilation perfect, the cold winds finding egress from all points of the compass. This may have cooled the enthusiasm of both teacher and scholar.

Grafton Pond was also among the first of the schools in the district to be closed. If there were such barriers to his education, Gage overcame them. There is independent evidence that he read and wrote well enough to keep the records his occupation required.[6]

Working on the Railroad

We do not know what Phineas worked at prior to his employment on the construction of the Rutland and Burlington Railroad (R&BRR). His skills at farm work, including looking after cattle and horses and driving horse teams, survived his injury and are consistent with the New Hampshire milieu. The U.S. Census of 1840 also reveals that 23,434 of the 26,777 employed in Grafton County, or 87.5 percent, were then employed in agriculture. Further, because stone was so commonly used in constructing the foundations of buildings, the cellars, and even the fences on farms in that part of New England, the skills in selecting rock and drilling and blasting it may have been common enough for Phineas to have acquired them while working on the family farm or on others in the area. There is also the possibility that he acquired these skills on the building of one of the New Hampshire railroads that began construction ahead of the

R&BRR. For example, the Northern Railroad Company line, completed in November 1847, passed through or close to many of the towns, such as Grafton, Enfield, and Lebanon, in which members of his family lived. Phineas could also have worked in the isinglass (mica) mines and quarries for which Grafton was famous, some of which were only a short distance from his grandfather's farm. If so, he would have acquired exceptional skills in blasting because, in mining isinglass, it was important to recover the thin and fragile layers of mica imprisoned within the granite in sheets as large as possible.[7]

According to Thompson, the construction of various railways within and across Vermont had been proposed as early as about 1830, but although several companies had been incorporated by 1835, work did not commence until 1843. The Champlain and Connecticut River Railroad Company, later the Rutland and Burlington Railroad, was the more southerly of two planned to cross Vermont diagonally, in this case from Bellows Falls in the southeast, where it was to connect with lines to Boston and New York, through Rutland to Burlington on Lake Champlain, whence the St. Lawrence and the established routes to the West were readily accessible (figure 2.3). A few miles northwest of Bellows Falls, the surveyor for the Rutland and Burlington had determined that the line of the R&BRR would approach Duttonsville from the south and, a little less than half a mile from the center of the village, make a 90-degree turn to the west, toward Proctorsville. It is there that we first find Phineas Gage.[8]

To begin to understand Gage and what he was doing, we need to be guided by Harlow's clear statement that Gage was not employed directly by the Rutland and Burlington Railroad company. Rather he was employed by the firm of contractors, possibly Decker and Warner, who had won the tender for the preparation of the section of the bed of the railway that was to pass near Cavendish. Foreign as it may seem to our experience now, the foremen of such construction gangs were sometimes also independent subcontractors who had tendered competitively for the work to be performed by the gang they themselves had recruited. This tradition of so using contractors and subcontractors seems to have originated in the canal construction industries in Britain and the United States in the late 1700s and early 1800s, and to have then been adopted by the slightly later railway construction industry. Construction companies raised capital and employed engineers to survey routes and supervise work on the various sections of the canal or rail line. From the beginning

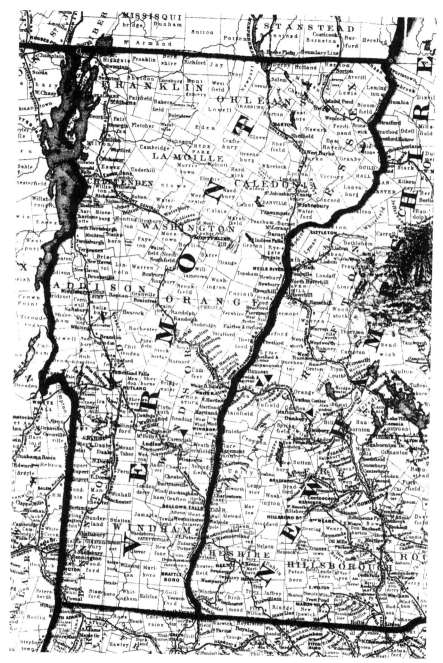

Figure 2.3
Vermont and the Rutland and Burlington Railroad
From Poor 1860 (foldout map in pocket).

of both industries, it was usual for different contractors to undertake work on different sections of the route and also usual for them to let out portions of their work to subcontractors. As had been the case when water transport began along the canals, the subcontracting system was continued in railway transportation after lines went into service. Significantly enough, the same system maintained itself in many New England factories until the end of the nineteenth century. At those places, the work the foreman had tendered for was performed under the very roof of, and with equipment supplied by, the factory owner.

At first, canal and railroad contractors, subcontractors, and laborers were alike in usually being resident near the construction site. Frequently all three groups were made up of local townspeople, farmers, or agricultural laborers seeking to make money in the nonagricultural seasons of the year. Several years elapsed before more or less stable firms of experienced contractors and subcontractors came into being, and with them, a class of more or less permanent wage laborers who, because they were tied neither to farm nor town, moved from one construction enterprise to another. Much of this evolution had already taken place among the canal workers but some aspects of it were repeated among the railroad workers of New England. The use of the canal worker term "navigator," abbreviated to "navvy," for those constructing the railways provides a not unimportant illustration of the overlap between canal and railway workers and their methods of work. The abbreviation is current in Australia and the United Kingdom and is still understood in some parts of the United States.

The literature on canal and railway construction makes it clear that social stratification among the different groups making up the workforce became more marked as work practices evolved. When the workforce was recruited from the immediate vicinity of the work site, its members retired to their usual housing at the end of the day's work. One presumes that even at that early stage, contractors drawn from the commercial classes in the nearby towns or the local farming community lived in greater comfort than the laborers from town or farm. The development of stable firms of contractors and permanent groups of laborers who moved with the construction accentuated the difference in living standards. Contractors rented accommodations, probably local houses, but among the navvies, those who did not sleep unsheltered, out in the open, lived in substandard temporary accommodation, such as tents, barracks, or crude huts made from material scrounged from nearby fields and forests.

We do not know where or how the contractors, subcontractors, and workers on the section of the R&BRR near Cavendish were housed. But it is likely that houses for the navvies were not very different from those described at about the same time in Pennsylvania by Charles Dickens:

The best were poor protection from the weather; the worst let in the wind and rain through wide breeches in the roofs of sodden grass, and in the walls of mud; some had neither door nor window; some had nearly fallen down, and were imperfectly propped up by stakes and poles; all were ruinous and filthy. Hideously ugly old women, and very buxom young ones, pigs, dogs, men, children, babies, pots, kettles, dunghills, vile refuse, rank straw, and standing water, all wallowing together in an inseparable heap, composed the furniture of every dark and dirty hut.

Up the line at Ferrisburgh, less than twenty miles south of the Burlington terminus of the R&BRR in the north, a paymaster saw the Irish workers thus:

I drove to a place in the forest, where nobody ever went, or goes except Railroad folks, when I found about 40 paddies at work & quite a settlement of Shantys. I had my horse put out & went into a Shanty, 6 inches by 4—where the goods are kept—& commenced posting up the paddies accounts, which occupied me until perhaps 8 o'clock ... I had a very polite & urging invitation to take some tea & spend the night among those *animals* congregated in the Shantys, but as I had in my possession 500 dollars ... I did not feel safe to accept of their very polite invitation.

If Gage was employed directly by his contractors, he would have been paid at least three to four times the rate of the navvies in his gang; if he was a subcontractor, he would have earned much more. Unlike the navvies, he could afford to live at some distance from the site, in Cavendish in an inn or tavern. His accommodations are consistent with his being at least separated socially from his men, and possibly a subcontractor.[9]

Whether or not Gage as foreman was also a subcontractor, he did have to plan and maintain an efficient work schedule. It may be only these features of his work that are reflected in Harlow's otherwise puzzling description of him in 1868 as a "shrewd, smart, business man." In the New England vernacular of the day, "shrewd" was synonymous with clever, keen witted in practical affairs, astute or sagacious in action or speech, and "smart" with being quick, keen, active, industrious, energetic, not lazy, clever, and intelligent. The unhyphenated term "business man" was just beginning to acquire its modern meanings and then still meant, as Mrs. Frances Childs (who described herself as "a Yankee from way back") told me, and as Mr. James Davidson of the Rutland Historical Society confirmed, "one who organized the work of others." Consistent with these definitions, Deanna Chiasson of Merriam-Webster's Language Research Staff found that the relevant meaning of "business" in the 1841 Webster was "employment," tending to refer simply to particular occupations. The dictionary observed that "business" was "a word of extensive use and indefinite signification," and gave no entry for "business man." I have found no exact dictionary instance of Harlow's phrase although three come close. Urdang, Hunsinger, and La Roche cite Mathews's older use of "Mr. A. was a prompt and successful business man, 'smart as a whip' as the Yankees say" for business man. Bartlett gives as his example of the use of "smart," "He is a smart business man," and the *Oxford English Dictionary* has "Directing the work, and, Yankee-like, 'doing right smart of it' himself as they say here" for the same word.[10]

Related to his men as employer or not, a foreman had to allot tasks to the men in his gang fairly, record accurately the time each man spent on each task, treat the men comprising the gang equally, and pay them properly. Foremen who did not meet these standards were necessarily unpopular, and violent attacks on them, some of which ended fatally, were not unknown, including some in the area around Cavendish. These attacks took place within something of a culture of violence, in which fights among different national, religious, and regional groups was not uncommon. The Vermont newspapers of the day contain many reports of such incidents, a large number involving the Irish workers who predominated among the navvies. In 1910, an observer recalled one such incident that had taken place at the small "tar papered wooden shack" village in Mt. Holly, deemed "Shanty Town," about fifteen miles west of Cavendish:

During the building of the Rutland and Burlington Railroad in the fall of 1849, I was called to assist in quelling a riot, in which, after much firing into shanties at night and frequent pugilistic encounters by day, more than 1,000 laborers from one district of Ireland, armed with all available weapons from muskets to pick-handles, came down from the Summitt in Mount Holly to drive from the rock-cut of Section Eight in Ludlow, some 400 of their countrymen from another part of "that Island," having brought with them and continued here feuds of the ancient petty kingdoms there.

The authorities were a deputy sheriff and a justice of the peace, both elderly men, and I was the sole representative of the posse-comitatus. We met the rioters as they came in squads, capturing some from each, while the rest ran away, and, finally, by a charge in a one-horse-wagon on the main body, put them to flight in all directions, their leader being brought down by a charge of buckshot in his leg from a fowling-piece with which Matthew Leonard was supposed to have been murdered in 1848, and four Irishmen were put to trial, in the hands of the youngest of the sheriff's party. Three other laborers on the road and one citizen received gunshot wounds; ten prisoners, mostly arrested by me, were sent to Woodstock jail, and this was the last similar act of violence on the road, attributed by railroad men to the buckshot treatment.

It seems very likely that such Irishmen formed a substantial part of Gage's gang.[11]

In this context, Harlow's 1848 testimony that Gage was a great favorite with the men in his gang complements perfectly the qualities of efficiency and capability his contractors noted. It is not too much to suppose that it was the combination of Gage's work skills and personal qualities that led him to the rapidly expanding and potentially rewarding railroad construction industry. Gage was certainly well-equipped physically and psychologically for railroad construction work. At the time of the accident, Harlow said he was of "vigorous physical organization," and twenty years later, Harlow added to this characterization by saying he was:

a perfectly healthy, strong and active young man ... possessing ... an iron frame; muscular system unusually well-developed—having had scarcely a day's illness from his childhood.

In 1848 Harlow had also said that Gage was psychologically of "temperate habits, and possessed of considerable energy of character." Harlow added in 1868 that Gage's temperament was "nervo-bilious," and that he had an iron will. By this characterization Harlow meant that Gage had an athletic frame that imparted energy and strength to his mind and body, making it possible for him to endure great mental and physical labor. And those temperamental characteristics are consistent with the first tangible piece of information we have about Gage: his position as foreman of a gang of men constructing the bed for the railroad.[12]

"Tamkin" and the Accident

On that cool day in early fall when Gage was "tamkin for a blast," he was tamping or packing the explosive charge in the place chosen for the explosion. Plausibly derived from the French *tampon* or *tapon*, the purpose of tamping is to obtain the greatest efficiency from the charge by

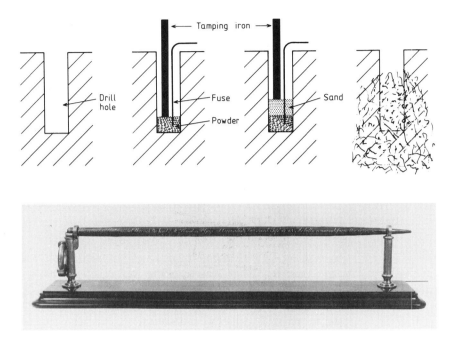

Figure 2.4
Tamping an explosive charge and Gage's tamping iron
Tamping iron reproduced by courtesy of the Warren Anatomical Museum, Harvard University.

confining the explosion to as small a space as possible. Tamping, now most often called "stemming," is carried out in two distinct phases: in the first the charge is packed into as small a space as possible at the actual point chosen for the explosion, and in the second it is confined there by being surrounded by some kind of explosively inert material (figure 2.4). In blasting of the kind Gage was undertaking, a hole was drilled in the rock by hand, a safety fuse (common from the 1830s) knotted at the end and possibly scored behind the knot, but without the yet-to-be-invented detonator, put into the hole, and an explosive powder consisting, one presumes, of a mixture of sulfur, charcoal, and a nitrate such as saltpeter placed over it. The powder would then be packed into the hole with a series of gentle but firm pats. Even though it contained a fuse, the charge so primed would usually be sufficiently stable not to be affected by the consolidation. Sand, clay, or other material would then be placed over the charge and tamped similarly, although more vigorously. The explosive force liberated when the fuse ignited a charge so confined would then be directed into the rock at the end of the drill hole rather than escaping ineffectually back along it.[13]

"Tamkin" is actually one of the more dangerous stages in blasting. Although blasting itself is not skilled work in the sense of requiring formal occupational training, it nevertheless requires considerable ability. The effect of the explosion has to be maximized by assessing the rifts or joints along which the rock will fracture, selecting the right sites for the holes to be drilled, and ensuring they are drilled at the correct angle and to the right depth. Then the right amount of powder has to be selected, packed into place, and fired safely. Incorrect judgments in planning or conducting the operations proper to any of these stages not only results in ineffective or dangerous explosions—and the history of railway and canal construction reveals many such—but errors in drilling or charging could result in too little removal of rock, its fragmentation into pieces too large for easy removal, or the scattering of whatever rock was obtained over too large an area. Work that required considerable labor might then have to be repeated. This was especially galling in drilling, where three men might take a whole day to drill a single hole one and three-quarters inches in diameter to a depth of twelve feet. Further, because blasting is carried out at successive sites, excessive damage at one could increase the amount of work required at the next.[14]

Tamping requires the use of a reasonably heavy implement, and crowbars were once commonly used for that purpose. When the crowbar was held at the pointed end, the flat, squared, and sometimes slightly flared other end provided a surface for packing both charge and plug at the bottom of the drill hole. Where the material being drilled is of a kind that the impact of an iron bar upon it is likely to generate a spark, and the explosive charge is susceptible to being so ignited, the use of a crowbar is somewhat imprudent. These elements were present in the accident: the tamping was being carried out with an iron rod resembling a small crowbar called a tamping iron, the rock being blasted was of an extreme hardness, and the explosive charge was a readily combustible powder.

By the time we first hear of Gage he had acquired a tamping iron rather different from most. Forged by a neighboring blacksmith, the iron was, Bigelow said in 1850, "unlike any other," having been made "to please the fancy of the owner." It was three feet and seven inches long, one and one-quarter inches in diameter at the larger end, tapering over a

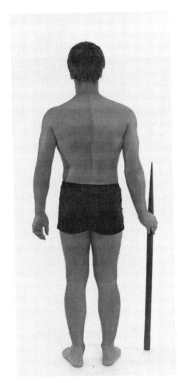 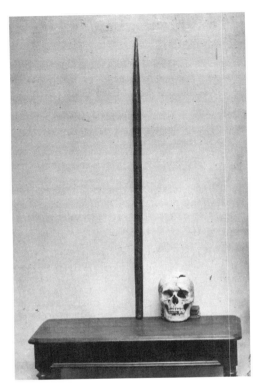

Figure 2.5
S. Webster Wyman's 1868 photograph of Phineas Gage's skull in relation to the
tamping iron and a "Gage" in relation to a replica of the iron
Wyman's photograph from the Glennon Archives, Woburn Public Library,
Woburn, Massachusetts, and reproduced by permission of the Trustees of the
Library.

distance of about twelve inches to a diameter of one-quarter of an inch
at the other, and weighed thirteen and one-quarter pounds. At the time
of the accident in 1848, Harlow gave no details of Gage's height and
weight, saying merely that he was "of middle stature." After Gage's
death, Harlow was more definite: Gage was five feet six inches tall and
had an "average weight" of 150 pounds. Gage was, therefore, about half
as tall again as his tamping iron, and about eleven and one-third times as
heavy, but the iron was some five and one-quarter times longer than the
height of his head. Some of these relationships are important when we
come to trace the journey that the tamping iron undertook (figure 2.5).

We have no contemporary record of precisely where Gage was "tam-kin" his blast. In 1938, nearly ninety years after the accident, Walton A. Green of the nearby village of Proctorsville wrote that in 1906 he and Joseph H. Adams (known as "Deaf Joe") were shown "the exact spot" by Christopher A. Goodrich, who had been nearby with his ox-team—"one of the best" in the town. Goodrich, twenty-four years old at the time of the incident, but then eighty-two, told Green that:

The accident took place at the second cut south of Cavendish where many pot-holes in the rock give evidence that black river once went this way near where Roswell Downer built his lime kiln.

Some doubt exists as to whether the cutting should be counted as the second and smaller of the two as one moves south from Cavendish, or the larger that is the second as one approaches the town from the from the south. The center of the larger is almost exactly three-quarters of a mile from the traditional site of the tavern in which Gage resided, but the smaller contains the potholes, and the remains of the lime kiln are about halfway between them (figure 2.6).[15]

When we turn to what took place at the site at 4 : 30 on the afternoon of 13 September 1848, we also find uncertainties about how the travels of Gage's tamping iron were initiated. According to Harlow, Gage was tamping the powder and fuse ("slightly" in the 1848 account) prior to the sand's being poured in when his attention was attracted by his men, who were loading excavated rock onto a platform car in the pit a few feet behind him. With his head still averted and while continuing to look over his right shoulder, Gage dropped the iron onto the powder again where, this time, it hit the rock, struck a spark, ignited the charge, and immedi-ately reversed its initial direction. Bigelow had it differently. According to him, the powder and fuse had already been "adjusted" in the hole, and Gage had instructed an assistant to pour in the sand. While waiting for this to be done, Gage turned his head away, and after an interval of a few seconds again dropped the iron, this time, as he supposed, onto the sand. However, no sand had been added, and, when the bar struck the rock, the charge exploded, driving it upward. There is also a slight but impor-tant difference in the descriptions of Gage's posture at the time of the explosion. Harlow's first account contains nothing on the subject, the second is quite definite: Gage was "sitting ... on a shelf of rock above the hole." Bigelow was equally definite: "Mr. Gage was ... standing above the hole, leaning forward, with his face slightly averted."[16]

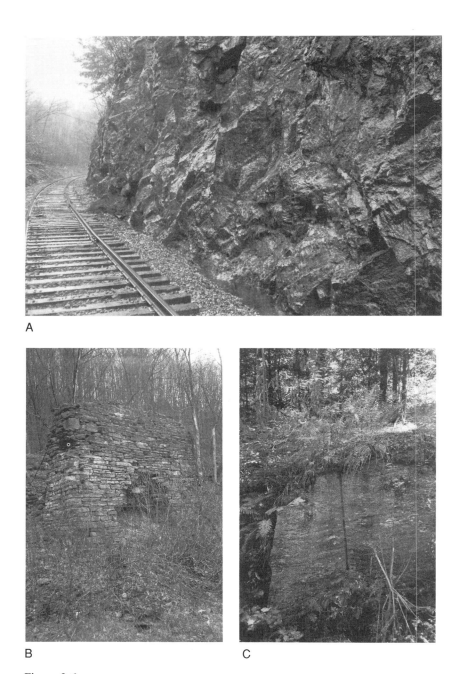

Figure 2.6
(a) The site (?) of the accident, (b) the remains of Downer's lime kiln, (c) a drill hole, all about 0.75 miles south of Cavendish, Vermont
Author's photographs.

Both Harlow's and Bigelow's accounts of Gage's posture and the cause of the explosion are internally consistent and, as we shall see, consistent with the pattern of injury. It is therefore impossible to say which is the more correct. For my part, I incline to Harlow. Although I find the sitting position an unlikely one, from my own experience it is much more unlikely that anyone knowledgeable about setting charges would deliberately place any part of their body, especially their head, directly in line with the tamping iron and the explosive, as Bigelow's description requires.

Whatever Gage's posture, immediately after the explosion the tamping iron was driven completely through his head, landing some four or five rods (between about twenty and twenty-five meters) behind him. Gage was thrown on to his back, gave a few convulsive movements of his limbs, and, possibly without losing consciousness, spoke in a few minutes. He either walked a "few rods" to the road by himself or was helped to do so by his men. There he climbed into Christopher Goodrich's oxcart, in which, while sitting down and supporting himself against the foreboard, he was driven three-quarters of a mile to where he resided, in the tavern of Mr. Joseph Adams a few buildings west of the intersection of Depot and Main Streets. On arrival, Gage stood up by himself, walked to the back of the cart, and allowed two of his men to help him down. They helped him up the steps to the piazza or veranda, where he sat himself on a chair to await medical attention.[17]

At about 5 P.M., some half an hour after the accident, Edward Higginson Williams, M.D., of Proctorsville, the first physician to see Gage, arrived. John Martyn Harlow came at about 6 P.M., that is, another hour later and about one and a half hours after the explosion. Williams does not mention any treatment of his own in his account and seems to have spent most of his time confirming the details of the accident. He also seems to have deferred to Harlow, because it was only after the latter's arrival that Williams mentions any treatment at all. What then happened seems to have been initiated by Harlow: Gage stood and walked with little or no assistance up an internal flight of stairs to his room, where Harlow examined him. Harlow and Williams then jointly cleaned and dressed the burns on Gage's arms and the wounds to his head. Directing the attendants to keep him in a sitting position, the pair left at about 7:30 P.M., and Harlow returned two and a half hours later.[18]

Between the time of the explosion and Williams's and Harlow's ministrations, Gage was fully conscious. He spoke rationally with those around him, describing the accident accurately and insisting he would be back at work in a day or two. His mind was "clear" and there was no impairment of "sensorial powers." At some point his mother, who was then apparently living in Lebanon, New Hampshire, some thirty miles away, had been sent for, and Gage had no difficulty in recognizing her or his uncle, who seems to have traveled with her, when the pair appeared at his bedside at 7 A.M. the next morning. Rationality is in fact the striking feature shown by Gage during his recovery, although there were, as we shall see, periods of delirium and coma. Even though Gage made remarkable progress over the next ten days, Harlow's prognosis was that it was not possible for him to recover, a view shared by his friends and relatives. Gage was actually measured by Thomas Winslow, the town cabinet maker, so that there would be a coffin "in readiness to use." Walton Green, the source of this detail, also gives the location of Winslow's workshop, where the coffin was made. In the event, Winslow's measurements were not needed.

Conclusion

Phineas Gage was in his mid-twenties when work on the Rutland and Burlington Railroad commenced in May 1847. He neither worked on it for very long nor saw much return for his labor. By the time the first section of fourteen miles was opened in June 1849, he was still too weak physically to be working, and by the time the two sections of the line, now totalling 105.5 miles, were joined at Mt. Holly on 18 December 1849, his fame as victim was practically all that was left to him. Close to that date, a professional Burlington man wishing to attend a meeting at the Massachusetts Medical College of Harvard University could board the 8 A.M. to Boston, pass through Cavendish, and arrive in Boston at 7 P.M. the same day. As he mounted the steps to the three-storied college building on North Grove Street, he would have had time, had Phineas still been sitting there, tamping iron in hand, to toss a few coins into his begging bowl.[19]

Notes

1. I am using the *Boston Post*'s reprinting of the report in the *Free Soil Union* because I have been unable to find a copy of this issue of the Ludlow paper. In fact, only two individual copies of the *Free Soil Union* seem to be held in the

United States, one by the Library of Congress, for 3 November 1848, and the other by the Vermont Historical Society, for 3 January 1849. The Library of Congress classes the paper as a weekly, but if they are correct in thinking it began on 1 September 1848, the 3 November issue could not be number 10, as they say. The paper ceased publication some time early in 1849. The 3 January issue carries an advertisement that its Ludlow printery is for sale.

2. Although I prefer the name-date system widely used in scientific writing for giving references, I know that general and specialist humanities readers find that this system makes reading difficult. I have therefore adopted a kind of hybrid method in which all the references to the topics discussed in a self-contained section of text, usually a paragraph, are given in a note at the end of the section. In the notes, the topics are referenced sequentially using the name-date system. Quotations will be found in these references, but I have given page numbers only for quotations that are difficult to locate. Generally that means I have not given page numbers for material quoted from book chapters and journal articles.

I quote frequently from three items: Harlow's two papers and Bigelow's confirmatory study. I believe the contexts in which they are quoted are usually clear enough for them not to be listed again in the notes. Harlow's papers are Harlow 1848 and 1868—the latter also appeared as a booklet in 1869—and there is also a short letter of 1849. Bigelow's paper and its booklet form are Bigelow 1850b and 1850c. All are reproduced in facsimile in Appendix A.

Harlow's second name often appears as "Martin," but "Martyn" is the correct spelling because that was his mother's family name.

3. For this geneology, see the first part of Appendix G.

4. Harlow (1868). The lineage of Phineas Gage is set out in Appendix G. I have to apologize for giving Gage's birth date as 9 September 1823 in my 1986 paper, especially for the implication that Leavitt's records may have been the source (see also Macmillan 1996a). That dating was careless, due only partly to my difficulties in translating the American date system into the Australian one of day, month, year. The farming background of the Gages comes from Child 1886, pp. 258, 285; Roberts 1957, pp. 399, 400; C. V. Gage 1964?, p. 53; Robert Leavitt; Marjorie Carr, Enfield Public Library; and Frances Childs, Enfield Historical Society, New Hampshire.

5. Documents located under the name "Gage" in the Grafton County Registry by Richard Henderson (Enfield, New Hampshire) and Robert Drake (Hanover, New Hampshire), together with the inquiries made by Pieter van Schaik (Cavendish, Vermont) and correspondence with Virginia Dennerley have been considered in trying to locate the farm in Lebanon or East Lebanon on which Phineas Gage may have grown up. However, no record has been found of a farm owned by Phineas's father, Jesse Eaton Gage, in either area in the 1820s—the places where Hannah Trussell Swetland resided and where they were married, respectively. However, Hannah's parents seem to have farmed in East Lebanon, and it is possible that Jesse worked on their property. The Phineas recorded in the 1840 Census is at Enfield, and is most probably our Phineas's grandfather. To confuse the matter, there is a second Jesse Gage who does not seem to be directly related

to this branch of the family. He acquired property in the town of Orford, New Hampshire, just north of Hanover, in 1834 and 1837, and was said to be resident there. He, but not a Hannah, was at Orford for the 1840 Census. However, the converse is true for 1850.

School attendance figures are from U.S. Census Office 1841, pp. 32–33, and 1853, pp. 18–19, and literacy estimates are from them and the U.S. Bureau of the Census 1960, p. 206, H407–411. In neither Census are the school attendance figures broken down by age. It is not possible, therefore, to subtract the number of scholars "over 15 and under 20" from the total number of scholars and, by comparing them with the similarly corrected population figures, obtain something like a true rate of school attendance for the over 5 and under 15 year olds. Naturally it should not be assumed that almost 100 percent of the potential scholars in the fifteen to twenty age range were actually at school.

6. Cushing 1992, p. 104 for Grafton schools.

7. Pieter van Schaik of Cavendish suggested the possibility that Phineas may have worked on a New Hampshire Railroad passing near these towns, and Poor (1860, pp. 37, 58–59) gives details for the Northern RR Co., Cushing (1992) for Grafton's isinglass mines, and Chowdhury (1941, especially pp. 58–73) for mining mica.

8. For Vermont railways generally, see Thompson 1842, p. 217, n.; Meyer 1948, p. 342; Poor 1860, pp. 69–70; and for the Champlain and Connecticut River Railroad Company, later the R&BRR, see Kirkland 1948, p. 167; Poor 1860, p. 74; and Baker 1937, pp. xviii–xix, 233–234.

9. Harlow, 1868. My thanks to Gerald (Jerry) Fox, railroad historian of Essex Junction, Vermont, for directing me to the literature on foremen, subcontracting, and the organization of work, working conditions, housing, and occupational hazards among canal and railway navvies (Clawson 1980, chap. 4; Chandler 1977, pp. 43–55, 94–98; Coleman 1965; Licht 1983; Patten 1968, pp. 12–16; and Way 1993). Peter Way and Jerry Fox have told me that they would allow that Gage could have been a subcontractor, and Walter Licht shares my belief that he actually was. Dickens is quoted in Way 1993, p. 144, and the Ferrisburgh incident is from Bassett 1992, p. 37.

10. For the possible meanings of the phrase and its constituent words, see Bartlett 1968; Craigie and Hulbert 1938; Mathews 1951; Mencken 1936; Oxford University Press 1992; Schele de Vere 1872; and Urdang, Hunsinger, and LaRoche (1985). Note also that "shrewd" and "business man" also have the slightly negative connotations of one who cheats or deceives.

11. Wheeler 1952 for attacks on foremen (quotation is on p. 26), and Fulham 1910 for the riot.

12. Temperamental characteristics in Buell and Sizer 1842, pp. 23–24, and Fowler 1839.

13. There seem to be no records for the weather in Cavendish on 13 September 1848, but three entries in diaries held at the University of Vermont allow us a reasonable basis for inference. William Henry Hoyt, writing in his diary from

across the border with New York state, said it was "beautifully fine clear weather with cool wind," Royal William Peake "Pleasant but cool" in Bristol, Vermont, and George Augustus Weeks in Bakersfield, Vermont, had his "pretty cold" of the 13th preceded by "rather cold" for the 12th and followed by a 14th that was "very rainy and cold," (Diaries at University of Vermont—Appendix H). The skills required in preparing for blasting, and how tamping and firing were carried out in Gage's time, can be inferred from the many nineteenth-century blaster's manuals. More convenient sources are the appropriate entries in Nelson 1964 and Du Pont 1969, pp. 1–4, 25–28, 187, 210–211, 221–222, 327–336.

14. The harshness of the working conditions and the dangers of blasting are from Way 1993, chap. 5.

15. Walton A. Green's statement is reproduced in Appendix C.

16. Details in Harlow 1848, 1868, and 1869 and Bigelow 1850b, 1850c.

17. The long since demolished Adams hotel can be identified as the "Hotel A. Walker" on Beers 1869 map (fig. 2.2) from the record of inns and hotels compiled by Wriston 1991, pp. 178–179. Linda Welch, the Cavendish historian, has told me that there was more than one Joseph Adams in Cavendish at the time, and that the one operating the hotel was doing so on behalf of Salmon Dutton (who himself ran what was known as the Stage-Coach Inn, since removed to the Shelburne Museum in Shelburne, Vermont). Joseph Adams's own house still stands on the east side of Depot Street immediately south of Black River. "Piazza" is still, my New England friends tell me, a not uncommon New England word for an ordinary veranda. It seems never to have been used there for the grand, spacious, open areas that it refers to in other versions of English and in other languages (see U.S. dictionaries like Webster's or Random House, and the complete *Oxford English Dictionary*).

18. In this paragraph and the text that follows I have referred directly to the papers by Harlow and Bigelow but sometimes drawn on yet-to-be-cited newspaper and other accounts, and on the letters from Williams and Adams that Bigelow reproduced. However, most of what I draw on is found in Appendix A.

19. Dates, timetable, and other details for the Rutland and Burlington from Rutland and Burlington Railroad Company 1850; Poor 1860, pp. 70–74; *Rutland Herald*, 22 August 1850, p. 4, col. 4; Meyer 1948, pp. 144, 340–342; Kirkland 1948, chap. 6; and Baker 1937, Introduction and chap. 10.

3

Early Receptions: Popular and Medical

For marvellous strangeness and wonderful termination it surpasses everything surgical that ever occurred.

—Dr. Alonzo Chapin, *Annual Address*, Middlesex East District Medical Society, 1870

From 1850 onward the medical literature devoted to Gage is replete with comments about the considerable interest his accident generated in lay and professional circles. Partly in the hope of determining what caught the minds of those who saw him, I tried to retrace his steps by visiting many of the places to which he is said to have gone. I looked in local newspapers, sought out handbills and broadsheets, and read the letters and diaries of those townspeople, such as teachers and physicians, whom one might have expected to be interested in him, and who might have recorded what they made of him.

Newspapers from September 1848 to March 1849

Given the supposed degree of interest, it is surprising that my researchers and I found a total of only five reasonably different newspaper reports and two letters describing Gage's accident. Although some of the more ignorant remarks about it claim otherwise, the Gage case made no headlines, mainly because headlines had hardly been invented in 1848. When coping with the real difficulties of locating newspaper reports on Gage, I actually drew some dark comfort from these fancifully uninformed claims. If only they had been true.[1]

Over time there is a clear shift in the emphasis of the small number of items that we did find. The first newspaper report seems to be the short, three-sentence account in the Ludlow, Vermont, *Free Soil Union* quoted in chapter 2. On Wednesday, 20 September, the *Boston Courier* and the *Boston Daily Journal* published identical second reports, which, although different from the *Free Soil Union* and not acknowledging it, were clearly based on it. The differences were that the two Boston papers named the railroad, located Cavendish in Vermont, replaced the phrase that had included the mysterious term "tamkin" with one more intelligible to readers, altered the text to match the different date of publication, and made some minor grammatical changes:

Horrible Accident. Phineas P. Gage, a foreman on the Rutland Railroad at Cavendish, Vt., was preparing for a blast on Wednesday last, when the powder exploded, carrying through his head an iron instrument, an inch and a fourth in circumference, and three feet and eight inches in length. The iron entered on the side of his face, shattering the upper jaw, and passing back of the left eye, and out the top of his head. Singularly enough, he was alive at two o'clock the next afternoon, in full possession of his reason, and free from pain.

This account was republished that day, with acknowledgment to the *Courier*, in the Boston *Daily Evening Traveller*, and what was clearly the same report also appeared but without acknowledgment later the same month in the *Herald* (Rutland, Vermont) and the *Green Mountain Freeman* (Montpelier, Vermont). The *True Democrat and Granite State Whig* (Lebanon, New Hampshire) concluded its unacknowledged report with a slightly altered last sentence and an exclamation mark, "He was alive at last accounts and hopes are entertained of his recovery!"[2]

What characterizes these Boston reports and the Ludlow original on which they are based is the use of simple capitalized or italicized side headings as introductions, their factual nature, and, except for the circumference of the bar being given as "an inch and a fourth" rather than the diameter, their accuracy. Only the exclamation mark used by the *True Democrat and Granite State Whig* can be thought of as marking Gage's case as unusual.

A third report in the *Vermont Mercury* (Woodstock) appears to have been written four days after the event:

WONDERFUL ACCIDENT

In the afternoon of Wednesday 13th inst., a foreman named Phineas P. Gage, employed on the Railroad just below Duttonsville in Cavendish, was tamping down a charge, preparatory to blasting, with a bar of round iron 1 1-4 inches in diameter, and 3 ft. 7 in. long. The bar tapered so that at the end it was but little more than 1-4 of an inch across. The charge in the hole exploded, and the bar entered the man's face just anterior to the angle of the lower jaw, passed up outside of the teeth of the upper jaw, entered the bone of the cheek on its under surface, without, however destroying the shape of the face, and passed out just behind where the frontal and two parietal bones meet, that is, near the top of the head. The bar went about five rods, and stuck in the road. The skull was fractured in every direction around the opening made by the bar. After the accident, the man walked some two or three rods to a cart, and rode to Mr. Adam's tavern in Duttonsville, when he got out of the cart, and went into the house. The doctors, who visited him, found him sitting in a chair, perfectly rational at that time, and he told them the particulars of the accident. His wounds were dressed, with, however, no hopes of success. When the surgeons left him that night, he was still rational, although somewhat faint from loss of blood, which he swallowed and vomited. The bleeding ceased at about eleven o'clock, and then he was quiet almost the whole remainder of the night.

Four days after the accident, Mr. Gage was alive and apparently better—though it seems impossible that he should survive.

Although the technical and medical details were accurately reported, and the conclusion pessimistic rather than sensational, this heading and conclusion are the first to emphasize anything about the case as amazing or improbable. Over the next two weeks The *Vermont Mercury* report was reprinted, exactly and with acknowledgment, in the *Vermont Chronicle* (Windsor), the *Caledonian* (St. Johnsbury, Vermont), and the *Vermont Gazette* (East Bennington).[3]

Our next item is a signed letter from the *Christian Reflector and Christian Watchman*, (Boston) that almost qualifies as a report that, were it so, has a date that would make it the fourth account of the accident. Its stress on the unusual is marked:

AN ASTONISHING FACT—One of the most singular and astonishing accidents occurred on the railroad in Cavendish, Vt., about three weeks since, that has ever been recorded. You may have seen some account of it, but you will be willing, I know, to have a short original article from one who has almost daily visited the bed side of the sufferer.

As Mr. Phineas P. Gage, an overseer on the road just below Duttonville [*sic*], Vt., was charging a rock for blasting, the powder ignited, throwing the tamping iron entirely through his head. The iron is three feet seven inches and a quarter *long*, and one and five sixteenths in *diameter*, not *circumference*, as reported, and weighs thirteen and a half pounds. It entered on the left cheek, just over the jaw bone, and under the cheek bone, and passed back of the left eye, and came out on the top of the head, a little forward of the centre, and almost precisely where the skull is found unclosed in an infant's head. The iron was considerably sharpened at the upper end, which prevented its tearing the head, as it otherwise would have done. It was found several rods off completely *smeared with brains*. Mr. Gage was immediately taken into a horse cart, rode without much assistance nearly

three quarters of a mile, to Mr. J. Adam's tavern, where he was boarding, got out nearly alone—sat up while his head was washed, and then walked up a flight of stairs without assistance, to his room. He seemed to have his senses all the while—said the iron had passed through his head, but thought he should get well. Dr. Harlow was immediately called to dress his wounds, which of course, he pronounced *mortal*. For sometime he continued to vomit large quantities of blood, which flowed into his mouth and passed into his stomach. No-one supposed he could live a day or an hour, but strange as it may appear, he is *yet alive, twenty two days from the time of the accident*. He has had his senses most of the time—recognizes all whom he has ever known, converses most of the time coherently, though often somewhat bewildered. The wound on his cheek has entirely healed, and the larger one on top of his head is apparently doing well—discharges freely, but has a healing and healthy appearance. A piece of the skull, larger than a dollar, is loose, and will have to be removed, should he live. Many, who have not seen him, think the *iron could not have passed through his head*, but no surgeon, or other person who has seen him, has the least doubt as to the fact of the *iron passing entirely through his head as above stated*. I have often been asked, "Do you think he will recover?" To this, I can only reply, it is *marvellous* that he could have lived a *moment*—it is *marvellous* that he has lived *so long*—it will only be *marvellous* if he should *recover*. Altogether, it is one of the strangest occurrences on record, and will form a subject of inquiry for the learned physiologist. We live in an eventful era, but if a man can have thirteen pounds of iron in the shape of a pointed bar, thrown entirely through his head, carrying with it a quantity of the brain, and yet live and have his senses, we may well exclaim, What next? And yet the facts above stated can be attested by hundreds.
A. Angier.
Cavendish, Vt., Oct. 3, 1848.

The fourth real newspaper report appeared at about the same time.[4] Although the *Vermont Mercury* (Woodstock) still used a simple side heading as introduction, the content of the heading, the comments correcting the size of the iron, the italics, and the concluding exclamation mark also drew attention to the sensational aspects:

THE "STRANGE CASE IN SURGERY."—We gave some account, a few weeks ago, of the wonderful case of Mr. Gage, foreman on the Railroad in Cavendish, who in preparing a charge for blasting a rock, had an iron bar driven through his head, entering through his cheek, and passing out at the top of his head, with a force that carried the bar some rods, after performing its wonderful journey through skull and brains. The iron was in *diameter* an inch and a quarter, and in length, three feet and seven inches; the upper end of the iron, however, tapering to the diameter of one fourth of an inch. We repeat the dimensions of the rod, as we observe some of papers, that copied the article, substituted the word *circumference* for *diameter*, thinking perhaps the story told in that way, would be quite as large as could well be believed. But we refer to this wonderful case again to say that the patient not only survives, but is much improved; the wound in his head has healed, the *scuttle* in his roof is closing up, and he is likely to be out again, with no visible injury but the loss of an eye!

Over the next month, this fourth account was reprinted in its entirety, sometimes with a small center heading and with the *Vermont Mercury* properly acknowledged, by the daily *Boston Journal*, the *Vermont Journal* (Windsor), the *National Eagle* (Claremont, New Hampshire), the *New Hampshire Patriot and State Gazette* (Concord), and the *Green Mountain Freeman* (Montpelier, Vermont). Only the *Caledonian* (St. Johnsbury, Vermont) altered the report by omitting the second-to-last sentence correcting the diameter of the tamping iron.[5]

The fifth report, from the *North Star* (Danville, Vermont), is throughout at least as sensational in content as its italics, exclamation marks, and center heading suggest:

ALIVE FROM THE DEAD, ALMOST.
Some of our readers may recollect the case of Mr. Phineas Gage, who was injured, supposed mortally, while blasting rocks at Cavendish, Vt., some four or five weeks since. On Wednesday evening, the 18th instant, we conversed with a gentleman who lives in that town, and who states that when he left, on Monday evening, the 16th inst., Mr. Gage was not only living, but bade fair to continue alive, and to some extent comfortable for a considerable time yet.

By the explosion of a charge in the rock, an iron bar 2 feet 9 inches [*sic*] in length, and 1 1-4th inch in *diameter*, not in *circumference*, as some of the papers had it, was forced quite through his head, and passing upward a considerable way, fell on a spot where it was picked up the next day. Striking him on the face, just below the cheek bone, it forced itself through the skull near the top of the head, passing directly through what phrenologists call the organ of *veneration*. When picked up it was found to be actually *greased* with the matter of the brain. Mr. Gage, upon meeting with the accident, *got into the cart and rode home*, first telling a man who was at work with him to be there the next day, as *he* should be there! Arrived at the house, he walked up one flight of stairs to his chamber. Word was immediately sent to his mother, who lived thirty miles off in New Hampshire, as nobody imagined he could live after what had befallen him. The physicians on dressing the wound, found the fractures of the skull to be fearful. The wound bled freely, which tended to prevent inflammation, and portions of the brain, intermixed with the blood, kept falling into the throat, causing vomiting.

Mr. Gage is an unmarried man, some twenty six or thirty years of age.—What is very remarkable is that he has been able to converse ever since his accident, and has in great part retained his reason. He desired to have his mother sent for. As she came having been told what had happened, she had not the least expectation of finding him alive.

This case is probably the most remarkable one on record. If read of for the first time in a romance it would appear ludicrously absurd. But,
—Truth is strange
Stranger than fiction.

I know this report only from the *North Star*, for although the Boston *Post* is given as its source, our search of the *daily* of that name failed to find it.[6]

To judge from a letter of the following year, this time in the *National Eagle* (Claremont, New Hampshire), the disbelief continued to grow after Gage had recovered:

INCREDIBLE, BUT TRUE EVERY WORD
Mr. Editor:—I saw the other day a man who has been the subject of a casuality [*sic*], the like of which probably no man now living on the earth has survived.

Phineas P. Gage, the individual referred to, is of stature thick, muscular form, and rather short; is 25 years of age, and has his home in Lebanon N. H. In the month of September last this young man, being overseer of a party of blasters on the Railroad in Cavendish, Vt. was in the act of tamping down a charge. The implement, which was employed in the operation and which was seen and examined by me, was a round bar of iron three feet and seven inches long—at one end five quarters of an inch in diameter, the same continuing for about two-thirds of the whole length, then regularly diminishing to the other end, which is one fourth of an inch in diameter. In the process of tamping a spark was struck, and an explosion followed—an occurrence, which proved of very serious importance to our young friend, the aforesaid overseer, for it drove his tamping bar, small end forward, right through his own head. Verily so!! The bar struck the left side of the operator's face, entering just above the upper teeth, about mid-way between the nose and the ear—passed under the cheek bone, back of the left eye which it destroyed, and came out on the top of the head at a point lying about an inch back of the centre of a straight line drawn from the middle of the top of the forehead to the left angle of the forehead.

Thus the entire length of this bar of iron, weighing not less than 12 or 13 pounds, passed through the man's head, went into the air no one knows how high, and was found the next day four or five rods from the spot whence it started, covered with blood and brains. Did death ever quit his hold on such a subject before? Still the man lives—restored to perfect health and soundness—and has gone back to resume his post of labor and peril on the road.

The scar on the cheek is not a very bad one—not in the least degree unsightly. The wound upon the top of the head appears not to have been carefully and skillfully managed; which he accounts for by stating, that it being thought absolutely impossible to save his life, nothing was attempted further than to make his remaining hours or days comfortable.

He thinks the wound must have discharged nearly his own weight of purulent matter. He informs me, that he was never at any time deprived of consciousness,

—that he knew immediately after the explosion what had happened to him—that he rose upon his feet and walked, telling the by-standers they need not carry him, —and that while riding to his boarding house he took his pencil and "time-book" from his pocket and made an entry. This is confirmed by witnesses.

So very remarkable is this case, that I have thought it worth while to be minute in the description. If your readers have doubts, say a corroborating word yourself; for the facts are known to you.

C.

Unfortunately there do not seem to have been any doubters, or at least not enough of them for the editor to take up "C"'s suggestion. Only in New Hampshire, but apparently not elsewhere, does the letter seem to have been reprinted. It appeared a week later, with acknowledgment but not "C"'s signature, in the *True Democrat and Granite State Whig* (Lebanon, New Hampshire).[7]

What is immediately apparent is how the reports successively emphasize the unusual aspects of the case. Restrained as they are when judged by modern journalistic standards, the later reports are sensational nevertheless. The same development characterizes the medical literature.

Henry Jacob Bigelow and the Medical Skeptics

One cannot say that Harlow's 1848 report attracted much more attention in the American and English medical press of the day than in the popular press. In fact our reasonably thorough search turned up a total of only five references, usually reprints or long summaries, none of which was accompanied by extensive comment. Thus the *North-Western Medical and Surgical Journal* reprinted Harlow's account in full with no comment at all. The *American Journal of the Medical Sciences*, the *Medical Times* (London), and W. H. Ranking's *Half-Yearly Abstract of the Medical Sciences* all noted the case as "remarkable": the first two directly and the second only indirectly in its index entry: "Harlow, Dr., remarkable case by." It was left to the *Buffalo Medical Journal*, which had also reprinted Harlow's paper a month before without comment, to raise, after reproducing a note from Harlow in January, the following:

Quere. Is there any ground to suspect that the medical attendant [i.e. Harlow] may have deceived himself as to the passage of the rod *through* the head?

Harlow reported in 1868 that the doubt had originally gone much further. Many of his metropolitan colleagues had then utterly refused to believe that the man had risen, until they had thrust their fingers into the hole in his head, and even then they required … attested statements, from clergymen and lawyers, before they *could* or *would* believe—many eminent surgeons regarding such an occurrence as a physiological impossibility.

Harlow found in Henry Jacob Bigelow, then about to become Professor of Surgery at Harvard Medical School, someone who turned out to be an unlikely ally against the skeptics. Although Bigelow also tended to confirm Gage as a mere curiosity, what he did was decisive in overcoming the doubters.[8]

Bigelow said he had become interested in the case "a few days" after the accident but was "at first wholly skeptical." He seems to have done five things to resolve his doubts. First, he wrote to Harlow seeking details of the case; second, he asked Harlow to collect statements confirming the circumstances of the accident; third, he obtained the iron and studied it; fourth, after Gage had recovered, he arranged for Gage to come to Boston, where he examined him; and fifth, by drilling holes in a skull he showed that the iron could have passed through Gage's. It seems to have been during that visit that Gage's life mask, now in the Warren Anatomical Museum, was made. Presumably "the top of his head" would have had to have closed before it could be made, a requirement consistent with J. B. S. Jackson's implying that Bigelow arranged for "the cast" to be taken during this visit.

Bigelow must have written to Harlow in late November or early December 1848, because the earliest of the statements Harlow obtained for him is dated 4 December 1848, and at the 11 December meeting of the Boston Society for Medical Improvement, just before Harlow's first paper was published—but after its completion on 27 November—the Secretary recorded Bigelow's first intervention:

Perforation of the Brain by a drill. Dr. H. J. Bigelow gave some details of the case which he had from the consulting physician, a more particular account of which will be found in the next number of the Boston Medical and Surgical Journal—a drill nearly three feet in length and averaging an inch in diameter passed in the region of the upper jaw, and out near the sagittal suture, being shot clear through—the patient is now well.

The following year, at the meeting on 14 May 1849, the Secretary recorded:

Tamping Iron passing through the head of a man. Dr. H. J. Bigelow exhibited the Iron weighing 13 1/2 lbs. The case, which has been *alluded* to at a previous meeting is reported in the Boston Med. & Surg. Journ.

It may seem odd that Gage would have allowed the tamping iron to be sent to Boston without his going with it. But it would have been just as odd that he should have been there and not been presented at the same time. According to Harlow, Bigelow's request to send Gage to Boston was made "soon after publication of this case." But not until Gage was quite well, "the top of his head being entirely closed," presumably some months after the request, did he go to Boston (at Bigelow's expense), where he remained for "eight or nine weeks."[9]

Bigelow's presentation of Gage and his tamping iron was at the 10 November 1849 meeting of the society:

Tamping Iron passing thro. head. Dr. H. J. Bigelow exhibited the patient the subject of the accident whose case he had mentioned before & which is recorded in full in Boston Med. Surgical Journal. Dr. B. also showed the Iron & a skull prepared to exhibit its course showing how the optic nerve might still be preserved intact.

Four days earlier, in his inaugural address at his installation as Professor of Surgery at Harvard, Bigelow had assured his audience that:

Now almost any thing may occur in medicine. The most fantastic possibilities actually do occur. For instance, a good sized crowbar was shot through a man's brain, and he recovered.

Bigelow first set about removing his own doubts. As soon as his inquiries and drilling had done so, he set about removing those of others.

The earliest of the statements Bigelow obtained through Harlow and reproduced in his 1850 paper was from Edward Higginson Williams of the nearby village of Proctorsville, the first physician to see Gage. Dated 4 December 1848, the statement indicated Dr. Williams found Gage some twenty-five to thirty minutes after the accident sitting on the piazza of Adams's tavern, where he greeted Williams with one of the great understatements of medical history, "Doctor, here is business enough for you." Throughout Williams's examination Gage continued to relate to the bystanders the manner in which he was injured, insisting that the tamping iron had passed through his head, and did so so rationally that Williams preferred Gage's account "to the men who were with him at the time of the accident." Although Williams had observed the top of Gage's head to have something of the appearance of "an inverted funnel," and that "the edges of [the] opening were everted, so that the whole wound appeared as if some wedge-shaped body had passed from below upward," he did not believe Gage's account. He thought Gage "was deceived" until Gage himself pointed out the entry slit on his cheek, "discoloured by powder and iron rust," and an Irishman standing by said, "Sure it was so, sir, for the bar is lying on the road below, all blood and brains."

Alerted by what an Irishman, whom he had seen riding rapidly in search of Harlow, had told him, the Reverend Joseph Freeman, also of the village of Proctorsville, wrote on 5 December 1848 that he joined the procession bringing Gage to the village. His observations, also passed on to Bigelow by Harlow, were:

I found him sitting in a cart, sitting up without aid, with his back against the foreboard. When we reached his quarters, he rose on his feet without aid, and walked quick, though with an unsteady step, to the hind end of the cart, when two of his men came forward and aided him out, and walked with him supporting him to the house.

I then asked his men how he came to be hurt? The reply was, "The blast went off when he was tamping it, and the tamping-iron passed through his head." I said, "That is impossible."

Soon after this, I went to the place where the accident happened. I found upon the rocks, where I supposed he had fallen, a small quantity of brains. There being no person at this place, I passed on to a blacksmith's shop a few rods beyond, in and about which a number of Irishmen were collected. As I came up to them, they pointed me to the iron, which has since attracted so much attention, standing outside the shop-door. They said they found it covered with brains and dirt, and had washed it in the brook. The *appearance* of the iron corresponded with this story. It had a greasy appearance, and was so to the touch.

On 14 December 1848, Joseph Adams, who was a Justice of the Peace as well as the proprietor of the tavern, wrote to Harlow confirming Freeman's account of Gage's arrival. He added that Gage was "perfectly conscious of what was passing around him" and described how on:

The morning subsequent to the accident I went in quest of the bar and found it at a smith's shop, near the pit in which he was engaged.

The men in his pit asserted that "they found the iron, covered with blood and brains," several rods behind where Mr. Gage stood, and that they washed it in the brook, and returned it with the other tools; which representation was fully corroborated by the greasy feel and look of the iron, and the *fragments of brain* which I saw upon the rock where it fell.

Although Bigelow said that Harlow had forwarded "about a dozen of similar documents," these three were the only ones he used.[10]

Bigelow seems to have overcome most of the skeptics. Of the five references I found to Bigelow's paper, the *London Journal of Medicine*, the

London Medical Gazette, and the *Dublin Medical Press* printed condensations of varying length, usually with some endorsing introductory or concluding phrase such as "this truly remarkable case." The *British and Foreign Medico-Chirurgical Review* went further: after dismissing the evidence of what it called "the bystanders" as of "very little value," it added, "the case must be received into the archives of medical science for what it professes to be, and therefore as one of the most extra ordinary on record." Only in the *Edinburgh Medical and Surgical Journal* was doubt expressed, and then politely: its heading read, "Case in which an Iron Rod is *believed* to have passed through the Skull, touching and wounding the Brain, yet terminating in Recovery" [emphasis added].[11]

There is another side to Bigelow's actions in quelling the doubts about Gage's injury. Despite Bigelow's giving the date for his presenting Gage to the Boston Society for Medical Improvement as January 1850, we have it in the handwritten minutes of the Society that Gage was presented to the 10 November 1849 meeting, and there is no record of any other appearance. From the minutes we learn that Gage had been immediately preceded by another exhibit of Bigelow's:

Remarkable Stalagmite. Dr. H. J. Bigelow exhibited the specimen sent from New York found on the borders of a pond. Remarkable for its singular resemblance to a petrified penis.

Whatever other effect Bigelow's action might have had on the skeptics, exhibiting what looked like a petrified penis before presenting Gage probably reinforced the picture of Gage as a mere curiosity, especially as Gage was followed by Dr. Strong's cure of an enlarged ankle by purgatives.[12]

Bigelow's introduction to the conclusions of his 1850 paper on the case, with its uncanny echo of the thought in the Danville *North Star* report of two years earlier, has the same quality:

The leading feature of this case is its improbability. A physician who holds in his hand a crowbar, three feet and a half long, and more than thirteen pounds in weight, will not readily believe that it has been driven with a crash through the brain of a man who is still able to walk off, talking with composure and equanimity of the hole in his head. This is the sort of accident that happens in the pantomime at the theatre, but not elsewhere. Yet there is every reason for supposing it in this case literally true.

The emphasis of the *Public Ledger and Daily Transcript* (Philadelphia) comment on Bigelow's paper shows the connection between popular and medical credulity in an especially clear form:

A MOST REMARKABLE CASE—The Journal of [the] American Medical Sciences contains an account of injury to the brain and recovery of the man, which draws considerably upon one's faith to credit. The story in brief is that the person injured was engaged in blasting and was tamping in the charge, when it exploded and the tamping iron, three feet seven inches in length and an inch and a quarter in diameter, weighing thirteen and a quarter pounds, passed through the left cheek, just behind and below the mouth, ascended into the brain behind the left eye, passed from the skull, which it shattered and raised up, "like an inverted funnel," for a distance of about two inches in every direction around the wound, flew through the air, and was picked up by the workmen, "covered with blood and brains," several rods behind where he stood. The man was placed in a cart and carried three quarters of a mile. He got out of the car [*sic*] himself, walked up stairs, and in ten weeks was nearly well, and though he lost a considerable portion of his brains he exhibited no difference in mental perceptions and power than before the accident. This case occurred in Vermont, upon the line of the Rutland and Burlington Railroad, in September, 1848, in the practice of Dr. J. M. Harlow, of Cavendish, Vt. The physician, in commenting on the case, says it is unparalleled in the annals of surgery, and that its leading feature is its improbability.

The first sentence is original with the *Ledger*. The rest, including the quoted statements and the concluding judgment, came directly from Bigelow.

The successive reports given the news of Gage's accident in both the popular and medical press show a similar increase of incredulity over time. Perhaps this is to be expected. John Barnard Swets Jackson found Gage was well known in Bellow's Falls because, presumably during his recovery, "ye tavern-keeper at Cavendish, where ye accident happened, beg. in ye habit of askg. persons up to see ye pt." The longer Gage lived, the greater the miracle. Had he died shortly after the accident, there would have been little at which to be surprised. Although that may be, the tone of the later reports, and in some instances the content, have a quality of special pleading. "C"'s appeal to the editor of the *National Eagle* to quell the doubts resembles Bigelow's appeal to Harlow: someone else, preferably someone of repute, was needed to confirm the basic facts of a curious and almost unbelievable story.[13]

The Tamping Iron and the Museum

A final point about Bigelow's treatment of Gage is not without its poignancy. In his 1850 paper, Bigelow announced the iron had "been deposited in the museum of the Massachusetts Medical College, where it may be seen, together with a cast of the patient's head." The tamping iron, now in the Warren Anatomical Museum of Harvard Medical School, is inscribed, and when the inscription is read carefully we make out the following:

This is the bar that was shot through the head of Mr. Phineluis P. Gage at Cavendish, Vermont, Sept. 14, 1848. He fully recovered from the injure & deposited this bar in the Museum of the Medical College, Harvard University. Phinehaus P. Gage Jan 6 1850

As now placed in its display case, Gage's "signature" and date are on the underside of the bar and, for that reason, are almost always overlooked. So, Phineas gave the iron to the Museum in 1850. But, according to the Editor of the *Boston Medical and Surgical Journal*:

It was Dr. Bigelow who ... had the inscription made on the tamping iron and persuaded the patient to allow it to be deposited in the Museum of the Medical College.

In his own footnote the editor added, "it was subsequently reclaimed by the patient," a fact consistent with reports that Gage had the iron when he was begging on the steps of the Massachusetts Medical College, and with Harlow's accounts of Phineas's having it with him when he later exhibited himself, and of his obtaining it from the relatives after Phineas's death.[14]

Poor Phineas. Not only was he of so little account to Bigelow that Bigelow managed to have the wrong date put on the tamping iron and have Gage's name misspelled twice, but he had also attempted to take away the only solid proof of his fame.

Notes

1. There are almost certainly more reports than we found. To begin with, there are very many more newspapers than we could have searched. For example, according to the Boston *Daily Evening Transcript* of 30 December 1850 (p. 1, col. 5), in Boston alone, fourteen daily, fifty-eight weekly, and nine semiweekly newspapers were published in 1850. For the period of the accident itself, we could search only a small number of mainly New England papers, mostly because the holdings are widely scattered and are often incomplete. Conducting an exhaustive search was well beyond our resources. Appendix H contains a list of newspapers searched by me or my various helpers. Second, subediting style in the 1800s was very different from our own. Use of a double-column spread was very rare and headings were minimal, if they were used at all. A given report was most frequently just another paragraph in a column of text set in the same font on a page in which all the columns looked very much alike. Reports as short as the

first two that we did find are easily overlooked, especially on a microfilm reader. Third, even when the holdings were apparently complete, it was often the case that pages and supplementary or other special editions were missing from both the original holdings and the microfilm copies of them (now the most commonly available form). These last two facts are mainly responsible for our failure to find those earlier reports that are so clearly implied in the later ones we did find.

2. *Boston Courier*, 20 September 1848, p. 2, col. 4, and *Boston Daily Journal*, 20 September 1848, p. 1, col. 7. Republished in Boston *Daily Evening Traveller*, 20 September, p. 2, col. 4 (*Courier* acknowledged); *Herald* (Rutland, Vermont), 27 September, p. 2, col. 3; *Green Mountain Freeman* (Montpelier, Vermont), 28 September, p. 2, col. 4; *True Democrat and Granite State Whig* (Lebanon, New Hampshire), 29 September, p. 2, col. 4 (all unacknowledged; the last has the new final sentence).

3. *Vermont Mercury* (Woodstock), 22 September, p. 2, col. 3; *Vermont Chronicle* (Windsor), 27 September, p. 2, col. 2; *Caledonian* (St. Johnsbury, Vermont), 30 September, p. 3, col. 3; *Vermont Gazette* (East Bennington), 5 October, p. 1, col. 2.

4. Angier's letter in the *Christian Reflector and Christian Watchman* (Boston), 12 October, p. 162, col. 6. It drew a rebuke from Harlow (1848) denying that there was a loose piece of skull.

5. *Vermont Mercury* (Woodstock), 13 October, p. 2, col. 4 (some pages of this edition are dated "November 13," but the volume/edition numbers as well as the contents, such as the Whig State Convention meeting announced in column 1 of page 2, make it clear that the paper was printed on 13 October). Reprintings with acknowledgment in *Boston Journal*, 19 October, p. 1, col. 3; *Vermont Journal* (Windsor), 20 October, p. 2, col. 5; *National Eagle* (Claremont, New Hampshire), 26 October, p. 1, col. 2; *New Hampshire Patriot and State Gazette* (Concord), 9 November, p. 3, col. 2; *Green Mountain Freeman* (Montpelier, Vermont), 16 November, p. 3, col. 2; *Caledonian* (St. Johnsbury, Vermont), 21 October, p. 3, col. 3.

6. *North Star* (Danville, Vermont), 6 November, p. 1, col. 2.

7. *National Eagle* (Claremont, New Hampshire), 29 March 1849, p. 2, col. 2. Reprinted in *True Democrat and Granite State Whig* (Lebanon, New Hampshire), 6 April 1849, p. 1, col. 7.

8. *North-Western Medical and Surgical Journal*, 1849, vol. 1, pp. 513–518; *American Journal of the Medical Sciences*, 1849, vol. 17, pp. 546–548; *Medical Times* (London), 1849, vol. 20, p. 9; Ranking's *Half-Yearly Abstract of the Medical Sciences*, 1849, vol. 10, pp. 181–184; *Buffalo Medical Journal*, 1848–1849, vol. 4, p. 584., cf. pp. 493–496; Harlow 1868, 1869.

9. Bigelow 1850b, 1850c; *Boston Society for Medical Improvement*, 1849, *Records of Meetings*, vol. 6, pp. 48, 75; Harlow 1868, p. 330, n.1, 1869; J. B. S. Jackson 1870, p. 149.

10. Bigelow's presentation of Gage in *Boston Society for Medical Improvement, Records of Meetings*, vol. 6, p. 103. Bigelow's address is Bigelow 1850a, p. 15. The statements of Williams, Freeman, and Adams are in Bigelow 1850b, and 1850c. They were gathered by Harlow.

11. *London Journal of Medicine*, 1850, vol. 19, pp. 1893–1894; *London Medical Gazette*, 1850, vol. 46, pp. 519–520; *Dublin Medical Press*, 1850, vol. 24, pp. 117–120; *British and Foreign Medico-Chirurgical Review*, 1850, vol. 6, pp. 543–544; and *Edinburgh Medical and Surgical Journal*, 1850, vol. 74, pp. 475–482.

12. *Boston Society for Medical Improvement*, 1849, *Records of Meetings*, vol. 6, pp. 103–104.

13. *Public Ledger and Daily Transcript* (Philadelphia), 3 July 1850, p. 2, col. 1; J. B. S. Jackson (1849, Case Number 1777).

14. Bigelow 1850b, 1850c; Bibliographical Notice, *Boston Medical and Surgical Journal*, 1869, vol. 80, pp. 116–117.

4

The Implications of Harlow's Treatment

The parts of brain that looked good for something I put back. Those that were too badly injured and looked as though they would be no good, I threw away. I kept the wound clean, sewed it up, and Gage got well.
—Norman Williams's account of his brother Edward's treatment, 1929

Once the medical profession or at least some of its members had accepted Harlow's description of the passage of Gage's tamping iron as accurate, two kinds of implication of the case could be explored: those for medical treatment, and those for understanding the functions of the brain. Here I take up the first.

Harlow's Treatment

Three phases in Harlow's treatment of Gage can be distinguished. In the first, the targets were the fracture and the hemorrhage, in the second a delirium and subsequent coma, and in the third a feverish condition that was not a direct consequence of the accident. Harlow's 1848 and 1868 accounts of his treatment of Gage are slightly different, and it is necessary to combine them to obtain enough detail to analyze what he did. My outline draws freely on both his accounts but, in a departure from the usual referencing system, I give dates for those quotations that refer to particular days of the recovery period.[1]

The First Phase (Fracture and Hemorrhage)
Harlow directed the first phase of treatment to the immediate arrest of the hemorrhage—Gage and his bed "were literally one gore of blood"— and to the repair of the damaged skull. He shaved the scalp, cleaned the wound of dried blood, and removed three small triangular pieces of

frontal bone and about an ounce of brain tissue that protruded through the fracture. Then, with one index finger in each of the openings, he searched inside the skull for other pieces of bone. Two pieces of frontal bone had been detached and Harlow replaced them before

the lacerated scalp was brought together as nearly as possible, and retained by adhesive straps, excepting at the posterior angle, and over this a simple dressing—compress, night cap and roller. The wound in the face was left patulous, covered only by a simple dressing.

The burns on hands and forearms were also dressed, and Gage was put to bed with his head elevated. Although the treatment may seem passive, what Harlow did was successful. Later that evening the hemorrhage was "abating," by the next morning it "continue[d] slightly," and it had ceased completely by the next day. However, by then other problems had supervened and a second phase of treatment began.

The Second Phase (Delirium and Coma)
The day after the accident, Harlow noted that swelling of the face was "considerable and increasing." The pulse was also up, from the 60 of a few hours after the accident to 75, and by the evening of the second day after the accident, 15 September, Gage had "lost control of his mind, and became decidedly delirious, with occasional lucid intervals." That change, together with a further increase of the pulse to 84, indicated the presence of what Harlow termed an "inflammation," "reaction," or "inflammatory reaction," that is, an infection (Harlow could not have used the term "infection," at least in its modern sense). The inflammation seems to have lasted for about nineteen days, causing two short periods in which Gage was delirious (15–16 September, 18–22 September) and a longer one during which he was comatose (25 September to 3 October).

Harlow began the second phase of treatment as soon as Gage became "restless and delirious." He first passed a metallic probe "into the opening in the top of the head, and down until it reached the base of the skull." Finding nothing, he prescribed a purgative of a half a fluid dram of vin. colchicum (1.85 ml of a purgative made from *Colchicum autumnale*, the autumn crocus) "every six hours until it purges him," and had the night cap removed. Although the purgative had not acted by the next morning, by which time Gage should have had two doses, the pulse was down and the delirium less. However, there was, Harlow said in 1868:

a fetid sero-purulent discharge, with particles of brain intermingled ... from the opening in the top of the head and also from the one in the base of the skull into the mouth.

What Harlow termed "a fungus" had also appeared at the external canthus of the left eye. Further repeated attempts at catharsis were made, this time with doses of magnesium sulphate (Epsom salts) every four hours. By the next morning Gage had "purged freely" and was rational. Although the wound in the face was healing, the discharge from that in the head continued.[2]

When the second short period of delirium began, on 18 September, the fifth day after the accident, Harlow again "passed a probe to the base of the cranium" and again prescribed a cathartic, this time unspecified. Otherwise he seems to have been content to wait, merely changing the dressings three times a day, regularly disinfecting the mouth and back of the throat, cleaning the face of the material discharged by the wounds, and keeping iced water on the head. Purgatives were not given again until, after three very restless days and nights, calomel (mercurous chloride) and rhubarb was given, possibly followed by castor oil, on the morning of the ninth day, the 22nd. By the afternoon Gage had "purged freely twice, and incline[d] to sleep." By the next day, the 23rd, he was markedly stronger and more rational. The discharge from the head wound was also smaller and less fetid. Consequently the scalp was reshaven and the edges of the wound brought closer together.

By the evening of the tenth day after the accident (23 September) Harlow began to entertain, for the first time, the possibility that Gage might survive. His optimism was to be dashed. Two days later, on the evening of the 25th, Gage became semicomatose: he was "stupid, did not speak unless aroused, and then only with difficulty." Over the next three days the coma deepened: Gage spoke only "when aroused," and then solely in monosyllables, and had to be "strongly urged" to take nourishment. By now, treatment consisted of the thrice-daily changing of the dressings, supporting Gage "with food and stimulants," and giving laxatives of an unspecified kind now combined with an "occasional dose" of the presumably stronger calomel. Nevertheless, the fungi from the eye now pushed out "rapidly" as did the "large fungi" from the brain, where emerging from "the opening in the top of the head," they prevented all but a "scanty" discharge from it. In addition, the tissues on the forehead under the frontalis muscle, between the lower edge of the fracture in the frontal bone and the left nasal protuberance, became "swollen, hot, and red."

The attendants and Gage's friends now despaired of his recovery and Thomas Winslow prepared his coffin. On the fourteenth day after the accident, the 27th, one attendant even urged Harlow to discontinue treatment so as not to prolong Gage's suffering. According to his 1868 report, Harlow appears to have been goaded into action by her adding the remark that it seemed as though Gage had water on the brain. Replying that "it is not water, but matter that is killing the man," and with

a pair of curved scissors I cut off the fungi which were sprouting out from the top of the brain and filling the opening, and made free application of caustic [crystalline nitrate of silver] to them. With a scalpel I laid open the integuments between the opening and the roots of the nose, and immediately there were discharged eight-ounces of ill-conditioned pus, with blood, and excessively foetid.

Over the next nine days (28 September to 6 October) there was profuse and fetid discharge "from the openings" and although Gage remained comatose, he was able to swallow well and "took considerable nourishment, with brandy and milk." By 5 October, twenty-two days after the accident, Harlow noted Gage was "improving" and the wound and sinus were discharging "laudable pus." On the 6th, he was able to raise himself into a sitting position for about four minutes and by the 7th, the twenty-third day, Gage took his first step.

Harlow published notes from only four of the days between the 7 October and 8 November. In all, the signs of continued healing are marked: the pus remained laudable, and the fungi gave way under the nitrate of silver until, by 20 October, after thirty-seven days, they had disappeared and the head wound began to close rapidly. The sinus had almost healed by 8 November, fifty-six days after the accident. By then Gage's appetite was "good," he digested food "easily," his bowels were "regular," and he was sleeping "well." He was also able to walk around the house, up and down the stairs, and into the piazza, and finally to venture into the street. Harlow, apparently judging him well enough, left Cavendish, enjoining Gage before he did so "to avoid excitement and exposure." The only other treatment Harlow mentions during this obvious period of recovery, is that he continued to keep Gage on "a low diet," or that he "was not allowed on a full diet," even though his appetite was "good."

The Third Phase (Chill and Fever)
Harlow returned on the evening of 14 November to learn that Gage had disobeyed his instruction and been out in the street "every day except Sunday." On the 14th he had actually:

walked half a mile and purchased some small articles at the store. The atmosphere was cold and damp, the ground wet, and he went without an overcoat, and with thin boots. He got wet feet and a chill.

When Harlow saw him, Gage had "rigors," was "depressed and irritable," his pulse up to 100, his skin hot and dry, his face and head painful, his tongue coated, and he was constipated. Harlow then began the third phase of his treatment by first prescribing cold to the face and head, and a cathartic ("a black dose"), which was to be repeated in six hours if necessary. Gage passed a "sleepless night" and the next morning, 16 November, although the cathartic had "operated freely," his symptoms were virtually unchanged. His pulse was now 120, the highest Harlow reported. Gage was thereupon bled of 16 fluid ounces of blood (about 500 ml) and prescribed a further purgative of 10 grains (650 mg) of calomel and 2 grains (130 mg) of the emetic ipecacuanha (a derivative of the root or rhizome of the South American *Cephaelis ipecacuanha*), with a follow-up dose of castor oil four hours later. By the evening Gage had "purged freely," his pulse was lower, his skin moist, and the pains in his head had "moderated." Harlow now prescribed a dessert spoonful of another emetic of 3 grains (195 mg) of antimony potassium tartrate in 6 fluid ounces (180 ml) of syrup simplex every four hours. During the night he again "purged freely" and woke on the morning of the 17th, sixty-five days after being injured, without pain and expressed himself as "feeling better in every respect."

Gage's recovery then continued without further interruption. On 27 November, Harlow completed the first of his papers and recorded that the portions of bone had "united firmly." By then, Gage had returned to Lebanon, leaving Cavendish two days earlier, only seventy-three days after the accident. When Harlow visited him a week later he found him "going on well." One hundred twelve days after the accident, on 3 January 1849, Harlow saw him in Lebanon, where he found him "walking about the house, riding out, improving both mentally and physically." The recovery seemed complete (see Appendices A and B).

Antiphlogistic and Other Therapies

In 1868 Harlow adduced four circumstances that had worked in Gage's favor. The pointed shape and smoothness of the tamping iron reduced damage to his brain by concussion and compression; his physique, will, and endurance made Gage "the man for the case"; the iron's entry through the base of the skull had created "a natural drainage point for the wound"; and "the portion of the brain traversed, was, for several reasons, the best fitted of any ... to sustain the injury."

The shape and smoothness of the tamping iron, as well as its probable velocity, undoubtedly reduced the injury to Gage's brain, but could not eliminate concussive or compressive damage entirely. If we grant that concussive damage may be indexed by loss of consciousness, the damage was probably slight. Although one notes the considerable agreement among the various accounts of the immediate effect of the passage of the iron, the statements that Gage did not lose consciousness at all seem to derive from Gage himself, and should perhaps be regarded with reserve. Whether and how much compressive damage there was is impossible to say—Gage's ultimate recovery cannot, of course, serve as the evidence for its being slight.[3]

Harlow's remarks about Gage's being the man for the case and the importance of the wound's being able to drain have be understood in relation to the *antiphlogistic* therapeutic or *depletion* regimen he practiced. It is usefully discussed in the general context provided by the analysis of common nineteenth-century U.S. medical practice by Warner, and the more specific one of the treatment of open head injuries in the United States between 1810 and 1880 that Barker documents so comprehensively. Antiphlogistic therapy was based on the belief that most diseases were *sthenic* (Gr. *sthenos*, "strength") and had overstimulated and unbalanced the patient. As can be seen from the discussions of Warner, Berman, and Carter, the physician's task was to reduce the inflammatory or *phlogistic* (Gr. *phlogos*, "flame", *phlogistos*, "inflammable") state associated with the sthenic condition and restore the patient to a healthy, natural balance. Bloodletting was one of the main therapeutic techniques available to physicians adopting the antiphlogistic regimen. Whether carried out by venesection, cupping, or the application of leeches, the main basis for its effect was almost self-evident: bloodletting removed the *plethora* or excess of blood found in sthenic conditions. Together with cathartics, emetics, diet reduction, and counterirritants (blisters), bloodletting also cleansed the patient's system of matter causing the inflammation and impeded its functioning.[4]

Many of Harlow's final comments nearly twenty years after the accident show the strength of his adherence to antiphlogistic principles. For example, he began his concluding remarks about treatment by saying:

The initiatory treatment, received from the iron, *though it might not be well received in this presence*, was decidedly antiphlogistic, a very large amount of blood having been lost. May we not infer that this prepared the system for the trying ordeal through which it was about to pass? (emphasis added)

Nash had made the same point about his case, seen at about the same time: "a large quantity of blood taken away at first will have more effect than frequent bleedings afterwards." Harlow's stresses on the regimen were as deliberate as they were significant. He was speaking at a time when antiphlogistic therapy was in decline generally, and to an audience drawn from an area (Massachusetts) in which, as Warner and Barker both show, the decline was especially marked.

When the delirium and coma of the second phase began, it would have seemed obvious to Harlow that Gage's system was "morbidly animated" to the point of being unbalanced. Harlow's general treatment in this phase, as well as in treating the feverish condition brought on by the chill, seems to have been to maintain Gage on a low diet and to prescribe cathartics and emetics when he was delirious or constipated. Venesection was used once, in the third phase. All this is in line with antiphlogistic doctrine and practice. So was Harlow's action during what he termed "the two critical periods," when he thought his treatment had "undoubtedly" prevented a fatal result. On the fourteenth day, he had drained a large abscess that he believed most probably communicated with the left lateral ventricle. A marked improvement in all the symptoms followed. And on the sixty-fourth day, after the chill caused Gage to become feverish, he had bled him of sixteen ounces.

When he gave credit to Gage's physique, will, and endurance, it seems that, even there, Harlow was crediting the constitutional and temperamental factors thought to interact with the antiphlogistic regimen. As Warner notes, it was generally believed that working men, particularly those living in rural areas, were more prone to inflammatory or sthenic diseases than those in the cities, and more so than the indolent middle and upper classes in either. But it was also not an uncommon view that at least some who worked with their hands, such as the peasants of England mentioned by Bodkin and Maunsell, also had a natural anti-inflammatory diathesis. Antiphlogistic remedies were therefore used more strictly for the strong and choleric than for the strong and phlegmatic, and the former corresponds to the bilious part of the "nervo-bilious" temperament Harlow ascribed to Gage.[5]

Adequate drainage of the wound, the third of the factors to which Harlow attributed Gage's recovery, was also part of the antiphlogistic regimen. Inflammation occurring after a head injury indicated the necessity of cleansing the system of accumulated pus if the symptoms of intracerebral compression were to be relieved. The remedies usually combined drainage, venesection, and purging. As Barker has shown, drainage was stressed in an antiphlogistic context in the teaching of Thomas Mütter, Professor of Surgery, and Joseph Pancoast, Professor of Anatomy, who were both at Jefferson Medical College when Harlow studied there. Barker points out that the cornerstones of Mütter's antiphlogistic therapy were vigorous bleeding, purgatives, and cathartics as well as proper draining of the head wounds. Barker also shows that Harlow saw a famous demonstration by Pancoast of the importance of drainage in a case of head injury treated almost as vigorously. Although the patient had died, death had been due an intracerebral accumulation of pus being unable to drain because of the formation of granulation tissue.

Here it is worth noting that Harlow did not apply rigidly what he had learned. Thus when Gage was comatose, Harlow made sure he was fed and, in giving brandy and unspecified substances, he was actually adding what were then regarded as stimulants. To this extent he drew on what was then regarded as the opposite to antiphlogistic therapy: treatment by *stimulation*. Further, immediately after the accident, when there was probably little more that Harlow could have done but arrest the bleeding and repair the skull, there is good reason for believing that even those essentially *passive* measures were based on a doctrine of natural healing that had been popular in New England medical circles even before its formal proclamation by Bigelow's father in 1835. At various places Harlow specifically attributed Gage's recovery to the very power criticized by those who advocated active medical intervention, the *vis vitae*, *vis conservatrix*, or *vis medicatrix naturae*.

As Harlow saw it in 1868, there were no contradictions between the components of his treatment:

I indulge the hope, that *surely but little if anything was done to retard the progress of the case, or to interfere with the natural recuperative powers*. Nature is certainly greater than art. Some one has wisely said, that vain is learning without wit. So we may say, vain is art without nature. For what surgeon, the most skilful, with all the blandishments of his art, has the world ever known, who could presume to take one of his fellows who has had so formidable a missile hurled through his brain, with a crash, and bring him, without the aid of this *vis con-servatrix*, so that, on the fifty-sixth day thereafter, he would have been walking in the streets again? (Emphasis added)

Harlow did not, as did many practitioners, prescribe his antiphlogistic remedies in a routine, preventive way. He intervened only when it seemed necessary to do so.[6]

Harlow's Treatment Compared with Others

My analysis of a large but somewhat unsystematically collected sample of nineteenth-century reports of the treatment of injury to the brain or fractures of the skull shows Harlow drew on his antiphlogistic remedies in moderation. Although those remedies were in reasonably wide use, he did not use them nearly as forcefully as his contemporaries.

In the medical literature up to and including 1849, the antiphlogistic regimen is most often described by that name or it is termed "depletion." And, if we define the antiphlogistic regimen by the prescription of combinations of at least two of the cathartics, emetics, enemas, bloodletting, or counterirritants, and a low diet, an absence of stimulants, especially alcohol, and rest in a dark or quiet room, the use of that regimen or some discussion of its desirability occurs in very many more reports of the treatment of brain injury, including those in which brain tissue was lost or destroyed. After 1849, it continued in use, albeit sometimes modified, until as late as the 1890s.[7]

When his treatment of Gage is measured against the standards of medical practice revealed by these pre-1850 reports, we see how moderate Harlow was. Armour, for example, took 10 fluid ounces of blood from William Park seven hours after his injury and another 15 ounces an hour later. Park was a fifteen year old who had had his frontal bone fractured above the right eye and his brain damaged by a kick from a horse. The next day, Park was bled three times for a total of 33 ounces and, when he began to convulse after the third venesection, ten leeches and a blister were applied. By that time he had also been given five boluses, each containing 3 grains of calomel and 5 of rhubarb, as well as an emetic! What Marvin described as a "violent reaction" as his twelve-year-old patient, John Wooster, recovered from a left temporal fracture with loss of brain tissue required "frequent and copious bleedings, together with cathartics and antimonials." Similar enthusiasm is found in other reports and recommendations in the use of antiphlogistics in the treatment of brain injury.[8]

Warner's investigations make possible some quantitative comparison of Harlow's therapy with that of his contemporaries. Warner found that between 1810 and 1860 the incidence of venesection in private practice "for the larger part of the American profession clustered between two percent and nine percent of recorded *visits*," with variation from as low as 0.7 percent to as high as 16.9 percent. If we count Harlow's visits as taking place only once per day and omit the six days he was away from Cavendish, we find he visited Gage 67 times and venesected on only one of them, a rate of 1.5 percent, well below the lowest percentage Warner found. Warner's calculations of prescription rates for *patients* (not visits) admitted to the Massachusetts General Hospital in the 1840s, at a time when it was staffed by physicians opposed to antiphlogistic practice, show calomel was prescribed for 31 percent, ipecacuanha for 17 percent, alcohol for 17 percent, tartar emetic for 12 percent, venesection for 6 percent, and low diet for 3 percent. Harlow prescribed cathartics on sixteen of his visits, including each of the ten when Gage was comatose, and emetics on two. Because it is very apparent from the cases already cited that Harlow prescribed small amounts relatively infrequently, these figures would be consistent with a much lower use of emetics and cathartics than at Massachusetts General.[9]

Harlow's low use of antiphlogistic remedies is also consistent with Warner's conclusions that there was a less aggressive use of depletive therapy in the New England medical community than elsewhere, and that a steady decline in the use of all of its components began there in the 1830s. Barker has since confirmed this declining trend in the treatment of open brain injury by a logistic regression analysis of the numbers of physicians using venesection as a treatment in 170 such cases over the period 1810–1880. By 1848 Barker estimates that only 30 percent of physicians would have used it. That percentage would not, of course, have put Harlow very much at odds with other members of his profession, even had his use of it and related techniques been more aggressive. That the treatment may have had some positive value has been suggested by Steegmann, who judged Harlow's use of cathartics and emetics, together with his single venesection, "may have favourably influenced the outcome" by reducing intracranial pressure through dehydration.[10]

Other aspects of Harlow's treatment show his skillful and imaginative adaptation of traditional methods. Approximating the edges of the scalp with adhesive bandages or a single suture and leaving a part of the wound open before applying a light dressing was a common method of ensuring that wounds drained freely, but Harlow added the semirecumbent position for Gage for the same purpose. He realized that although the iron's piercing the base of the skull had provided a "natural drainage point," that opening would not automatically function as such. His opinion was borne out by the formation of the abscess on the fourteenth day which he had had to drain so vigorously and dramatically. In reuniting the two pieces of frontal bone and applying light dressings to promote their growth, he seems to have followed Mütter and Pancoast. But it may also have been because he believed that fungi would then be less likely to form.[11]

On two details in his treatment that were matters of some controversy, Harlow took the progressive view. The first was whether all the bone fragments should be removed from the wound or not. Most physicians seem to have taken the view that the "inflammation" that usually occurred when pieces of bone were left in the wound or in the brain itself was deleterious, but some seem to have believed any discharge so created actually aided healing. There was also the problem that an exhaustive search for bone fragments might cause hemorrhaging or other direct injury to the brain. Harlow's cautious initial search for fragments seems to show a divergence from Mütter.[12]

The second detail was about how the fungi should be treated, if at all. The disagreement sprang from differences of opinion about their nature. Some thought fungi were structurally sound brain tissue that had been extruded from the wound as true *hernia cerebri*. The extrusion was seen as a consequence of arterial pressure acting either by itself or in conjunction with the loss of the support the unbroken bone and tissue surrounding it normally gave the brain. Others regarded fungi as an admixture of fragmented blood vessels and broken down brain substance, sometimes speaking of "putrid" brain, or observing it was brain "so altered in its character" that they would "not venture to return it into the cranium." Occasionally there was recognition that there might be more than one type of fungus, but Abernethy's view that they were *always* new living tissue formed from or around coagula seems to have been rarely endorsed.

Were fungi considered to be sound tissue, it was appropriate to use pressure, most often from special forms of bandaging, to force them back inside the skull. Alternatively, as "disorganised" substance, they were to be removed by being cut away from the opening. Removal could cause fatal hemorrhage, but replacement had the potential for causing equally dangerous brain compression. Applications of caustic compounds avoided both risks at the cost of possibly destroying sound brain substance.[13]

Harlow's methods were not very different from those of his predecessors and contemporaries, even allowing for his emphasis on cleanliness and the use of disinfectants. They should not be counted as unusual factors and Harlow thereby placed well in advance of his time. True, Lister's advocacy of aseptic surgery dates from 1867 and, true, many surgeons did operate in their ordinary clothes, often without washing their hands, and after only a perfunctory rinse of their instruments in the buckets of cold water standing beside them that had been used previously for the same purpose. But this was not true of all; the same stress on cleanliness, perhaps not always to the same degree, is to be found in most of the reports on similar cases that I have cited. But although not different in their fundamentals concerning treatment, Butler was probably not exaggerating when he asked whether the credulity of a Pott (whom he credited, with good reason, for revolutionizing the treatment of fractures of the skull) "would not have been somewhat taxed" had he been able to read of the successful treatments of "modern times." Butler was commenting upon a case reported by Fitch in which the right temporal and parietal regions were injured following a skull fracture caused by a kick from a horse. The modern instance with which Butler illustrated his point was none other than Harlow's treatment of Gage.

On my analysis, Blakemore's description of Harlow's treatment as confined to "liberal doses of calomel, rhubarb and castor oil" is a gross caricature. Harlow skillfully adapted conservative and progressive elements from the available therapies to the particular needs posed by Gage's injury. Harlow's 1868 summary was therefore far too modest: "I can only say ... with good old Ambro[i]se Paré, I dressed him, God healed him."[14]

Acknowledgments of Harlow's Experience

During what may be termed the post-Gage era, the treatment of other cases was sometimes compared with Harlow's, especially those cases in which the premature explosion of muskets or guns damaged the frontal areas. One of the most striking is Noyes's case of Lewis Avery. In September 1881, as Avery was aiming his musket, it exploded in his face. Unknown to him, the breech pin was driven through the skull above the right eye, lodging in the right frontal lobe, destroying the tissue around it. By November of that year his recovery seemed complete, and in February 1882 he sought to have his disfiguration repaired. Only during the preliminaries to that operation was the breech pin discovered. It was removed four days later. The pin was found to be $4\frac{7}{16}$ inches long, about $\frac{1}{2}$ inch broad, and weight 2 ounces, 5 drachms, and 25 grains (figure 4.1). Technically the operation was successful but a few days later an infection

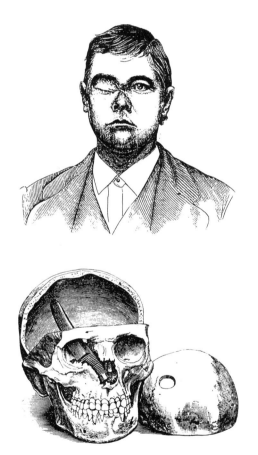

Figure 4.1
Lewis Avery before the attempted facial repair and the post-mortem location of the breech pin
From Noyes 1882.

set in, and Avery died, thirty-nine days later, on 29 March. Post mortem study enabled the breech pin to be accurately located within the skull and the considerable damage to the right frontal lobe and other structures assessed. Death seems to have been due to the formation of an abscess that could not be adequately drained, partly because of its position and partly because the patient could not be dissuaded from lying on his left side. Noyes stressed the need to provide for the best drainage possible, citing Harlow's opinion in a letter from him that "it was due in great measure to the free outlets through the skull below and above that the man Gage owed his life." When concluding his report of a very similar but completely successful case, Kemper, perhaps not surprisingly, quoted these views of Noyes and Harlow and endorsed them completely.[15]

Injury and Resistance

Thirty years before Gage's accident, Wharton set out what he regarded as the major superstition about injuries to the brain as

the long received opinion among mankind, learned as well as illiterate, that the slightest injury of the brain was followed, *in all cases* by death.

Stated so extremely, Wharton was correct in concluding that the complete recovery of his fourteen-year-old patient after the loss of an amount of tissue "about the size of a large garden pea" from what seems to have been the left frontal lobe "plainly prove[d]" the opinion fallacious.

Although it is true that at the end of the eighteenth century and the beginning of the nineteenth there was much superstition about the effects of injury to the brain, even before Wharton's opinion there were a number of reports of complete recovery following quite extensive loss or destruction of brain substance. When Tyrrell discussed Rogers's case of Mark George, one could say that he summed up those reports, even though he made no reference to other authors. George was also injured by the bursting of an overcharged gun. In his case the breech pin was driven into his left frontal and left temporal regions. Rogers described the amount of tissue that then escaped as "considerable," judging also that as much "as a table-spoonful adhered to the hair and integuments around." However, the pin itself was not discovered to be in the brain until nearly four weeks after the accident. Removed during an operation, it consisted "of solid iron, three inches in length and exactly three ounces in weight." Tyrrell began his comments by saying:

Many cases are recorded in which large portions of the cerebrum have been lost without any immediate or subsequent derangement of the mental and corporeal functions; but I am not aware that any case has been attended with the lodgement of so large a foreign body in the cavity of the cranium, for so long a period as twenty seven days, with the production of so little mischief.

Rogers observed that "the smell and hearing are both perfect" and that there was no defect "in regard to his memory or general mental faculties." Six months after the accident, George's recovery was complete except for the loss of sight in the left eye. Despite this and other post-Wharton cases in which there was also loss of brain, Guthrie could still open a major work on head injury with this assertion:

Injuries of the head affecting the brain are difficult of distinction, doubtful in their character, treacherous in their course, and for the most part fatal in their result.

Consequently, it is not surprising that when Butler came to comment on the relation between Gage and Fitch's case, we find Wharton's "superstition" still alive virtually in the middle of the century:

It is a popular notion, and even some of the profession are involved in it, that injuries to the brain, more especially where any portion of its substance has been lost, necessarily involve loss of life.

Fitch's case, like Wharton's, was of a fracture of the skull caused by a kick from a horse. The right temporal and parietal regions had been injured with "portions" of the brain being lost.[16]

By 1860 Brown expressed the opinion that "sufficiently numerous cases are on record of perfect recovery after dangerous and extensive injury of the brain from mechanical causes" to require more than a mere report of another to justify publication. Twelve years later, Dupuis expressed similar sentiments, and the same conclusion can be seen in Wharton's tabulation of the consequences of 316 cases in which foreign bodies remained in the brain. Of course, all the other cases I have cited who recovered despite the loss of brain tissue also support the conclusion.[17]

Remarks conveying surprise that the brain could resist serious injury are best thought of as variants of the "superstition," albeit a more optimistic one. They seem to be first made in the 1820s but are sometimes found even in the twentieth century. Maunsell put the variant best when said his case of bilateral frontal damage taught, among other things, "how much this organ can bear under peculiar circumstances." Sometimes, as with Bodkin, Maunsell was explicitly endorsed but more frequently it was a similar sentiment that was expressed or subscribed to.[18]

Gage the Standard

The amount of cerebral damage caused by Gage's tamping iron soon became the standard against which other injuries to the brain were judged. Some of the comparisons were competitively lighthearted. Writing from Georgetown, Kentucky, Sutton concluded his account of the nonfatal course of a revolver bullet by saying:

If you Yankees *can* send a tamping bar through a fellow's brain and not kill him, I *guess* there are not many can shoot a pistol bullet between a man's mouth and his brains, stopping just short of the medulla oblongata, and not touch either.

Butler's classing Fitch's case, in which "portions" of the brain were lost, with Gage was a completely serious comparison, however. Butler granted of Gage that there was probably "not on record a case of recovery from such an extensive lesion of the brain."

Quite serious competition is evident in some of the comparisons, that of Jewett for example. Jewett's case was that of Joel Lenn, a French or French Canadian miner working in Ohio, who had had a blasting barrel, consisting of a four-foot-long gas pipe five-eighths of an inch in diameter shot for about half its length through his head, from the external angle of the right superciliary ridge to a point about one and a half inches above the left ear. The pipe passed through the right frontal and left temporal lobes, lacerating the longitudinal sinus on the way. Eight months after the accident Jewett said that Lenn was physically as well as ever. Although Jewett conceded that the bar that injured Gage was much larger than the blasting barrel, he did emphasize that it traversed a much smaller portion of the brain than in Lenn's case.

Folsom's report added an element of grim humor to the competition. His case was of a Mr. Chase, a foreman at a sawmill, whose head had been cut open by a circular saw, about an eighth of an inch thick, spinning at some 2,000 rpm. The cut extended from one-half inch above the nose for a distance of about nine inches to the "occipital protuberance" and was about three inches deep. Five or six weeks after the accident, the victim resumed work. Folsom thought the case to be "second to none reported, save the famous tamping iron case of Dr. Harlow." He said he understood why his report might not be believed and would be happy to give more information but added "I cannot well gratify the desire of my professional brethren to possess Mr. Chase's skull, until he has no further use for it himself."

Conclusion

Despite competition, including that provided by injuries from other tamping irons, from axes, from bolts, from accidents with bridges, and even falling gum tree branches, the status of Phineas Gage's injuries was maintained. At the end of the century it received a kind of official recognition when Gould and Pyle, in their encyclopedic *Anomalies and Curiosities of Medicine*, placed Phineas first among the class of head injuries with loss of cerebral substance, offering the opinion that his was "possibly the most noted" of them.

Subsequent to Gould and Pyle, only the case reported in 1981 by Stone, Rifai, and Moody challenges Gage's preeminence. In that case, a tunnel worker was struck from above by a falling, star-ended, hexagonal drill bit 3.0 cm in diameter, 1.8 m long, and weighing about 7.5 kg that:

penetrated the man's helmet and then his skull to the left of the midline at the coronal suture. It passed through the left frontal and anterior temporal lobes and emerged through the left temporal fossa. It shattered the left zygoma as the metal rod penetrated the face several centimetres anterior to the left tragus.

As can be appreciated, the drill bit traversed much the same path as Gage's tamping iron, although slightly more posterior, and from above downward. Its velocity, estimated at 38 m per second, was possibly less than that attained by Gage's iron: at least it did not pass completely through the head. Stone et al. describe the type of injury as "remarkable," saying that Gage was "the only similar injury which we have found in a search of the literature."

Stone has subsequently described twelve other cases (thus making a total of fourteen) in which there was survival of transcranial injury caused by rods and bars of one kind and another, the earliest in 1810 and the last in 1994. Consideration of these cases does not require much amendment of the judgement with which Harlow had introduced Phineas in 1848 when he described him as a "hitherto unparalleled case." Although all of the cases Stone described were clearly also "remarkable instances of survival," it was his own case of 1978 that most closely resembled Gage. The passage of time has therefore not required much revision to Harlow's estimate: only one really similar case 130 years later.[19]

Notes

1. Appendix B sets out thematically three different records of the case and the notes: those from Harlow's 1848 report, those from Bigelow's 1850b paper, and those in Harlow's final report of 1868. For the most part, Bigelow simply reprints Harlow's first set of notes, but does add some observations of his own that are different. On the whole the day-to-day variation between the 1848 and 1868 notes is not great, but their mainly chronological ordering allows for the ready identification of such differences as do exist.

2. The appearance of "fungi" was regarded as predicting an unfavourable outcome. What they might have been is discussed later.

3. The four "circumstances" are in Harlow 1868, 1869. Dr. Al Reubens, Chief of Neurology in the Medical Center of the University of Arizona, pointed out to me that the relatively low velocity of the tamping iron would also have minimized damage due to shock waves being transmitted through the substance of the brain, and Ordia 1989 makes the same point about velocities less than 1,000 feet per second.

4. Warner 1986; Barker 1993; Berman 1978; Carter 1982.

5. Nash 1847 for his not dissimilar case. See Warner 1986 and Barker 1993 for the antiphlogistic decline and Warner 1986, pp. 65–68, on diathesis generally. Bodkin 1830 and Maunsell 1830 for peasants. For the temperaments, see chapter 15 and note 7.

6. Barker 1995 for Mütter and Pancoast. Warner 1986, pp. 17–31, for stimulation. Harlow's flexibility may also be behind his defending himself against the criticism that he had not, during this first phase of treatment, passed a probe "through the entire extent of the wound." He explained he wished not to risk disturbing the already lacerated blood vessels that were near to being stanched (Harlow 1848). In similar cases the probe was used to map the extent of the fracture and to locate pieces of bone and other loose foreign bodies.

7. For the use of antiphlogistic or depletion regimes, see Leny 1793; Pott 1808, case 24; Harrup 1814; Peake 1820; Sewall 1828, case 1; Maunsell 1830; Fitzpatrick 1840; and Shipman 1848, case 4. For the use of various combinations of the constituents of the antiphlogistic regimen, see Baine 1742; French 1792; Scott 1796; Barlow 1802; Pott 1808; Crawford 1816; Wharton 1818; Edmondson 1823; Corban 1825; Crowfoot 1825; Jones 1826; Rogers 1827; Sewall 1828, case 2; Heustis 1829; Bodkin 1830; Armour 1831; Davidson 1838; Marvin 1838; Janson 1840; Carmichael 1841, case of Byrne; O'Callaghan 1845; Harvey 1846; Harris 1847; Nash 1847; Horlbeck 1848; Shipman 1848, cases 2, 3, 5; Forbes 1849; Fox 1849, case 3; Rice 1849; and Walke 1849. For late continuations, see Fitch 1852; Mackay 1853; Cabot 1856–1857; Spence 1856–1857; Chance 1858; McRae 1858; Porter 1858; Rose 1858; Smith 1858; Brown 1860; Cabot 1860; Gaffney 1860; Brooke 1861; Hargrave 1861; Quain 1861; Maclaren 1861–1862; Heard 1863; Hamilton 1864; MacGillivray 1864; Martin

1864; Ashhurst 1865; Bird 1865; Moon 1866; Cheney 1867; Croker 1867; Gray 1868; Jewett 1868; Alford 1869; Downs 1871; Howard 1871; Dupuis 1872; Morgan 1875; Kebbell 1876; Annandale 1877; Bolton 1878–1879; Capon 1879; Elcan 1880; Barton 1881; Boon 1881; Hunter 1881; Le Page 1881; M'carthy 1882–1883; Humphreys 1885; Molony 1887; Leishman 1890–1891; and D'Auvergne Collings 1893.

8. Armour 1831 and Marvin 1838. For other examples of the vigor with which the antiphlogistic regimen was adopted, see Corban 1825; Crowfoot 1825; Davidson 1838; Forbes 1849; Dupuis 1872; Edmondson 1823; Fitzpatrick 1840; Gray 1868; Guthrie 1842; Hamilton 1864; Maunsell 1830; Peake 1820; Pott 1808, case 28; Rogers 1827; Sewall 1828; and Shipman 1848, cases 3 and 4.

9. Warner 1986, pp. 95–96, 115–135, and table 1. Because Harlow sometimes visited as many as three times in a day, my 1.5 percent may overestimate Harlow's *per visit* venesection rate. However, although the rate would roughly double if only the thirty-one days on which something was definitely wrong were used as a base, he would have venesected on only 3.2 percent of the days.

10. Barker 1993; Steegmann 1962.

11. Pancoast in Barker 1995; fungi are discussed by "Review of Guthrie's" 1843 and Martin 1864.

12. Compare the discussions by Peake 1820; Carmichael 1841; Shipman 1848, case 6; the Editorial Note to Fitch 1852; Martin 1864; Moon 1866; and Guthrie 1842.

13. Fungi as normal tissue: Crawford 1816; Armour 1831; Davidson 1838; Stanley, cited in Guthrie 1842; Harvey 1846; Mackay 1853; Stapleton 1858; and Evans 1865. Fungi as breakdown products: Bodkin 1830; Carmichael 1841, case 2; Harvey 1846; Martin 1864. Different types of fungi: Carmichael 1841; Guthrie 1842; and Cabot 1856–1857, 1860. Abernethy is criticized in Heustis 1829. Caustic in treatment: Heustis 1829 and "Review of Guthrie's" 1843.

14. Butler in Fitch 1852; Blakemore 1977. Ambroise Paré (1510–1590), "the father of French surgery," who remarked on the successful outcome of his treatment in 1536 of an ankle wound "Je le pensay, et Dieu le guarist" (Paré 1580, *Le voyage de Thurin*, p. 689, in Malgaigne 1840, vol. 3, pp. 689–692. cf. Hamby 1967). Paré also seems to have made the remark at other times.

15. Noyes 1882; Kemper 1885.

16. Wharton 1818; Tyrrell in Rogers 1827; Guthrie 1842, p. 1; Butler in Fitch, 1852. Pre-Gage cases of brain injury with loss of tissue: Paré's cases 71–73 from Malgaigne 1840, vol. 2; Baine 1742; French 1792; Leny 1793; Scott 1796; Barlow 1802; Harrup 1814; Home 1814, sec. 8; Crawford 1816; Peake 1820; Edmondson 1823; Corban 1825; Crowfoot 1825; Jones 1826; Sewall 1828; Bodkin 1830; Green 1832, cited in Steegmann, 1962; Maunsell 1830; Marvin 1838; Roberts 1838–1839; Janson 1840; and Adams and Hargrave in Carmichael 1841.

17. Brown 1860; Dupuis 1872; Wharton 1879, cited in Steegmann, 1962.

18. Maunsell 1830 and Bodkin 1830. Other nineteenth-century expressions of the sentiment are Corban 1825; Williams 1835; Roberts 1838–1839; M'Coy, comment in O'Callaghan, 1845; Nash 1847; Mackay 1853; Shipman 1848; Smith 1858; Hamilton 1864; Martin 1864; Babbit 1867–1868; Croker 1867; Molony 1877; Parsons 1884; Humphreys 1885; Anderson 1888; Smith 1892; Michelmore in Cullin, 1893; and Fenner 1899.

19. Sutton 1850–1851; Butler in Fitch 1852; Jewett 1868; Folsom 1868–1869; Gould and Pyle 1896; Stone, Rifai, and Moody 1981; Stone 1999.

5

The Wonderful Journey

... cette observation remarquable et authentique, bien qu'americaine ...
—Eugene Dupuy, *Examen de quelques points de la physiologie du cerveau*, 1873

For as long as Phineas Gage lived it was not possible to be certain about what damage his tamping iron had done to his skull and brain. After his death there was no greater certainty. His brain was not then examined, and which parts were damaged and how the damage had been caused were not determined. Nor, I believe, can it be determined now. In this chapter I set out as systematically as I can the attempts to determine the damage to Gage's skull and brain between Harlow's first report and the present.

The year 1880 marks the end of the early period of this study. By then Gage's skull had become available and some consensus had been reached on what it showed. Although 1880 ends the first period, it cannot be said to mark the start of the modern era. Nearly sixty years were to elapse before further consideration was given to establishing just what damage the tamping iron had done. Then, presumably in response to the surgical and experimental studies of the effects of frontal lobe ablation conducted over about the previous ten years, Gage came back into the spotlight. Only then did the modern era begin.

The pre-1880 data about the damage to Gage's skull and brain come essentially from four kinds of examination: that of the live Gage (Harlow, Bigelow, and Phelps), of a skull drilled to cause damage resembling Gage's (Bigelow), of Gage's own skull (Harlow, J. B. S. Jackson, Dupuy), and of illustrations of the skull Bigelow had drilled (Dupuy) or photographs of Gage's skull (Ferrier). The modern era has seen two rather different types of methods: Cobb's somewhat impressionistic one in the

1940s as well as the technically based methods of the CT scan in 1982 by the Tylers and the 1994 computer-based study by Hanna Damasio and her colleagues.

This chapter has two main parts, one devoted to the damage to the skull, the other to that of the brain. Each contains a sequential discussion of the conclusions the pre-1880 investigators reached. The discussion of the technically rather more advanced methods of the twentieth century follows a similar chronological pattern. The difficulties in determining the passage of the tamping iron from the skull damage will be seen to be equivalent to trying to solve an equation with two unknowns: neither the place of entry nor exit can be determined with any real precision.

The Damage to Gage's Skull

Estimating the damage to Gage's skull requires considering the general direction of the tamping iron, the place of entry into the skull, and the place of exit. Even though details of most of the methods on which these estimates are based are lacking, the clinical-descriptive reasoning behind them can be followed reasonably easily.

The General Direction

In his 1848 paper Harlow described Gage as standing above the hole containing the charge, but in 1868 he had him sitting there. In both instances Gage's head was turned away from the hole and he was looking over his right shoulder. In 1848 Harlow described the general direction of the tamping iron as "upward and backward toward the median line," and later as being projected "obliquely upwards," so that it traversed the skull "obliquely upwards and obliquely backwards." Bigelow, who had Gage leaning forward with his face slightly averted, had the projection as "directly upwards" but the wound itself as "oblique." All three accounts result in the same general direction of the passage of the tamping iron through the skull. Even David Ferrier, who judged that Bigelow had represented the passage as more vertical than was warranted, would probably not have quarreled with "oblique" as a general indicator of direction. To establish more than this general trajectory, the places of entry and exit need to be found.

The Entry Area

However, when we turn to the problem of determining the entry point, we find that all we can ever determine is an area within which such a point might lie, that is, a point of entry is inherently indeterminate. The tamping iron was one and a quarter inches in diameter at its largest point and, after Gage's wound had healed, the hole it left where it had entered the base of the skull behind the eye was not much bigger. But it is bigger, a feature that means that a "true" entry point cannot be placed with exactitude. Damage to the surrounding structures, especially to the zygomatic arch, reduces the uncertainty somewhat but does not eliminate it. Considerable variation is therefore possible in placing a point of entry within the area of entry. The variation affects two things: the obliqueness of the passage of the iron through the skull and the placement of its exit relative to the coronal suture and the midline, that is, how far to the front of the skull or on its left or right side it emerged.

Because Harlow and Williams were the only persons to have examined Gage at the time of the accident, I start with their 1848 descriptions. Harlow's is dated 27 November and Williams's 4 December, about twelve and thirteen weeks after the accident, respectively. Harlow's account, the fuller, describes the entry as follows:

the powder exploded, driving the iron against the left side of the face, immediately anterior to the angle of the inferior maxillary bone. Taking a direction upward and backward toward the median line, it penetrated the integuments, the masseter and temporal muscles, passed under the zygomatic arch, and (probably) fracturing the temporal portion of the sphenoid bone, and the floor of the orbit of the left eye, entered the cranium.

In summary, as the iron entered, it probably fractured the temporal or outer portion of the sphenoid bone and the floor of the left orbit. Williams said only that the length of the wound in Gage's cheek was "about one and half an inch." What Harlow found in examining Gage's skull in 1868 can be considered as confirming his 1848 supposition about the entry. New bone had reduced the size of the opening but it was still one inch in its lateral and two inches in its antero-posterior dimension. Nevertheless, Harlow was quite precise about where the iron had entered: it was at a point the center of which was one and one-fourth inches from the median line in the junction of the lesser wing of the sphenoid with the orbital section of the frontal bone.

From his examination of Gage in Boston in November 1849, Bigelow judged the entry as "in a straight line from the angle of the lower jaw on one side" (i.e., the left). From his demonstration that the passage of the iron was possible he went further. He had taken a "common skull" in which the zygomatic processes were not very marked and drilled through it from "the left angle of the lower jaw" in the direction of where, on the basis of his examination of Gage, he presumed it had emerged. When enlarged to take the bar, Bigelow found he had removed "from the coronoid process of the lower jaw ... a fragment measuring about three-quarters of an inch in length" and that the hole entered "obliquely beneath the zygomatic arch, encroaching equally upon all its walls." Note however that Bigelow's drill made clean holes in the skull: there were no fractures in the bone around the entry point.

When David Ferrier compared photographs of Gage's skull with Bigelow's illustration, he concluded that Bigelow had represented the entry hole "a little further outwards from the middle than the photograph warrants" but, unlike Harlow's "one and one fourth inches from the midline," gave no estimate of the distance. Except for placing the entry point one inch to the left of the median line, instead of one and a quarter inches, J. B. S. Jackson drew almost identical conclusions to Harlow's. The variation seen in these nineteenth-century placements of the entry point within the area where the tamping iron had clearly entered persisted into the twentieth.

The Exit Area

The problem of an "area" versus a "point" particularly dogs the issue of where the tamping iron emerged from the top of Gage's skull. In fact, because so much of the bone there was totally destroyed, the indeterminism is greater. In 1848 Williams said in his letter to Harlow only that that the opening through the top of the skull "was not far from one and half inch in diameter." Harlow wrote that the tamping iron "made its exit in the median line, at the junction of the coronal and sagittal sutures, lacerating the longitudinal sinus, fracturing the parietal and frontal bones extensively ... and protruding the globe of the left eye from its socket, by nearly one half of its diameter." But by 1868, Harlow had become less precise, the iron "emerged in the median line, at the back part of the frontal bone, near the coronal suture."

The early disagreements with his estimate match Harlow's own seeming uncertainty. John Barnard Swets Jackson recorded Phelps's opinion from seeing Gage about six weeks after the accident. Phelps thought:

ye centre of ye wound on ye top of ye head must have been abt $\frac{1}{2}$ inch in front of coronal suture & 1 inch to ye left of ye median line (Dr. H. says at ye juncture of ye sutures).

Phelps also thought that "ye long. sinus was not wounded (as acc. to Dr. H.)." From his examination of Gage in 1849, Bigelow also concluded that the tamping iron had emerged at "the centre of the frontal bone ... near the sagittal suture," and his drilling had the iron emerging at "the median line of the cranium just in front of the junction of the sagittal and coronal sutures." However, he described the exit hole more precisely. It was "two-thirds ... upon the left, and one-third upon the right of the median line, its posterior border being quite near the coronal suture." As with the entry hole he had drilled, there was no mimicking of the destruction of bone at the exit, mainly on the left side of the top of Gage's skull. Nor did his drilling create a flap of frontal bone hinged on the right side. And although J. B. S. Jackson emphasized the left-sided location of the major damage, he pointed out that the inferior line of fracture extended "somewhat over the median line." He made no estimate of the center of the area of exit.

When Ferrier compared the photographs of Gage's skull with Bigelow's illustration, he suspected that Bigelow had represented the passage of the tamping iron "a little too much towards the middle line & beyond it & also somewhat nearer the coronal suture than was actually the case." As he wrote to Bowditch, it seemed that "from the opening at the left-side of the middle line [probably the large one to which Jackson had also drawn attention] that the bar did not cross the middle line at all, & that it emerged more in front raising the flap of bone hanging on the line of fracture on the right side of the frontal." As the tamping iron had emerged on the left side, it had raised the flap of bone hinging on the line of fracture on the right side of the frontal bone.

What is most interesting about Ferrier's attempt at precision is that it is not reflected in the use he eventually made of the photographs and woodcuts that Bowditch sent him. In his *Gulstonian Lectures*, he said, correctly, that Harlow did not describe the exit. It seems to me that by that time Ferrier also would have realized how impossible it was to say exactly where the iron had emerged. J. B. S. Jackson was similarly circumspect. In his examination of the skull, he noted that the exit fracture was "situated in the left half of the frontal bone, but, inferiorly, it extends somewhat over the median line." Although Jackson went on to comment on how the pieces of frontal bone had healed, he did not venture an opinion about where the tamping iron had emerged.[1]

Although these nineteenth-century descriptions reveal that there was no consensus about the precise point of exit, there was little disagreement that it lay to the left of the midline (see table 5.1). Conclusions consistent with these opinions are also found in the first of the technically based

Table 5.1
Estimates of the exit point in Gage's skull

Examiner and date	Material examined	The tamping iron's exit points in relation to	
		Coronal and sagittal junction	Median line
Harlow 1848	Gage	at	in
Phelps 1849	Gage	0.5″ in front	1″ to left
Bigelow 1850	Gage and drilled skull	front	right
Harlow 1868	Gage's skull	front, near	in
Jackson 1870	Gage's skull	front	?left
Dupuy 1873	Warren catalogue ? illustration	frontal	?left
Dupuy 1877	Gage's skull	?behind	?left
Ferrier 1877	Bigelow's illustration	more frontal	left
Ferrier 1878	Harlow's illustration and photos of Gage's skull	near but "frontal"	not stated
Cobb 1940, 1943	Gage's skull	between frontal bones	right
Tyler and Tyler 1982	CT scan of Gage's skull	not stated	not stated
H. Damasio et al. 1994	Gage's skull and 3-D computer model	front	right

studies conducted in this century, the CT scans by H. R. Tyler and K. Tyler. The complete set of images is reproduced in Appendix E and the more significant of them here as figure 5.1. Figures 5.1a and 5.1b are a lateral scan, showing the left side of the skull, and figures 5.1c and 5.1d are frontal scans showing the skull in coronal section. Figure 5.1d shows the largest of the openings in the base and the top of the skull. Imaginary lines joining the right and left sides of the upper opening with the corresponding sides of the lower will be found to constitute an inverted funnel, narrow at the base and wide at the top. If this funnel is taken as defining the horizontal limits of the path of the tamping iron, it will be seen that most of the skull damage is to the left of the midline.

H. R. Tyler noted an asymmetry of Gage's skull such that on the side of the lesion there is more prominent parietal bowing and the temporal fossa is smaller. Tyler's impression is that the right half of the skull case is slightly larger than the left—not a striking difference and one more likely to be present before the accident than caused by it. He thought the asymmetry would make only differences of millimeters to any precise estimates of the passage of the tamping iron.

From his direct examination of the skull and the scans of it, H. R. Tyler summarized the damage as follows:

Entry area

There is minimal damage to medial and lateral pterygoid lamina, lateral and pterygoid canal.

There is damage to the tip of the greater wing of the sphenoid (and anterior temporal fossa) with damage of the mid and lateral lesser wing of the sphenoid. The medial sphenoid bone and clinoids are spared. The orbital plate of the frontal bone posteriorly is damaged, as is the posterior portion of the orbital surface of the maxilla and the lamina papyracea of the ethmoid. The temporal base, foramina spinosum, ovale, and rotundum [are] spared. The zygomatic arch on the left is bowed outward.

Exit area

There is a defect which is partially overlain by a fragment of bone which has healed like an anterior flap. There is a posterior defect about 25% of the total area. The defect goes to slightly across the midline and is about 1″ or more in front of the coronal sulcus. The flap of bone clearly crosses the midline.

There is a crack in the frontal bone above the frontal sinus. The optic foramen on the left cannot be identified.

The conclusion from this aspect of the Tyler study is that precise points of entry and exit cannot be determined. Their work favors the path from an entry in the area nominated by Harlow to an exit closer to the point described by Bigelow than Harlow.[2]

Hanna Damasio and her colleagues attempted to estimate the damage to Gage's skull by generating a three-dimensional computer model of the skull from measurements, X-rays, and photographs of it. She and her colleagues then mapped possible exit points for the tamping iron onto the model. They produced possible trajectories by projecting lines connecting those exit points with the midpoint of the hole in the base of the skull and then projecting them down to the entry area between the upper jaw and cheek bone. They then selected entry points consistent with the known anatomical damage at that lower level and further examined trajectories from them to the exit points. They chose a "most likely trajectory" from among them and simulated the passage of the tamping iron along it through a computer model of Gage's brain.[3]

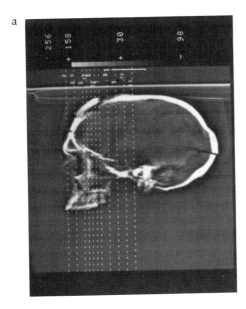

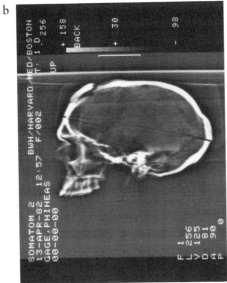

Figure 5.1
The CT scans of Phineas Gage's skull (see also appendix E)
Scans by courtesy of Dr. H. Richard Tyler and Dr. Ken Tyler, Boston, Massachusetts.

c

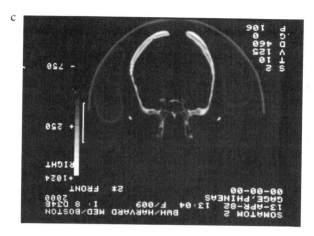

d

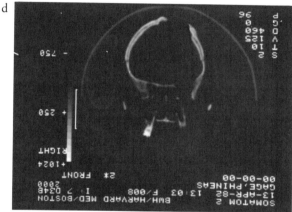

Figure 5.1 (continued)

   This first thing to ask is whether Damasio et al. resolved the uncertainties over the tamping iron's entry and exit. They begin by selecting an "a priori" most likely exit point and then define an area around it within which other exit points might lie. Damasio et al. called this region the area of "bone loss." It included the area of *total* bone loss, that is, the hole over which Gage's scalp had regrown *and* the flap to the right and front of it that had reunited with the skull. It did *not* include the reunited rear flap. We see immediately that the area they defined as "bone loss" is only about half the total area in which bone was either completely destroyed or detached.

Damasio et al. went on to define an exit area by considering the diameter of the tamping iron in relation to the side and front margins of their region of "bone loss." No part of this exit area could be closer than 1.5 cm, or half the largest diameter of the iron, from the margins. Within that area Damasio et al. mapped fifteen other points. They then connected those points to the center of the hole in the base of the skull and projected the lines down to the entry area under the cheekbone, or zygomatic arch. The shape of this area, situated to the side of what is known as the mandibular ramus, meant that no entry point could be closer than 1.5 cm from the mid-thickness of the arch, 1 cm from the intact tooth socket for the last upper tooth, or superior molar, and 0.5 cm from the coronoid process of the upper jaw. The lines from the exit points projected on to nineteen points within a 1.5 cm radius of the point that Damasio et al. considered the a priori most likely entry point to the side of the mandibular ramus.

Only seven of the trajectories so produced seemed possible but, on closer examination, Damasio et al. rejected two that would have hit the front, or anterior horn, of the left lateral ventricle under the assumption that Gage, living in the pre-antibiotic era, would not have survived the massive infection caused by such an injury. They then simulated the passage of the iron along all of the remaining five. Damasio et al. then chose as the most likely trajectory the one that best met the entry point constraints.

Damasio et al.'s figures show all five of their exit points lying further forward and more to the right of the one they initially nominated as the a priori most likely exit. Similarly, all five of their chosen entry points under the zygomatic arch lie to the left of their a priori most likely one, and come from among those furthest to the left of the mandibular ramus. Consequently, all five trajectories appear to pass under the cheekbone at a more obtuse angle, enter the base of the skull farther to the left, and emerge at the top of the skull farther to the right and front than in previous estimates. These estimates of Damasio et al. and earlier ones are summarized in table 5.1.

How likely are any of the Damasio et al. paths? Recall they *began* at the top of the skull, at the area of exit. Damasio et al. gave no basis for characterizing the a priori exit point there. It is virtually on the front border of the area of total bone loss, rather than somewhere toward the *center* of that hole, or even about midway between the two flaps of reunited bone. Further, inspection of the skull itself shows that all but a small triangular segment of the area of the hole lies to the left of the midline. Additionally, as their photograph of the underside of Gage's skull shows, the rear flap lies almost entirely to the left of the midline. Thus, well over half of the area of loss and damage is *left-sided*. Even a good part of the frontal flap lies to the left. However, one sees from their computer model that almost all of the rectangular area within which they searched lies to the right of the midline. Of the points they examined within that area, four are behind the a priori most likely, one is approximately level with it, ten are forward of it, and these forward points are much closer together than those behind it. It may not be surprising that the exit point Damasio et al. most favor is not only right and frontal; but it is surprising that it is actually *under* the right frontal flap where no hole was created.

The second step of Damasio et al.'s reconstruction of the trajectory began from their estimated exit points. They "drew" lines from each to the center of the hole where the tamping iron entered the base of the skull. Where was this center? The healed entry hole is irregular in shape, being about one inch wide and two inches long, but the original was obviously larger. How did Damasio et al. determine its center? Now, imagine two lines, one drawn across the opening and the other along it. The "center" could be thought of as their point of intersection. But should it? And, if it is, where should the lines be placed? Damasio et al. do not tell us. Pretty clearly, there is room for variation in the placement and intersection of any lines so placed, and the same indeterminacy is true of any method for determining the center. But however determined, any forward-backward variation in placing the center affects the location of the exit point relative to the coronal suture, and any side to side variation affects its relation to the midline.

When Damasio et al. examined the entry area under the zygomatic arch to see which of their initial trajectories were compatible with the anatomical damage at that site, that procedure not only did not provide data for choosing between possible trajectories, it added a third unknown to an equation that already contained two: the point within the exit area, and the center of the opening in the base of the skull.

Damasio et al.'s third step was to reject two trajectories because they presumed Gage would not have survived infection resulting from the tamping iron damaging the anterior horn of the left lateral ventricle. However, Harlow believed that precisely that damage had occurred: as he said, the abscess he drained on the fourteenth day "probably communicated with the left lateral ventricle." Bigelow concurred: his reconstruction led to the conclusion that "the anterior extremity of the left lateral ventricle" must have been laid open. Gage's survival surprised neither Harlow nor Bigelow in this respect, possibly because it matched earlier reports of recovery from such damage, one of the most notable going back to the eleventh century. Antibiotics were not necessary to Gage's survival. A tamping iron following either of the two trajectories would probably have emerged closer to the coronal suture and more to the left of the midline. Either trajectory would probably have been more like that described by Harlow in 1868. More particularly, it is unlikely that either would have emerged *under* the frontal flap, as did most of Damasio et al.'s choices.

Finally one notes that because the anatomical constraints define the area under the zygomatic arch within which the entry point must lie better than any other, it would have been more logical for Damasio et al. to have started there. Lines projected from likely entry points there could have been passed through a variety of "centers" of the hole in the base of the skull, and the most likely exit points determined relative to what the *total* pattern of bone loss and damage on the top of the skull suggested.[4]

The Damage to Gage's Brain

Indeterminacies about where the tamping iron entered and left the skull imply indeterminacy about its passage through the brain. To this uncertainty we have to add another. Individual differences in the position of the brain inside the skull are marked enough for such external features of the skull as the junctions of the sutures not to provide exact guides to the parts of the brain that lie beneath them. In brains of about the same overall size, particular convolutions may vary by as much as half an inch from the skull landmarks. Certainty about the passage of the tamping iron through the brain does not necessarily give us certainty about the parts of Gage's brain that might have been damaged.

Harlow was very brief in 1848 about the supposed brain damage. The tamping iron had passed through "the anterior left lobe of the cerebrum ... breaking up considerable portions of the brain." In 1868 he was more expansive:

The iron, as you will perceive, entered the left cerebrum at the fissure of Sylvius, possibly puncturing the cornu of the left lateral ventricle, and in its passage and exit must have produced serious lesion of the brain substance—the anterior and middle [i.e., temporal] left lobes of the cerebrum—disintegrating and pulpifying it, drawing out a considerable quantity of it at the opening in the top of the head.

If Phelps said anything to J. B. S. Jackson in 1849 about which parts of Gage's brain he thought were damaged, Jackson did not record it. Neither did Jackson say anything on his own account in 1870. Bigelow's 1850 inference was, however, very definite and very specific:

a considerable portion of the brain must have been carried away; that while a portion of its lateral substance may have remained intact, the whole central part of the left anterior lobe, and the front of the sphenoidal or middle lobe must have been lacerated and destroyed. This loss of substance would also lay open the anterior extremity of the left lateral ventricle; and the iron, in emerging from above must have largely impinged upon the right cerebral lobe, lacerating the falx and the longitudinal sinus.

Harlow had said nothing about injury to the right hemisphere in his summary, but in his discussion he was quite specific: it had been "left intact."

William Hammond and Eugene Dupuy used J. B. S. Jackson's description of the skull damage to estimate the damage to the brain. Both discussed the Gage case in the debate over whether a language function was localized in the brain. Hammond believed Gage's left frontal lobe to have "suffered severely," but that the third left frontal convolution, the location of the language area being debated, was left intact. On the other hand, and also on the basis of Jackson's *Catalogue* entry, Dupuy, a French neurologist, testified that in "this remarkable and authentic observation, even though it is American," there had been absolute destruction of the left frontal lobe. Four years later Dupuy measured the skull himself and claimed that the Island of Reil had been destroyed along with the Sylvian artery that nourished Broca's language area. Shortly after, Dodds cited the Gage case (although not by name) in the same context only to reject Dupuy's conclusion that either structure had been destroyed or damaged.[5]

Cobb began the modern era of the study of the damage to Gage's brain with a diagram of the parts of it he thought to have been affected. His drawing shows damage and destruction of both frontal lobes, more on the left than the right. He did not describe how he had arrived at his diagram other than to say it was based on the skull damage that he had apparently assessed for himself at the Warren. He cites Harlow on the pattern of skull damage but is a little imprecise. Thus the tamping iron made its exit, according to Cobb, "between the frontal bones" and "a little to the right of the midline."

The Tylers' 1982 CT scan of the skull was the first use of modern techniques to determine the iron's entry and exit points and from them to assess the brain damage more accurately. Their conclusions, which have not been published in full, were that the damage was to the left anterior frontal lobe, part of the tip of the left temporal lobe, part of the anterior horn of the left lateral ventricle on the left, the head of the caudate nucleus and the putamen, the superior sagittal sinus, and the right hemisphere, including parts of the right superior frontal and cingulate gyri. With the exception of right hemisphere involvement their conclusion is similar to Harlow's, and on the right-sided damage it is very similar to Bigelow's.[6]

Damasio et al. employed a standard measuring system used in CT scan work to build up their model of Gage's brain from the measurements of his skull and to compare the model with twenty-seven normal brains. These comparisons led them to identify seven brains having two of their three main dimensions within millimeters of Gage's, and in each they simulated the passage of the tamping iron along all five of the trajectories they identified as possible. In the simulations, the areas of the brain that were damaged were similar in all seven. Damasio et al. concluded that the damage to Gage's left hemisphere involved "the anterior half of the orbital frontal cortex ... the polar and anterior mesial frontal cortices ... and the anterior-most sector of the anterior cingulate gyrus." Right hemisphere damage was similar but less marked in the orbital frontal region. Table 5.2 summarizes the various estimates of the damage to Gage's brain.

Conclusion

Three general problems can be identified in those studies that focus on the damage done to Phineas Gage's brain by the passage of his tamping iron. They would remain even were there no indeterminacies about the entrance and exit of the iron. First, such estimations take no account of the damage from hemorrhaging that Harlow said was "very profuse." Blood also flowed into Gage's mouth and stomach, causing him to vomit several times, and before Harlow's arrival, Williams had observed that the first time this happened, "the effort of vomiting pressed out about half a teacupful of the brain." Pieces of bone from the opening in the base of the skull probably caused additional damage. Harlow seems to have found only five pieces of frontal bone, so that the pieces clearly missing from the base must have been driven through the brain by the tamping iron or carried away during the hemorrhaging. Neither do these studies make allowance for the further loss of brain substance through the infection, nor take into account damage to the brain from concus-

Table 5.2
Estimates of the damage to Gage's brain

	Parts of the brain affected	
Examiner	Destroyed	Damaged
Harlow 1848	left frontal	not stated
Phelps 1849	not stated	not stated
Bigelow 1850	central left frontal front of left temporal	left ventricle medial right frontal
Harlow 1868	left frontal only	left lateral ventricle part left temporal
Dupuy 1873	"absolue" left frontal	not stated
Dupuy 1877	Broca's area Sylvian artery Island of Reil	not stated
Ferrier 1877	left frontal only	not stated
Ferrier 1878	left prefrontal	tip of left temporal
Hammond 1871	left anterior only 3rd frontal convolution and Island of Reil escaped	not stated
Cobb 1940, 1943	large parts of left and some right prefrontal	large parts of left and some right prefrontal
Tyler and Tyler 1982	left anterior frontal tip of left temporal anterior horn of left lateral ventricle head of caudate nucleus and putamen right hemisphere, including right superior and cingulate gyri	
H. Damasio et al. 1994	anterior half of left orbital frontal cortex polar and anterior mesial frontal cortices anterior-most part of anterior cingulate gyrus right hemisphere similar, but less marked in orbital frontal region	

sion. At the John Martyn Harlow Frontal Lobe Symposium held in Cavendish on 12 September 1998 as part of the 150th commemoration of the accident to Phineas Gage, Dr. H. R. Tyler expressed the view that these factors make it impossible to know with any exactitude which areas of Gage's brain were affected.[7]

Second, using the damage to Gage's skull to identify the areas of his brain that might have been damaged assumes that his brain occupied a kind of "average" position within the skull. Yet we know that there is considerable variation in the relation between landmarks derived from the skull and the structures of the brain. Third, relating the supposed damage to the structures to the changes in Gage's behavior overlooks the fact that the same functions may be localized at different places in seemingly similar brains. The kind of knowledge that we would like to have about the damage done to Phineas Gage's brain seems still beyond our reach.

In 1868, Harlow said it was a "fact" that the right lobe "was left intact." We will see that this may reflect his phrenological belief about how functions were localized, but it may also reflect his very privileged observation. During his 1848 examination he had explored the wound by placing one index finger in the opening in the skull until it "received the other finger in like manner" from the wound in the cheek. Further, the quadrangular opening in the front and top of the skull before the larger pieces of bone were replaced was almost three and a half by two inches. Virtually the whole of the front of the skull was open. It is just possible that Harlow could have sensed whether the right hemisphere was intact, and perhaps, although less likely, what other parts had been damaged. He may also have been able to observe the brain when he changed the dressings and when he removed the "fungi." Before alighting, Williams had observed from his carriage the brain pulsating, and Harlow reported the pulsations could still be seen in April 1849 beneath the two-inch by one-and-a-half-inch depression left on the top of the skull.

Parts of Harlow's 1848 conclusions were clearly based on what he could see and feel, some parts were clearly supposition, and some were probably a mixture. We cannot make the observation-supposition differentiation about all that he wrote. Neither can we say how much time elapsed before he came to his conclusions. He could have reached them within hours of the examination or during the weeks in which he had time to reflect on what he knew had happened.

Thus although we have Gage's skull and can specify the damage to it very accurately, what we learn from it is problematic: the bone damage, which is patent, does not tell us the path of the tamping iron with the precision needed to make an accurate estimate of the brain damage. And the tamping iron was not the sole agent of damage; what the others did can never be known. Even were we able to resolve the uncertainties about the damage to Gage's brain, there are equally insurmountable obstacles to our relating the changes in his behavior to them.

Notes

1. Exit and entry areas: Harlow 1848, 1868, 1869; Bigelow 1850b,c; Phelps in J. B. S. Jackson 1849, case Number 1777; J. B. S. Jackson 1870; Dupuy 1873 and 1877; Ferrier 1877–1879, 1878a, 1878b.

2. Tyler and Tyler 1982, and personal communications from K. L. Tyler, 8 October 1993, and H. R. Tyler, 12 September 1998, and during January, March, and May 1999. I am very much indebted to both Drs. Tyler for they way they have shared this and other information with me.

3. H. Damasio, Grabowski, Frank, Galaburda, and A. R. Damasio 1994. See also A. R. Damasio 1993, 1994, and Blakeslee 1994.

4. Theodoric [1267] 1955, vol. I, p. 109, and Whitaker and Luzzatti 1997 for recovery from ventricular damage in the preantibiotic era.

5. Hammond 1871, pp. 174, 179–180; Dupuy 1873, pp. 31–33, 1877, and Dodds 1877–1878, p. 470.

6. Cobb 1940, 1943 for his reconstruction; Tyler and Tyler 1982 and note 2 above.

7. For details of the Symposium and the commemoration, see either of Macmillan 1999 or 2000b, or the 'Anniversary' section of the website ⟨http://www.hbs.deakin.edu.au/gagepage/pgage.htm⟩

6

The Damage to Gage's Psyche

... the above wonderful case ... far transcends any case of recovery from injury of the head that can be found in the records of surgery.
—J. B. S. Jackson *Warren Museum Catalogue*, 1870

Even were the uncertainties over the damage to Gage's skull and brain resolvable, there would be insurmountable obstacles to our relating the changes in his behavior to them. Establishing just what psychological damage the tamping iron did to Phineas Gage requires us to compare a range of his behaviors before it began its journey and after it landed. In Gage's day not only was there nothing like a modern neuropsychological assessment, of course, but there was no discipline of neuropsychology. The conceptual tools from which that field would emerge lay some seventy years in the future, and its own parents, neurology and psychology, had barely been conceived. But the fetal state of these disciplines is not responsible for the absence of adequate pre- and postaccident evaluations in Gage's case. Rather it is that although the psychological consequences of his injury were clearly major, there is almost no information about his personality and behavior before the accident and very little description of it after. Even an idealized modern neuropsychological assessment would need more. It would begin with a good baseline from which the changes could be assessed and use adequate methods for evaluating the altered behaviour itself. In Gage's case there is a further limitation to the picture we have of him. Those few descriptions of what he was like beforehand are very general, rarely contemporary or even independent of those set down after it. Most are implicit components of the postaccident descriptions. Nor do they seem to have reached us free of filtering.

In this chapter I begin the examination of these problems by setting out as systematically as I can the facts and presumed facts about his behavior as it was understood up to 1880. The approximately 300 words in which Gage's behavior is described derives from direct observation (Harlow, Bigelow, AMA *Report of the Standing Committee on Surgery*, the *American Phrenological Journal*, and Channing), from discussions with Gage's relatives (J. B. S. Jackson), or from Harlow's summaries of his now lost case notes and correspondence between him, Gage's relatives, and possibly with Gage.

Psychological Change

Although assessing the effects of the damage to Gage's brain on Gage's behavior is an almost impossible task, I set out as much as can be gleaned from the various sources of what we do know about him under the four headings of his (1) preaccident psychology and behavior, (2) behavior during the immediate postaccident period, (3) short-term postrecovery behavior, and (4) psychology and behavior in the long term.

Preaccident Psychology and Behavior

Harlow's first report of 1848 contains very little about Gage's behavior and mental qualities before the accident. He was of "temperate habits, and possessed of considerable energy of character." There was not much more in his second report of 1868: Gage was "strong and active," of "nervo-bilious temperament," and possessed of "an iron will as well as an iron frame." Educationally and psychologically:

although untrained in the schools, he possessed a well-balanced mind, and was looked upon by those who knew him as a shrewd, smart business man, very energetic and persistent in executing all his plans of operation.

We have seen that he probably attended primary school and, as "C"'s letter in the Claremont, New Hampshire, *National Eagle* seems to attest, he could write well enough to make entries in his time book. A report that appeared about eighteen months after the accident said he had been "quiet and respectful" before it. Twenty years after the accident, Harlow said Gage had not been prone to swearing before it, and that Gage's contractors had then "regarded him as the most efficient and capable foreman in their employ."[1]

Immediate Postaccident Behavior

By combining the slightly different selections from the original case notes as Harlow presented them in his 1848 and 1868 reports, we can form some picture of the significant behavioral and mental changes in Gage during the first two months after the accident. I have combined the two sets of case notes in Appendix B, and it is clear that these changes were minimal. On the evening of the accident, Harlow noted that Gage's "sensorial powers" were unimpaired, his mind was "clear," that he did "not wish to see his friends as he shall be at work in a day or two," and could give details of relatives in Lebanon. Early the next morning he recognized his mother and uncle and was "rational." Apart from the episodes of delirium and coma, the most striking feature in Harlow's notes, especially in the 1848 selections, is Gage's rationality.

However, about three weeks after the accident, shortly after the effects of a frontal abscess had subsided, some ominous signs emerged. On the 5 and 6 October, Harlow recorded:

Calls for his pants and wishes to get out of bed, though he is unable to raise his head from the pillow.... Appears demented, or in a state of mental hebetude.

The extract for the 6th in the second paper is somewhat more foreboding:

General appearance somewhat improved ... calls for his pants, and desires to be helped out of bed, though when lying on his back cannot raise his head from the pillow. By turning to one side he succeeded in rising, and sat ... for about four minutes.... Appears demented, or in a state of mental hebetude.

Then, only five days later on 11 October, exactly twenty-eight days after the accident:

Intellectual faculties brightening. When I asked him how long since he was injured, he replied, "four weeks this afternoon at $4\frac{1}{2}$ o'clock." Relates the manner in which it occurred and how he came to the house. He keeps the day of the week and time of day in his mind. Says he knows more than half of those who enquire after him.

But admixed with this more positive picture there appears the first hint of a cognitive deficit quite distinct from any other consequence of infection:

Does not estimate size or money accurately, though he has memory as perfect as ever. He would not take $1,000 for a few pebbles which he took from an ancient river bed where he was at work.

Two days later, on the 15 October, thirty-two days after the accident, the ominous features began to predominate:

Remembers passing and past events correctly, as well before as since the injury. Intellectual manifestations feeble, being exceedingly capricious and childish, but with a will as indomitable as ever; is particularly obstinate; will not yield to restraint when it conflicts with his desires.

On the thirty-seventh day, 20 October:

Improving. Gets out and into bed with but little assistance. Sits up thirty minutes twice in twenty-four hours. Is very childish; wishes to go home to Lebanon, N. H. And

Improving; gets out and into bed with but little assistance.... Sensorial powers improving, and mind somewhat clearer, but very childish.

As Gage regained physical strength, the problem of controlling him seems to have become greater. By 8 November, on the fifty-sixth day:

He walks up and down stairs, and about the house, into the piazza, and I am informed this evening that he has been in the street to-day.—I leave him for a week, with strict instructions to avoid excitement and exposure.

During the following week Gage systematically disobeyed Harlow's injunction, disregarded the attempts of others to control him, and displayed another instance of his inability to appreciate the value of money. On 15 November, Harlow wrote:

Returned last evening, and learn that Gage has been in the street every day during my absence, excepting Sunday. Is impatient of restraint and could not be controlled by his friends. Making arrangements to go home. Yesterday he walked half a mile, purchased some articles at the store, inquired the price, and paid the money with his habitual accuracy; did not appear to be particular as to the price, provided he had money to meet it. The atmosphere was cold and damp, the ground wet, and he went without an overcoat, and with thin boots; got wet feet and a chill. I find him in bed, depressed and very irritable.

The effects of the chill lasted three days. Harlow then noted, Gage "appears to be in a way of recovering if he can be controlled." In 1868, Harlow revealed that when Gage left for Lebanon on 25 November 1848, a week after recovering from the chill, he had traveled "in a close carriage," that is, in an enclosed and sometimes padded vehicle of the kind used for transporting the insane.

Short-Term Postrecovery Behavior
Gage never regained his job as foreman. Twenty years after the accident Harlow explained that his contractors:

considered the change in his mind so marked that they could not give him his place again.

In about 160 words, Harlow set out the basis for their decision:

The equilibrium or balance, so to speak, between his intellectual faculties and his animal propensities, seems to have been destroyed. He is fitful, irreverent, indulging at times in the grossest profanity (which was not previously his custom), manifesting but little deference for his fellows, impatient of restraint or advice when it conflicts with his desires, at times pertinaciously obstinate, yet capricious and vacillating, devising many plans of future operation, which are no sooner arranged than they are abandoned in turn for others appearing more feasible. A child in his intellectual capacity and manifestations, he has the animal passions of a strong man. Previous to his injury, although untrained in the schools, he possessed a well-balanced mind, and was looked upon by those who knew him as a shrewd, smart business man, very energetic and persistent in executing all his plans of operation. In this regard his mind was radically changed, so decidedly that his friends and acquaintances said he was "no longer Gage."

When summing up, Harlow added:

Mentally the recovery was only partial, his intellectual faculties being decidedly impaired, but not totally lost; nothing like dementia, but they were enfeebled in their manifestations, his mental operations being perfect in kind, but not in degree or quantity.

It was as if the more ominous of the changes Harlow had observed during the two-month recovery period had finally come to dominate.

Except for reports or comments from three sources close to Gage or his family, we learn very little of these mental manifestations in anything written between 1848 and 1851. Dr. John Barnard Swets Jackson traveled from Boston to Lebanon in early August 1849 to see Gage. From Gage's mother and brother-in-law he learned only of one residual cognitive defect. Gage had been

weak and childish on getting home but now appears well in mind, exc. that his memory seems somewhat impaired; a stranger wd notice nothing peculiar.

Jackson obtained this information from the relatives because Gage himself was in Montpelier attempting, they told him, "to get work on the Rail Road."

Two anonymous 1850 reports agreed with J. B. S. Jackson that something had changed. One, a letter from someone who seems to have been close to Gage's family, was included in the American Medical Association's *Report of the Standing Committee on Surgery*. It was rather general:

A friend writes us, April 27th., 1850, that it is certain his mental powers are greatly impaired. This is stated by the family to which he belongs, and it is their belief that this degenerating process is still going on. He has also lost bodily powers although this fact is not so clearly manifested as the deficiency of his mental faculties.

The other came from the *American Phrenological Journal* and was rather more specific. It was in a comment on Bigelow's 1850 claim that Gage had "quite recovered in his faculties of body and mind, with the loss only of the sight of the injured eye." The phrenological view was very different:

The statement relative to the wound and recovery is correct. But that there was no difference in his mental manifestations after the recovery, is, however, *not* true … after the man recovered, and while recovering, he was gross, profane, coarse, and vulgar, to such a degree that his society was intolerable to decent people. Before the injury he was quiet and respectful.

Bigelow's opinion that Gage was unaffected was based on some eight weeks of close contact with Gage that began toward the end of 1849. Although he represented the significance of the case as showing how a grave lesion could coexist with "an inconsiderable disturbance of function," we can see that deleterious psychological and behavioral changes had actually been very apparent in the first few weeks of the recovery phase.[2]

Longer-Term Changes

In April 1849, about six months after the accident, Gage returned to Cavendish. Harlow then said, "His physical health is good, and I am inclined to say that he has fully recovered." Although Harlow's opinion is consistent with what Gage himself told "C" about being "restored to perfect health and soundness," and that he had resumed his work on the railroad, it is clearly not correct. J. B. S. Jackson's record of what he learned about Gage's physical condition from his family at about the time of these other reports indicates diminished physical capacity:

abt. February he was able to do a little work abt. ye horses & barn, feedg. ye cattle &c.; that as ye time for ploughing came he was able to do half a days work after that & bore it well.

Depending on the weather, ploughing would normally begin on farms near Lebanon in May or June. And as we saw from the letter included in the American Medical Association's *Report of the Standing Committee on Surgery*, even twelve months later, there was still considerable physical weakness.[3]

Subsequent History

Almost all of what we know about Gage's history subsequent to his recovery comes from Harlow, who differentiates five periods in Gage's postrecovery history: first, Gage exhibits himself and his tamping iron while traveling in New England; second, he does the same with Barnum's Museum in New York; third, he works in a livery stable and coaching business in Hanover; fourth, he looks after horses and drives coaches in Chile; finally, he works as a farm laborer in California, and there he dies. Following the order in which Harlow (1868, 1869) sets out his account, I now describe what I have found that expands on Harlow's history.

Traveling and Visiting Boston

According to Harlow, after he had recovered Gage "took to travelling, and visited Boston ... exhibiting himself and his iron." Documenting more than what is probably the beginning of this part of Gage's post-accident history has not proved possible. We know Gage was in Boston being examined by Bigelow in November 1849, because his being presented to the Boston Society for Medical Improvement on the 10th of that month is recorded in the minutes of the meeting. But apart from J. B. S. Jackson, Channing, and Holmes, no member of the society seems to have written anything then or subsequently about the event or about Gage himself. As we have seen, in 1849 Jackson recorded Phelps's inferences as well as what the family told him. The long entry he prepared on Gage for the *Catalogue* of the Warren Museum was based mainly on Harlow, but did include some minor points of his own. Walter Channing II made passing mention of Gage in a lecture delivered to an unspecified audience and entitled "Life and living. An address about 1860." Channing used Gage to illustrate how recovery was possible even after very serious injury: the "case in which a tamping iron passed through the brain without killing is one of these. In this case recovery was perfect. I have seen the man and the tamping iron."

The absence of any mention of Gage in the collection of John Collins Warren's papers at the Massachusetts Historical Society is especially significant. Much of Warren's correspondence, diary entries, and so forth, from September 1848 to the end of 1850 record his discussions with people like Jackson, Henry Jacob Bigelow, and Henry Pickering Bowditch about establishing the Massachusetts General Hospital and the medical museum. During January 1850, Bigelow, who was being treated medically by Warren, actually gave Warren an old tourniquet as a specimen for the museum during that month, but the topic of Bigelow's obtaining the tamping iron for it does not seem to have arisen. The absence of Gage's name in Warren's and other written records might be due to Gage's being talked about rather than written about. Most of the members of the society met frequently at work and professional meetings and socially at the regular weekly meeting of the informally constituted and named Warren, or Wednesday Evening, or Thursday Evening Club (all three names are used). None of "the medical class at the hospital," that is, the medical students enrolled at Harvard during the relevant terms, recorded Bigelow's presenting Gage. Nor did any of them write anything about Gage then or later.[4]

Apart from these largely unrecorded "official" engagements, what did Gage do in Boston? There are persistent reports of his begging outside the Massachusetts Medical College, but there is no eyewitness account of anyone seeing him do so. The letters from the 1850s of the notable Bostonian Louisa May Alcott have not survived, but if she did see Gage then, she wrote nothing about him in later life. Neither did she add a recollection in 1868, the year of Harlow's second paper. Emily Dickinson contrived her diaries and letters rather too poetically for her to squeeze in many everyday events, but even she noted a notable Boston murder trial and the visit of Jenny Lind, although not Gage. He does not appear to have included Amherst, where she lived, in his New England travels and by 1851–1852, if she knew about Gage at all, his novelty may have worn off sufficiently for her not to have commented on it after her visit to Boston in September 1851. But neither her brother Austin, resident in Boston since mid-1851, who seems to have written frequently and on everyday matters, nor her many New England correspondents, nor her father's cousins who visited from Hanover (New Hampshire?) in April 1852, seem to have conveyed news of Gage. Caroline Bennett White recorded much about her frequent visits to Boston and travels throughout New England between 1848 and 1852 but wrote nothing about Gage. Neither is his name to be found in the diary entries made by Anne Cushing, who lived in Dorchester, then just outside of Boston and a Ward of it since 1864. She was the wife of a physician, and between late 1848 and mid-1850 noted many newsworthy Boston events and described her frequent visits to that city or those of her friends from it, but said nothing about Gage (but her diary for the second half of 1850 is missing). Even Benjamin Eddy Cotting, intimately involved with the affairs of Massachusetts Medical Society for more than twenty years and its President from 1874–1876, made no mention of Gage. Perhaps of greater relevance, young Stephen Salisbury, who at nearly 17 years of age drove into Boston from Worcester on 6 April 1850 specifically to visit the medical school at a time when Gage himself could have been in Boston, possibly still begging on the steps of the medical school, wrote in his diary only "went to see the Médical College and examined the premises."[5]

Nor is there confirmation of Blackington's account placing Phineas in "a small tent on Boston Common" where he "exhibited his head and the bar which had passed through it," and was so loudmouthed, boisterous, and profane that eventually "the police drove him from Boston Common." While Blackington's clearly semifictional account contains many errors, much of his detail is factually accurate. However, none of the many Bostonians who made their way across the Common daily seems to have recorded seeing him, no newspaper appears to mention the events on the Common, and such police records as I have found are silent.[6]

Around the Larger New England Towns

According to Harlow, Gage's travels included "most of the larger New England towns," where he also exhibited himself and his tamping iron. What were these in the 1850s? They can be established fairly easily from sources like the U.S. Census and gazetteers and from the opinions of workers in local New England historical societies. In the mid-nineteenth century, as one traveled west and then south from Boston, they included the Massachusetts towns of Worcester, Amherst, and Springfield, the Connecticut towns of Hartford, New Haven, and Bridgeport, and the Rhode Island town of Providence. Traveling to the north and the northwest they included Salem in Massachusetts, Bangor in Maine, Manchester, Andover, Concord, Lebanon, and Hanover in New Hampshire, and the Vermont towns of Bellows Falls, Burlington, Montpelier, Rutland, Windsor, and Woodstock.

On the assumption that Gage would have sufficiently impressed someone in these towns to have made some record of his exhibition, I visited almost all of them and searched or had searches made of the local newspapers and the surviving diaries, letters, and journals of those local residents such as doctors and schoolteachers who I thought would have been especially interested in him. But there was absolutely no trace. Neither Luther V. Bell nor Judith Almira Upham Bell of Andover, the former an important businessman connected with the railroad industry and the latter a lively schoolgirl with a wide range of interests, remarks on Gage. Nor if he saw or heard of him at any of the many lectures and demonstrations he attended, mainly in Bangor, did young Benjamin Browne Foster of Orono, Maine, record anything about Gage in his diary, and Foster's curiosity was enormous, encompassing a huge range of general popular science subjects, the effects of laughing gas, electropsychology, animal magnetism, phrenology, and circuses.[7]

At Barnum's in New York

After concluding his travels in New England, Harlow said Gage went to New York, "remaining awhile in the latter place at Barnum's, with his iron." This is, of course, Barnum's famous American Museum in New York on Broadway at the corner of Ann Street that he purchased from Scudder in 1840. Harlow does not give dates for the time Gage is supposed to have been with Barnum, and apart from Blackington's account, we have no description of what Gage did there. Remembering that Blackington is semifictional and sometimes factually incorrect, there are nevertheless some interesting features in his portrayal:

He joined Austin and Stone's Museum, moving on from that show to New York where the ubiquitous P. T. Barnum didn't let the fact that Phineas' skull was healed stop him from advertising: THE ONLY LIVING MAN WITH A HOLE IN THE TOP OF HIS HEAD. The posters and one-sheets depicted a husky young man smiling broadly in spite of a huge iron bar which stuck out of his head. Actually, of course, the iron bar no longer protruded from Gage's head but he had it with him, and another skull, also perforated. During his side-show performances, he would shove the long iron rod through the holes in his extra skull to demonstrate just how he was injured. All the details were to be found in a pamphlet he sold, and by paying ten cents extra, skeptics could part Gage's hair and see his brain, what there was left of it, pulsating beneath the new, thin, covering.

If this portrayal is factual, one can see immediately how limited an attraction Gage would have been among the many thousands of Barnum's other oddities that in 1850–1851 included orangutans; monster snakes fed live prey daily; Miss Clofullia, the "Swiss Bearded Lady"; the exotic Miss Pwan Tekow from China; General Tom Thumb; General Frémont's Nondescript or Woolly Horse; and a negro whose skin was turning white because of a weed he was eating. The appeal of a hole that had already healed could offer little competition, either as instruction or entertainment.[8]

Although we shall see that it is commonly believed that Gage toured with a circus, possibly Barnum's, Harlow does not even hint that this was the case. Nevertheless, I considered whether Gage might have appeared with Barnum's Traveling Exhibition, which began touring in 1848, or its successor, Barnum's Great Asiatic Menagerie and Caravan, which toured from 1851 to 1854 (although this latter period is when Gage was working for Currier). The Menagerie and Caravan included the ubiquitous General Tom Thumb; Mr. S. K. G. Nellis, the Armless Wonder who played the accordion and the cello with his toes; and many other of Barnum's New York Museum attractions. In August 1851, its itinerary included Lebanon, New Hampshire, and Rutland, Vermont, the latter an important junction for the R&BRR only some twenty-five miles from Cavendish. However, if Gage did travel with the Menagerie and Caravan, we have to assume that Harlow's dates for his being with Barnum are incorrect. Perhaps Gage traveled with the circus of G. C. Quick, which advertised Bennington, Manchester, Rutland, Brandon, and Middlebury as part of its late August and early September 1850 itinerary for Vermont. But if Gage was with either Barnum or Quick, the main Lebanon and Rutland newspapers failed to single him out.[9]

An illustration of Gage with the tamping iron poking through his head does exist, and it may be based on a poster or leaflet for a museum or something similar (figure 6.1). Russell Windsor made this, the only reasonably early pictorial representation of Gage I have seen, for the book on phrenology published by her husband William Windsor some seventy years after the accident. Although Windsor's references to the work of Bernard Hollander, a British physician who defended phrenology well into this century, and who frequently referred to the Gage case, seem to provide a context for the picture, a search of Hollander's works has not

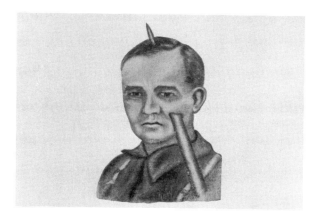

Figure 6.1
The only known early pictorial representation of Gage
From Windsor 1921, p. 507. Copy by courtesy of Carole Hughes, Dana Medical Library, University of Vermont, Burlington.

found it there. Nor has it turned up in the museum and circus literature. It may not be modeled on a poster after all but be original with Russell Windsor.[10]

Working in Hanover for Jonathan Currier

Harlow then tells us that in 1851, Phineas "engaged with Mr. Jonathan Currier, of Hanover, New Hampshire, to work in his livery stable." Hanover, where Jonathan Garland Currier conducted his livery stables and stagecoach business, is about ten miles north of Lebanon, and the businesses were situated to the side of the Dartmouth Hotel of which Currier was then also the proprietor (figure 6.2). Currier had been a mail contractor and stage driver for about twelve years before buying the hotel and leasing it while at the same time continuing the stage and livery

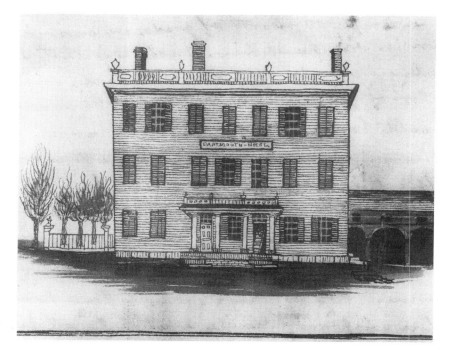

Figure 6.2
Jonathan Currier's Dartmouth Hotel in 1826 (stables on the right)
From drawing on a letter of 25 March 1826 by John Willard. Mss 826225, Special Collections, Baker Library, Dartmouth College, Hanover, New Hampshire. Reproduced by permission of Baker Library Special Collections.

business and running a large farm that he owned. Some of Currier's ledgers survive, but only for 1838–1850; even had they covered the period after 1850, they do not record wage payments and would probably have told us little about the time and regularity of Gage's employment. All that we know of his work with Currier comes therefore from Harlow: "He remained there without any interruption from ill health for nearly or quite a year and a half." We may presume he looked after the horses and that he also drove coaches.

Given that Gage worked continuously in Hanover for about eighteen months, one would think some of its citizens, especially those associated with Dartmouth Medical College, might have noted his presence during that time. A short walk from the front entrance of the livery stables of the hotel, where the Hanover Inn is now situated, takes one across the green to the college at which Edward Elisha Phelps was then Professor of the Theory and Practice of Physik and Pathological Anatomy. Here, then, was a medical school adjacent to the place of Gage's labors, one from which one of its senior members seems to have traveled to Cavendish to examine Gage only weeks after his accident and about two years before Currier engaged him. Did Phelps or other students and teachers from Dartmouth's famous medical school refer to him? It does not appear to be the case. None of Phelps's manuscripts refers to Gage, and the one set of lecture notes by one of his students to have survived makes no mention of Gage. Neither do the letters and manuscripts of medical and other instructors and students who were in Hanover at the time. Nor did Benjamin Hatch Bridgeman, a Dartmouth doctor who practiced for many years in both Grafton, Vermont, and Hanover itself, including the period of Gage's accident and employment by Currier, record anything about him. During 1851–1852, young Willis R. Peake records many visits from his Vermont home to Hanover to attend "negro shows" and the circuses, but does not seem to have seen Gage. Finally, no Hanover newspaper seems to have reported anything about Gage during 1851–1852 or around the time of his accident and recovery, either.[11]

One possible reason for the absence of Gage's name from the newspapers and manuscripts that have been searched may be that at the time, there were actually other and more interesting or important things by which one could be diverted. In Boston, for example, a considerable cholera epidemic raged over much of the summer of 1850. Were that not enough, the murder of Dr. Parkman on 23 November 1849 by John W.

Webster, the Professor of Chemistry at Harvard occupied the public's attention considerably. Boston newspapers devoted entire pages to the investigations, the arrest, the trial, and Webster's execution on 30 August, 1850. Some of the most intriguing detail, although neither reported nor given in evidence, was well enough known to consume what time there was for gossip. Henry Jacob Bigelow, for example, had become suspicious of his colleague Webster because of what he heard about the odd behavior of Parkman's dog from workers in a nearby foundry. They told him that the dog had followed Parkman to Webster's laboratory on the day of his disappearance but had been unwilling to move from the spot where it had been left. It was in the laboratory that some of Parkman's remains were later found. Louisa May Alcott, Emily Dickinson, Anne Cushing, and young Stephen Salisbury all recorded something about the trial, and Salisbury followed it with sufficient interest to devote one of his frequent visits to Boston to attending the court and listening to Webster's defense. But none of them seems to have noticed Gage.

In Boston and elsewhere at that time much attention was also being paid to Barnum. However, the reports of his doings centered on his promoting Jenny Lind, "The Swedish Nightingale," who drew unprecedented audiences to her concerts as well as huge crowds to her appearances in public. During the early part of 1850, Barnum devoted most of his considerable talents to maximizing publicity about her and was so successful that an estimated 30,000–40,000 of New York's population of slightly more than half a million turned out to greet her when her ship docked on 1 September 1850. His success continued with massive public interest over the ten months she toured under his auspices, including the approximately three weeks after her concerts began in Boston on the 27th of that month. So great was what was called "Jenny Lind mania" in New York that there were Jenny Lind polkas, gloves, pianos, cigars, riding hats, sofas, and unbelievably, Jenny Lind chewing tobaccos. Bostonians had all these, of course, as well as a massive fireworks display, a torchlight procession, their very own "Jenny Lind Tea Kettles" that "sang" on boiling, and unimaginably, "Jenny Lind sausages."

Throughout this time, the abolitionist movement was gaining strength, particularly in New England. Many of its residents would have little time for something as minor as the injury to Phineas Gage. Then there was the gold rush. The influence of California was everywhere. The New England newspapers were full of reports of the gold discoveries, of companies of men banding together, pooling their capital, purchasing mining equipment, outfitting themselves, and arranging travel overland by wagon, or by sea, or by combined sea and land travel if going via the isthmus of Panama. Among these other and more stirring events, is it surprising that no one seems to have noticed Gage?[12]

To Valparaiso with the Founder of a Coachline

The gold rush may even be responsible for what Phineas did in August 1852, when Harlow said "he engaged with a man who was going to Chili, in South America, to establish a line of coaches at Valparaiso." In the 1850s Valparaiso was popular as a first port of call on the western seaboard for ships from the eastern United States going to California via South America. As supplies were being replenished, passengers would take a few days' rest, during which time they often traveled the approximately seventy-five miles to the Chilean capital, Santiago. Consequently coach lines were most frequently established in Valparaiso in association with shipping lines. A shipping company setting up a new service to San Francisco might well have planned to establish a line of coaches to carry its passengers between the port and Santiago.

Harlow tells us that Gage embarked from Boston in August 1852 and that he suffered much from seasickness on the voyage. This and his coach line employment is the sum of what we know about Phineas's journey from New England and the reasons for it. Foreshadowing Phineas's eventual reunion with some of his family in San Francisco, I find it not unreasonable to speculate that he began his journey with them. Repeated earthquakes and fires have destroyed many of the records, such as those of birth, marriage, and death, ordinarily available in cities the size of San Francisco. Among the losses, those hampering my inquiries the most are the records of passenger arrivals.

By the time Gage left Boston in August 1852, twenty-two-year-old David Dustin Shattuck, soon to become his brother-in-law, was already in business at 93 Front Street, San Francisco, as a provision dealer. We have only a hint of the arrival of Phineas's mother and possibly his father in San Francisco, and none at all of the arrival of David Dustin Shattuck and Phebe Jane Gage in Rasmussen's laboriously compiled ship passenger lists. Rasmussen gives a "J. F. Gage" and a "Mrs. J. F. Gage" as arriving from Panama on the *California* on 6 October 1852. Could this initial be in error and really stand for Jesse *Eaton* Gage? There would have been time for the pair to have begun their journey in Boston in August, crossed the isthmus by coach, and completed the Panama section of it by the time the *California* left Panama for San Francisco on 20th. September. Had Phineas and his erstwhile employer accompanied them, they may have separated in Panama to continue to Valparaiso, possibly arriving there at the beginning of October, about the same time as Gage's mother and father disembarked in San Francisco. On the other hand, if Rasmussen's J. F. Gages were not Phineas's parents, there may just have been time for the otherwise unrecorded party to have left Boston via the Horn for Valparaiso and San Francisco but to have separated in Valparaiso before the parents went on to California.

Once he arrived in Valparaiso, we know almost nothing about Phineas's responsibilities to his employer or how he met them. Harlow said in 1868 that Gage was "occupied in caring for horses, and often driving a coach heavily laden and drawn by six horses." A Phineas so engaged would have been a novelty in Valparaiso at that time. Enos Christman described Valparaiso in the November of 1849 as "of a mean appearance" with narrow winding streets and its people having to rely on jackasses to tote water from the mountains to the city, rather than on other transport. Little development had occurred by June 1852, when Marcellus Bixby observed the same reliance on mules for bringing produce over the mountains.

J. B. S. Jackson described the vehicle Phineas drove as a "stage-coach," which, if this is true, was most probably a Concord coach of the kind shown in figure 6.3. By the mid-1800s, Concord coaches were in wide use around the world, and they, American coachlines, and American coach drivers, most of the latter from New England, struck George Augustus Peabody as a prominent feature of life in Santiago and Valparaiso when he was there in May 1858. Quite apart from that and the evidence of figure 6.3, I consider that the wide geographical distribution of Concord coaches, especially their suitability for rough terrain, makes it likely that Gage's employer would have used them on the Valparaiso-Santiago route.

By the time of the visit of the Peabody party, coaches seem to have replaced mules and parts of the mountainous sections of the route between Santiago and Valparaiso were "climbed by an excellent zigzag road." However, those sections over the plains country were a different

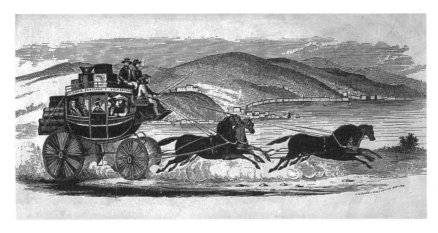

Figure 6.3
A Concord Coach on the Valparaiso-Santiago route
Prints s1994-546-036 of the Abbot-Downing Collection, Tuck Library, New
Hampshire Historical Society, Concord, New Hampshire. Reproduced by kind
permission of the Society.

matter. They were "heavy from recent rain," and the last part into Valparaiso required such "a long descent over a bad road" that Peabody said it was "no wonder that the inhabitants do not ride or drive much."[13]

If Phineas had been driving Concord coaches over such terrain, something of the great cognitive and motor skills demanded of him can be inferred from what we know of what was required of the drivers of the teams that drew those coaches for Cobb and Co. in Australia. Austin said the drivers not only had to look after their horses properly, they especially had to have "a genuine liking for horses, and ability to understand them." As for controlling the teams, Austin noted that:

Although much of the technique could be taught, the ability to achieve the necessary rapid co-ordination of brain, hand, and eye was instinctive rather than acquired. Merely to hold the reins or "ribbons," as they were sometimes called, in the "Cobb and Co grip" was an art. The four running reins (two for the leaders and two for the wheelers and polers from which check reins ran to each horse) were held in the left hand, with the reins through the fingers in such a way that the driver could slide his hands along the reins to get a better grip, and still keep each rein separate. So held, by day or by night, the driver could easily pick out the reins of the near or off-side horses with the right hand, and thus steer the team.

Bends and turns in the road required the driver to make the horses on the inner side move more slowly than those on the outside, an especially difficult task if there were an uneven number of horses in a span, as each "row" of horses was called. Handling the whip accurately, using its twelve to thirteen feet of lash to produce a crack just above the ears of a particular horse without tangling the whip in the harness, especially in wet weather, was a further skill. Night driving required a considerable and flexible memory; acetylene lamps were of such limited use that drivers had to memorize the details of tracks and of an ever-changing route. Drivers also had to be reliable, resourceful, and possess great endurance. But above all, they had to have the kind of personality that enabled them to get on well with their passengers.[14]

We know neither how long Gage continued in the employment of the man who had engaged him, nor how much driving he did relative to caring for the horses. Harlow says only that he carried out this work for "nearly eight years [actually seven] in the vicinity of Valparaiso and Santiago," a phrasing that can be interpreted as readily as meaning he stayed with the one employer the whole time as that he moved around.

Some time in [1858 and 1859], Harlow says Phineas's "health began to fail, and in the beginning of the latter year he had a long illness, the precise nature of which, I have never been able to learn." His mother added that he had "many ill turns while in Valparaiso, especially during the last year, and suffered much from hardship and exposure." Not recovering fully, "he decided to try a change of climate and in June, [1859], left for San Francisco."[15]

A change of Climate in San Francisco

The reasons that keep us in ignorance about the arrival of Gage's family in California also prevent us from documenting the date on which Phineas was reunited with them. On the more than reasonable assumption that some of the dates his mother gave Harlow are in error by a year, we can place Phineas's leaving Valparaiso in June 1859 and have him arriving as Harlow says "on or about July 1," but of that year. Rasmussen lists no one by the name of Gage arriving in San Francisco in either 1859 or 1860. Gage was, his mother told Harlow, "in a feeble condition, having failed very much since leaving New Hampshire."[16]

It must have been at about this time, so Harlow tells us, that his mother first had the opportunity of observing how

Phineas was accustomed to entertain his little nephews and nieces with the most fabulous recitals of his feats and hair-breadth escapes, without any foundation except in his fancy. He conceived a great fondness for pets and souvenirs, especially for children, horses and dogs—only exceeded by his attachment for his tamping iron, which was his constant companion during the remainder of his life.

Although some aspects of this behavior may have been present in New Hampshire during 1849–1852, Phineas then had few nephews and nieces, and little real background from which to fabulate his adventures.

We do not know how long he took to recuperate, but Harlow says that eventually:

his health improved, and being anxious to work engaged with a farmer in Santa Clara, but did not remain there long. In February, [1860], while sitting at dinner, he fell in a fit, and soon after had two or three fits in succession. He had no premonition of these attacks, or any subsequent ill feeling.

If Phineas's recovery took say, two to three months, that is, from July to September, it is not unreasonable to construe Harlow's "did not remain there long" as meaning that he worked for the one farmer for four to five months until the first convulsion in February.

What Harlow emphasizes and quotes verbatim from a letter by Gage's mother or brother-in-law seems to indicate that after the first convulsion, Phineas became less stable in his work:

"Had been ploughing the day before he had the first attack; got better in a few days, and continued to work in *various places*;" could not do much, *changing often*, "and always finding something that did not suit him in every place he tried."

This, the only part of Harlow's report in which Gage is said to have had difficulty in maintaining a job, conveys to me that only after this first seizure did he become successively dissatisfied with his employers. This concurs with what J. B. S. Jackson says in the Warren Museum *Catalogue*: after his arrival in San Francisco, Phineas "went to work upon a farm" (note the singular), but that after the convulsion, "In a few days he was better, and did at different times, various kinds of work" (note the plural: more than one kind). Because Jackson's account contains other detail not in Harlow's account, it is possible that he clarified Harlow's original description with him. It is also consistent with Jackson's practice of including unpublished detail in other *Catalogue* notes.

Four months later, on 18 May, after definitely becoming unsettled in his employment, something persuaded Phineas to leave Santa Clara to return to his mother. Two days later, at 5 A.M., he had a severe convulsion. Despite his being bled, the seizure turned out to be the first of a series that heralded the end. Over the next day and night the convulsions recurred frequently, and Phineas Gage expired, Harlow says, at 10 P.M. on 21 May 1861.

Despite the authority of Harlow's source, Phineas died in 1860, not 1861. No death notice appeared in a newspaper, and if a death certificate was issued it seems to have been destroyed. What, then, grounds my certainty? Two documents that I have examined personally. First, the Interment Records of the Laurel Hill Cemetery give the date of death of "Phineas B. Gage" as 20 May 1860 and the burial date as 23 May 1860. Second, N. Gray & Co.'s *Funeral Record 1850 to 1862* for the Lone Mountain Cemetery, reproduced here as figure 6.4, also gives 23 May 1860 as the date of the funeral. Both give the cause of death as "epilepsy."[17]

The only really peculiar feature of these records reflects on the date we have for Phineas's birth. Interment records and newspaper announcements at that time customarily gave the age at death in years, months, and days. Consequently, if Phineas really was born on 9 July 1823, he would have been 36 years, 10 months, and 14 days at the time of his death. What actually appears as his age on the Laurel Hill interment record is 36 years, 0 months, and 0 days. If the subtractions by which this figure was reached are accurate, the true date of his birth must have been 20 May 1824, that is, about ten months after that recorded by C. V. Gage. Did no one, including his mother, know the correct date? Or was it being hidden? What we can be sure of here is that Phineas survived the severe damage to his brain by nearly eleven and a half years, not the twelve and a half given by Harlow in 1868.

What Harlow Most Desired to See

Up to the time Phineas left Chile, Harlow implies that he had occasionally obtained news from him. After that he "lost all trace of him." Except, then, for his "good fortune" in July 1866 in learning the address of Phineas's mother, we might never have extended our small stock of facts much beyond Hanover, and we would certainly not have been able to see what damage had been done to his skull.

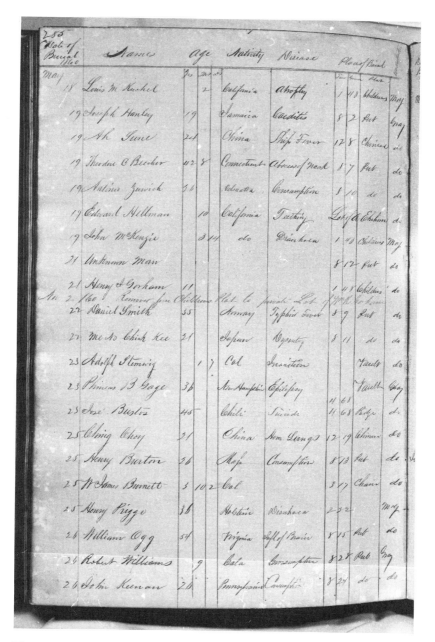

Figure 6.4
The date of Phineas Gage's burial: 23 May 1860
From N. Gray and Co.'s *Funeral Record 1850–1862*, p. 285, beginning 18 May 1860.

After finding that Gage was dead, Harlow's correspondence with his mother and David Dustin Shattuck seems to have been directed to one main purpose. Regretting "that an autopsy could not have been had, so that the precise condition of the encephalon at the time of his death might have been known," Harlow persuaded them to allow an exhumation. Gage's head, or rather what remained of it, was then removed and the skull made available for Harlow to study. The remains of the corpse were reinterred, almost certainly in the original grave, but when Harlow had finished with the skull, he deposited it in what is now the Warren Anatomical Museum of the Harvard University Medical School.

No record of the exhumation has survived, of course. It is not noted on the surviving documents at Cypress Lawn in Colma, California, no item was found about it in any San Francisco newspaper, and Michael Svanevik, a notable historian of San Francisco's netherworld, was unable to obtain any leads that might have dated it for me. Sibyl Semites, reference librarian, found no record at all of Phineas Gage, and none to any exhumation attended by Coon and/or Stillman at or about the time in question in the California history section of California State Library's extensive guide to official records known as the "California Information File: 1846–1985."

According to J. B. S. Jackson's notes about the skull in his *Catalogue* of Warren exhibits, "The cranium arrived in this city [Boston], with the bar, in 1868." That date, and some other details, allow us to infer that the exhumation took place in November or December of 1867. We note that the three people Harlow thanked "for their kind coöperation in executing my plans for obtaining the head and tamping iron, and for their fidelity in personally superintending the opening of the grave and forwarding what we so much desired to see" immediately helps fix the time. The three were David Dustin Shattuck, Gage's brother-in-law; Dr. Henri Perrin Coon, the mayor of San Francisco; and Dr. J. D. B. Stillman. Coon was mayor for two terms, from 1864 to 1867, and his mayoralty ceased on 2 December 1867. David Dustin Shattuck was elected to the San Francisco Board of Supervisors as member for the Sixth Ward in 1867, taking office on 2 December, at the same meeting at which Coon had retired. Only three weeks later, at a regular meeting of the Board of Supervisors, Shattuck asked for leave of absence. The *Alta California*, one of the city's main newspapers, reported the suddenness of the request thus:

CHRISTMAS EGG-NOG.—The attachés of the ALTA office desire to acknowledge the receipt of a huge bowl of creamy egg-nog, from the Pony Saloon, Kearny street, which was sent in just at midnight, and duly enjoyed. A careful analysis of the beverage failed to detect the slightest trace of any deleterious substance in its composition. We pronounce it good to take.

A DEPARTING SUPERVISOR.—At the last meeting of the Board of Supervisors, Mr. Shattuck, member from the Sixth Ward, was unanimously granted leave of absence for the next four months. Imperative business demands Mr. Shattuck's presence in the Atlantic States. He contemplates leaving for New York on the next Panama steamer.

NOTICE.—The undersigned will continue the Auction Sales of Watches, Jewelry, etc., at the store of Messrs. Joseph Brothers, 607 Montgomery street, every evening, commencing at 7 o'clock, until further notice.   R. D. W. DAVIS, Auctioneer.

Joseph Brothers will also continue the business at private sale during the day, as usual.   de25-tf

Although the *San Francisco Examiner* gave Shattuck's request a commercial or mercantile cast by saying Shattuck required leave because of "his business necessarily calling him to the East," the *Daily Morning Call* confirmed the less commercial *Alta* version by saying he "was obliged to go East on business of importance and asked for leave of four months."[18]

Clearly, Shattuck's request for leave was unexpected. If he was able to procure a passage "on the next Panama steamer," how soon could he have reached New York? Provided he left almost immediately, a steamship could have delivered him to Panama in time to cross the isthmus and connect with another that would have him there before the end of January 1868. No passenger ships left San Francisco between 24 December and 1 January, but on New Year's Day 1868, the Pacific Mail S.S. *Montana* departed for Panama, to be followed on the 4th by the North American S.S. *Nevada*. No list of the passengers carried on the *Montana* was published in any paper, and only two lists for the *Nevada* appeared. Shattuck's name is not on either of the latter but, since these lists were usually prepared in advance of sailing, that lack does not rule out his traveling on one of them. Either would have allowed him to deliver his brother-in-law's skull to Harlow by the end of January.[19]

The Reception Given Harlow's History

Harlow presented his "history and sequel of a case of severe injury of the head, followed by recovery, which, so far as I know, remains without parallel in the annals of surgery" at the annual meeting of the Massachusetts Medical Society on 3 June 1868. If Shattuck did arrive in January, Harlow's absences from the January and May meetings of the Middlesex East District Medical Society held in Woburn in the first half of 1868 are worth noting. His attendance had been reasonably regular the previous year, but if Shattuck brought the skull in January, it would seem to follow that Harlow's absences were because he was busily studying Gage's skull and preparing his report on the postaccident history of his patient.

Except for including extracts from the case notes conveying the more ominous features, Harlow's report of the course of Gage's recovery to the end of 1848 was very similar to that given nearly twenty years earlier. Four other things were new. The first, the result of an examination conducted in April 1849, described Gage's physical condition at that time but was relatively unimportant prognostically. Second, there was the evaluation, already considered in chapter 4, of the factors Harlow thought had aided recovery. The third was the description of the damage to the skull, and the fourth the summary of the psychological consequences through which the medical profession was to learn that after the accident he "was no longer Gage."

As we have seen, what the damaged skull showed Harlow was that the tamping iron had entered the base of the skull "an inch and a fourth to the left of the median line in the junction of the lesser wing of the sphenoid bone with the orbitar process of the frontal bone," that is, just behind the orbit of the left eye, and that it had emerged "in the median line, at the back part of the frontal bone, near the coronal suture." Consequently, Harlow believed it entered the left side of the brain:

at the fissure of Sylvius, possibly puncturing the cornu of the left lateral ventricle, and in its passage and exit must have produced serious lesion of the brain substance—the anterior and middle left lobes of the cerebrum—disintegrating and pulpifying it, drawing out a considerable quantity of it at the opening at the top of the head.

Harlow said nothing direct about what the damage to the skull revealed about damage to the right hemisphere. However, in his concluding remarks, he was quite specific: it had been "left intact."

Many points in Harlow's report were applauded. But Bigelow managed to steal much of Harlow's credit. After expressing "his full concurrence" with Harlow on the authenticity of the Gage case, Bigelow not only adduced Jewett's case of Joel Lenn in corroboration but actually produced Lenn in person and introduced him to the audience. Jewett was also present and, according to the *Medical and Surgical Reporter*, his statement of his treatment of Lenn "commanded the close attention of the Society." As the anonymous author of the *Memoir* on Bigelow said, it was "one of those *coups dramatiques* which were now and then incidents of his [Bigelow's] surgical communications." Bigelow's action may also have diverted attention from the fact that Gage had changed. In the four abstracts of Harlow's address in other medical journals known to me, only the *Medical and Surgical Reporter* provided detail on the "mental manifestations." Two others, although basing themselves on the same account, said merely that "his intellect was somewhat affected." Basing itself in turn on one of these, the other obliterated the change completely: it claimed Gage's "mental and bodily functions [were] unimpaired."

Barker has shown that this trend to minimize the consequences of Gage's injury was already evident in the pre-1869 U.S. periodical literature. Of the fourteen comments on Gage he found from that period, eleven quoted from or made explicit reference to Bigelow's 1850 version of the case. None of these mentioned any mental changes. Only the AMA Standing Committee on Surgery's report of 1850 did so. Barker also shows that some members of the medical community believed Gage to be alive in 1860 and that this information probably came from Harlow. Even so, and even though Harlow's address was given in 1868, Barker notes that the post-1868 literature also tends to deny the mental manifestations. He attributes this striking feature to the pervasiveness of Bigelow's view.[20]

Most of the newspaper accounts of Harlow's address also neglected the psychological consequences of Gage's injury. One exception is the report in the *Daily Evening Traveller* (Boston), which is almost word-for-word the same as that of the *Medical and Surgical Reporter* quoted above, but published nearly three weeks earlier. It began with the by now standard emphasis on the astonishing aspects:

A WONDERFUL SKULL
STORY OF A REMARKABLE CURE
A Present to the Mass. Medical Society
At the meeting of the Massachusetts Medical Society this morning, Dr. John M. Harlow, physician and surgeon, of Woburn, but formerly of Cavendish,

Vermont, read a paper containing the history of a most interesting case of injury to the head, and presented to the meeting the veritable skull which sustained the injury.

The rest of the relatively long article (about four-fifths of a column), a mostly accurate summary of what Harlow had said, included the following:

The subsequent history of the case is interesting. Gage came back to Cavendish in April, in fair health and strength, having his tamping iron with him, and he carried it with him until the day of his death, twelve years after. The effect of the injury appears to have been the destruction of the equilibrium between his intellectual faculties and the animal propensities. He was now capricious, fitful, irreverent, impatient of restraint, vacillating, a youth in intellectual capacity and manifestations, a man in physical system and passions. His physical recovery was complete, but those who once knew him as a shrewd, smart, energetic, persistent business man, recognized the change in his mental character. The balance of his mind was gone. He used to give his nephews and nieces wonderful accounts of his hair-breadth escapes, without foundation in fact, and conceived a great fondness for pets.

The *Traveller* article seems to have been reprinted in other newspapers and books, even in faraway California.

Two other newspaper accounts of Harlow's address failed to mention the change or did so inadequately. The emphasis on Bigelow and the errors of date and name in one of them, the *Woburn Journal*, must have been particularly galling:

At the session of the Massachusetts Medical Society in Boston, recently Dr. John M. Harlow, of Woburn, gave the history of a man named Gage, who while blasting rocks at Cavendish, Vt., in 1847 had a tamping iron, three feet seven inches long and one and one quarter inches thick, and tapering to a point, forced through his head, it entering the left cheek and coming out about the centre of the top of his head. Dr. Harlow, who attended the man, gave in detail the daily symptoms of his patient, and said that in fifty-nine days he was able to walk and ride, and was soon nearly as well as before, although his intellect was somewhat affected. This is considered the most remarkable case of the recuperative powers of nature, and has been doubted by many prominent surgeons. Gage died May 21, 1861, twelve years, six months, and eight days after the injury. Dr. Harlow procured the head, and has presented the skull to the Warren Museum of the Harvard Medical College. Dr Bigelow said he saw Gage twenty years ago, and was then satisfied of the reality of this wonderful case. He also said a tube of iron five-eights of an inch in diameter and about five feet long passed through a miner's head, while blasting coal in Ohio, and was pulled out by a fellow miner. The injured man was introduced to the audience, and Dr. Jewett, the attendant physician, recounted the case in detail. The young man's mind has not been fully restored.

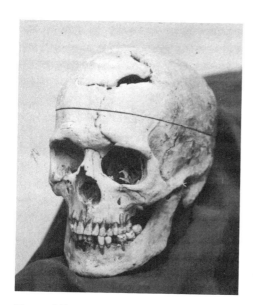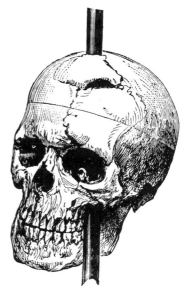

Figure 6.5
S. Webster Wyman's 1868 photograph of Phineas Gage's skull and the woodcut Harlow used as illustration (see appendix A)
Wyman's photograph from the Glennon Archives, Woburn Public Library, Woburn, Massachusetts, and reproduced by permission of the Trustees of the Library.

We have seen a photographic likeness of the skull of Mr. Gray, which shows the exact state of the skull after the bar of iron had passed through it. It was taken by our townsman, S. Webster Wyman, and is attracting much attention. Copies can be obtained of him.

The other, in the Burlington, Vermont, *Daily Free Press* was devoted solely to Bigelow's presentation of Joel Lenn and contained nothing at all about Gage.[21]

Despite the photographs and Harlow's illustration (figure 6.5) professional people as well as ordinary citizens showed a similar indifference. Anne Cushing's diary records her physician husband's driving in to Boston with friends and other medical colleagues to attend the meeting of the Massachusetts Medical Society at which Harlow spoke. Although she records nothing about Harlow or Gage, she did note that one of the family's friends, Robert Edes, had won the first of three prizes for an article awarded by the society. A week later Edes and another friend who had been at the meeting came to dinner, but if they mentioned Gage or

Harlow, she wrote nothing of what they said. Neither did Benjamin Eddy Cotting.[22]

Additions to the History

Many who knew of Gage's case did not allow that there had been any significant change in his behavior after the accident. Some of the few who did add to Harlow's postaccident history had first-hand knowledge of him or were close to those who had. For example, J. B. S. Jackson's entry in the Warren *Catalogue* said Gage was still as obstinate as ever. The attribution of obstinacy as a permanent characteristic is otherwise found only in Harlow's general reference to Gage's iron will and in his mentioning Gage's peculiar obstinacy. This latter reference is in the case notes and occurs in the context of his will being as indomitable as ever. Harlow may be read as referring to a temporary quality, but Jackson is clearly talking about a permanent one. It is also Jackson who has Gage working as a hostler, or stablehand, for Currier, driving a stagecoach in Chile, and only after Gage's first seizure does he have him moving from job to job.

Cobb, on the other hand, has Gage leading a roving life and working at small jobs here and there. His seems to be among the earliest of such characterizations. A precursor to one aspect of Cobb's interpretation is found in one of the two writers who give Gage a drinking problem. Wilson asserted in 1879 that Gage was finally beset by drinking habits, and in 1897 Hughes added that intemperance had played a part in Gage's irregular life. Otherwise, as we shall see in detail in chapter 14, what has been said about Gage subsequent to his physical recovery is mostly fable. Table 6.1 summarizes the various accounts of the changes.

Several aspects of the post-Harlow fables have been incorporated into the recent accounts by H. Damasio, Grabowski, Frank, Galaburda, and A. R. Damasio, and by A. R. Damasio. Between them, these authors have a preaccident Gage who is responsible, intelligent, socially well-adapted, and a favorite with his peers and elders and who had made progress and shown promise. After the accident his new learning is intact, and neither his memory nor his intelligence is affected. However, he has become irreverent and capricious, abundantly profane, and his respect for social conventions has vanished. He has lost his sense of responsibility, and cannot be trusted to honor his commitments. The "mental degradation" with which David Ferrier was to characterize the effects of frontal

Table 6.1
The psychological damage

Examiner	Comments
Harlow 1848	a great favorite with his men
	temperate habits
	considerable energy of character
	mental hebetude
	inaccurate estimation of size and money
	memory as perfect as ever
	intellectually feeble: capricious and childish
	uncontrollable behavior (including desire to return home)
	habitually accurate use of money in making purchases but not particular about price
	foreshadows report on mental manifestations
Jackson 1849	well in mind but memory seems somewhat impaired
Bigelow 1850	quite recovered in faculties of body and mind
Standing Committee of the AMA 1850	mental powers greatly impaired
	degenerating process still going on (psychological?)
American Phrenological Journal of 1851	was quiet and respectful
	now gross, profane, coarse, and vulgar
	animal propensities in control
Channing 1860?	recovery was perfect
Harlow 1868	nervo-bilious temperament, iron will
	the most efficient foreman employed by his contractors
	well-balanced mind, shrewd smart business man
	energetic and persistent in his plans
	balance of animal and intellectual faculties destroyed
	fitful, irreverent, profane
	little deference for fellows
	impatient of advice, obstinate, and capricious
	readily forms plans and abandons them
	a child in intellectual capacities with the animal passions of a strong man
	entertains nephews and nieces with fabulous recitals of his wonderful feats and escapes
	conceives great fondness for pets and souvenirs, especially children, horses, and dogs
	1849–1851 travels, visits Boston and larger N.E. towns, joins Barnum's Museum in New York
	1851–1852 in Hanover, N.H., works for Currier
	1852 in Chile, works as coach driver until 1859?

Table 6.1 (continued)

Examiner	Comments
	1859? in San Francisco, works as farm laborer, seizures begin 1860, continues to work after them but unable to settle at any one place
Jackson 1870	was not profane before
	still obstinate, fitful, vacillating, profane
	1851–1852 hostler in a stable
	1852–[1859] stagecoach driver, Chile
	[1859] on a farm
	[1860] seizures, then various jobs
Wilson 1879	finally beset by drinking habits
Hughes 1897	intemperance played part in his irregular life
Cobb 1940	roving life/small jobs here and there
H. Damasio et al. 1994	responsible, intelligent, socially well adapted
	a favorite with his peers and elders
	had made progress and showed promise
	new learning intact, neither memory nor intelligence affected
	irreverent, capricious
	respect for social conventions had vanished
	lost his sense of responsibility
	could not be trusted to honor his commitments
	life of wandering for a dozen years
	never returned to a fully independent existence
	neural basis of moral sense destroyed
A. R. Damasio 1994 (adds to H. Damasio et al. 1994)	Gage takes jobs on horse farms, works at one place or another briefly, quits capriciously
	featured at Barnum's, shows wound vaingloriously
	goes to South America to work on horse farms, eventually becomes a coach driver
	returns to San Francisco, farm worker, no one job for long, moves around a lot
	drinking and brawling in questionable places
	"collector" behavior (pets, souvenirs, etc.)
	parades his self-misery
	not independent, no secure job
	no concern about future, no sign of foresight
	probable reduction in emotional reactivity
	invents tales without foundation except in his fancy
	implicit parallel with psychopathic personality

damage, including those in Gage, came about because the neural basis of his moral sense had been destroyed.

The Gage of H. Damasio et al. leads a wandering life for a dozen years, never returning to a fully independent existence, never holding a secure job or holding one for long, and moving around a lot. He works on horse farms, usually at one place or another briefly, only to quit capriciously. When he goes to South America, it is to work on horse farms, but he eventually becomes a coach driver. On return to San Francisco, he is under the custody of his family, but moves around often, occasionally working as a farm laborer.

A. R. Damasio's Gage becomes a braggart, showing his wound vaingloriously at Barnum's, and takes to drinking and brawling in questionable places. He also invents tales without foundation except in his fancy and paraded his self-misery. He shows no concern for his future, displays no foresight, and probably suffers a reduction in his emotional reactivity. Here A. R. Damasio implies that there is a parallel between Gage and the typical psychopathic personality. Elsewhere, in a contemporaneous interview-report in the Science section of the *New York Times*, Damasio makes the parallel quite explicit: the postaccident Gage begins lying to his friends, not honoring his commitments, and behaving socially "like an idiot."[23]

A Kind of Conclusion

What almost everyone had first learned about Gage was that he had been unaffected by his injury, and Harlow's report of 1868 did little to disturb that memory. The same peace was not accorded the remains of Gage's body in San Francisco's Lone Mountain Cemetery. Established in 1854, the complex of four cemeteries at the base of the hill was renamed Laurel Hill in 1864. By 1912 pressure on land within the city boundaries, coupled with neglect of the older cemeteries, led the Board of Supervisors to vote to disinter the bodies and remove them to Colma. Resistance was fierce but gradually subsided by 1937, when voters decided in favor of the move. So on 17 May 1940, what was left of Phineas's body was taken to the Cypress Abbey's receiving vaults in Lawndale together with the remains of his mother and brother-in-law. On 24 September 1946, the remains of the two Gages were placed in vault number 962 of the massive underground facility that, marked by the Laurel Hill Mound and the Pioneer Monument atop it, provides "final resting place for approximately 35,000 San Francisco pioneers."

Many individual grave sites are now not marked:

Only those monuments and headstones transported at public expense were brought to Lawndale. All others were removed by San Francisco contractor Charles L. Harney. Priceless crypts, tombs and mausoleums were unceremoniously dumped in San Francisco Bay to create breakwaters.... In spring when the sand level along the beach is low, marble and granite monuments, still easily legible, surface.

One day, perhaps someone strolling along the beach will discover the inscribed stone that once marked Lone Mountain's Lot 433 where Phineas and his relatives originally rested. Remote as that possibility may seem, I believe it much more likely than our finding Harlow's case notes or the correspondence between him, Gage, and his relatives that would allow us to learn in more detail what happened after 13 September 1848 and correct the fables that have grown up since then.[24]

Notes

1. Harlow 1848, 1868. The eighteen-month report is "A most remarkable case," 1851.

2. Short-term changes: Harlow 1868, 1869; J. B. S. Jackson 1849, case Number 1777; Standing Committee on Surgery 1850; the *American Phrenological Journal* report (reproduced figure 15.2) is "A most remarkable case," 1851; and Bigelow 1850b, 1850c. Dr. Fred Barker found the Standing Committee on Surgery's report.

3. "C" in *National Eagle* (Claremont, New Hampshire), 29 March 1849 (p. 2, col. 2), and *True Democrat and Granite State Whig* (Lebanon, New Hampshire), 6 April 1849 (p. 1, col. 7). J. B. S. Jackson 1849, case Number 1777, records what the family told him.

4. Channing's lecture is among the Walter Channing II papers held by the Massachusetts Historical Society. The search for comments by members of the Society for Medical Improvement and the students in the medical class was based on those Countway Library and Harvard University Archives holdings listed under "Massachusetts" in Appendix H. Cushing's collection of material on Henry Jacob Bigelow in the Yale Medical Library and the other manuscripts held elsewhere at Yale on him and Phelps were equally unrevealing. Holmes's (1891) memoir of Bigelow contains no more than Bigelow's own account.

5. The letters and/or journals of Louisa May Alcott (Stern 1987) and Emily Dickinson (Johnson and Ward 1965). For manuscripts searched at the American Antiquarian Society, see Appendix H. For Cotting and the Massachusetts Medical Society, see Burrage 1923.

6. Blackington 1956, pp. 78, 80; Savage 1873. Blackington's sources are not documented directly and the fate of his manuscripts is, as John Fleischmann,

features editor of the magazine *Yankee* (Dublin, NH), told me on 20 October 1999, a "painful story." Almost all of the papers and photographs acquired by the founder of *Yankee* from Blackington in about 1965 (the *Blackington Collection*) were "not stored properly and were thrown out in a company house-cleaning" some time before 1970. Although Blackington did embellish his stories, the one file of his material that has survived shows him to have been meticulous about recording and storing the original information.

7. For the search for Gage's travels in New England see under the states listed in Appendix H. Note that Benjamin Browne Foster's diaries for late 1849 and the second half of 1850 are not included in the printed edition because they have not survived (Foster 1975).

8. Blackington 1956. John Fleischmann, of *Yankee* (Dublin, NH), has told me that Austin and Stone's Museum did not come into existence until 1883. See note 6.

9. For Barnum, see Appendix H under that heading and the *County Herald* (Rutland, Vermont), 18 July 1850 and 15 August 1851, and *True Democrat and Granite State Whig* (Lebanon, New Hampshire), 15 August 1850. During September 1850, the latter carried a detailed advertisement for the Boston Museum but the advertisement did not mention Gage.

10. The illustration (number 56 in Windsor 1921, p. 570) is assumed to be by Russell Windsor because her initials can be seen just below Gage's left collar. Robert Young, the historian of localization, who has read almost everything written by Hollander, does not know of Hollander's using it. Neither he nor any other notable historians of phrenology such as Madeleine Stern and Anthony Walsh have told me that they recall having seen it in other collections of phrenological material.

11. For searches relating to Hanover, New Hampshire, see under the Dartmouth College Libraries heading in Appendix H. Other material on Currier is in H. Child 1866, p. 326; F. Childs 1961; Currier 1984, p. 185; and the illustration of the Dartmouth Inn, seen originally in Childs 1961, was found in the Dartmouth College Library Archives by Barbara Krieger. Benjamin Bridgeman is among the physicians indexed at the Connecticut Historical Society; Willis R. Peake's diary is held by the University of Vermont.

12. Bigelow on Webster in *A Memoir of Henry Jacob Bigelow*, 1900, pp. 117–118; Barnum in Werner 1926 and Saxon 1989; Lind and Barnum in Ware and Lockhard 1980, chapters 1 and 2; Louisa May Alcott (Stern 1987); Emily Dickinson (Johnson and Ward 1965). Cushing (*Diary*, March) and Salisbury (*Diary*, 19 and 30 March) held at American Antiquarian Society.

13. Perhaps a Mr. James McGill was Gage's employer. The records of the Concord coach manufacturing company, Abbott-Downing of Concord, NH, are held by the New Hampshire Historical Society but are not complete for the early period. One coach was ordered from Valparaiso in 1860 by McGill. D. D. Shattuck's business and business address comes from the Great Register of Voters, San Francisco (his partners were then Hendley and Noyes). The ship passenger lists are from Rasmussen 1965–1969, vol. 1, p. 729, in which the names refer

to entry number 7162 on pp. 137 and 139 respectively. J. B. S. Jackson 1870, p. 147, for the "six-horse stage-coach" amendment, and the diaries of Enos Christman 1931 and Marcellus Bixby 1927, for life in Valparaiso, and George Augustus Peabody 1937, for Santiago as well.

14. The famous Australian coach line of Cobb and Co. was founded in Victoria in 1850 by four U.S. citizens, who imported Concord coaches to provide some of the earliest coach services to that state's gold fields, and the company eventually expanded across Australia. Two of the founders were New Englanders, one, John Murray Peck, actually having been born in Lebanon, New Hampshire, in 1830. These details, the drivers' skills, and the road conditions are from Austin 1977, pp. 127–128 and 129–132.

15. Because the date Harlow gives for Gage's death is in error by a whole year, I have usually placed what I believe must be the correct date or dates in square brackets, for example, the year he returned from Chile as [1859].

16. William Kooiman of the J. Porter Shaw Library of the U.S. Department of the Interior's National Maritime Museum in San Francisco tells me that after 1858, passenger arrival lists were rarely published in the *Daily Alta*, the main source, and when they were, they included only the cabin passengers and not those traveling steerage.

17. J. B. S. Jackson 1870, p. 147, for Gage's work before and after the seizure. Another addition may be his saying that Gage was "still very obstinate, as he always had been" after the accident. N. Gray & Co.'s bound, ledger-sized book recorded funerals in chronological order of year, month, and day, so that the page recording Gage's funeral cannot possibly be in error by a year. N. Gray & Co is now Halstead–N. Gray and Co.–Carew, and English, and is situated at 1123 Sutter Street, San Francisco. The 1860 date is also confirmed by the (admittedly) loose-leaf Lone Mountain/Laurel Hill record now in the care of Cypress Lawn Memorial Park in Colma. I had not seen the original records in 1986 but Marian Marquand, who found them for me in 1985, sent a sworn and notarized certification of the Gray entry, together with a photocopy of the Lone Mountain/Laurel Hill Record, in time for me to publish the correct date in 1986.

18. None of the papers or publications of the doctors Henry Perrin Coon and Jacob Davis Babcock Stillman in the San Francisco Public Library or the Bancroft Library, University of California, Berkeley, mention the exhumation or refer to Gage in any other way. Stillman was an important figure in Californian medical life (e.g., he founded the Medico-Chirurgical Association) and wrote much on Californian history, but the exhumation is not mentioned in anything he wrote or in the many references to his work (e.g., Lyman 1925). Stillman edited the *California Medical Gazette*, but Harlow's second paper on Gage is not mentioned in either of the only two volumes that seem to have been published (vols. 1 and 2, 1868 to 1870). In his second term, Coon was also ex officio President of the Board of Health. For the circumstantial evidence cited here, see San Francisco mayors and supervisors in Shuck 1894; the Board of Supervisor's meetings in *Alta California*, 25 December 1867, p. 2, col. 4; *San Francisco Examiner*, 24

December, p. 3, col. 3; and *Daily Morning Call*, 24 December 1867, p. 3, col. 1. For other material searched concerning Gage's exhumation, see Appendix H under the San Francisco heading.

19. Ships' departures and passenger lists, such as there are, appear in *Alta California*, 29 December 1867, p. 1, col. 2, and 4 January 1868, p. 1, col. 2, and the *San Francisco Examiner*, 29 December 1867, p. 1, col. 2, as well as in other papers.

20. Bigelow and Lennin *Medical and Surgical Reporter* (Philadelphia), 1868, vol. 18, pp. 533–534; *A Memoir of Henry Jacob Bigelow*, 1900, p. 123. Intellect somewhat affected: *The Medical Record*, 1868–1869, vol. 3, p. 276; and *Medical Record* (New York), 1868, vol. 3, p. 324; unimpaired: the *New York Journal of Medicine*, 1869, vol. 9, pp. 69–70, based on the New York *Medical Record*. Barker 1995 for the minimizing trend; Standing Committee on Surgery 1850.

21. *Daily Evening Traveller* (Boston), 3 June 1868, p. 2, col. 2; Shuck 1869, pp. 395–399; *Woburn Journal* (Woburn, Massachusetts), 13 June 1868, p. 2, col. 4; *Daily Free Press* (Burlington, Vermont), 5 June 1868.

22. American Antiquarian Society: Cushing Diaries, vol. 29, entries for June 1868, and papers of Benjamin Eddy Cotting. Robert Edes's prize essay in Edes 1868.

23. Jackson 1870, p. 147; Cobb 1940. H. Damasio, Grabowski, Frank, Galaburda, and A. R. Damasio 1994; A. R. Damasio 1994; Blakeslee 1994. Some years before the Damasio et al. study, Changeux ([1983] 1985, pp. 158–159) had anticipated A. R. Damasio in at least one respect: even though he then said nothing about Gage's "moral" behavior, he classed the changes in Gage as being of the "psychopathic" type. What A. R. Damasio here says about Gage's behavior matches what he has found in his own cases with the kind of frontal mesial damage attributed to Gage in Damasio et al.'s 1994 reconstruction.

24. For the Lone Mountain and Laurel Hill cemeteries, the transfer of the remains to Cypress Abbey and Cypress Lawn, their reinterment in the Pioneer Monument vaults, and the dumping of the headstones and other grave markers, see Svanevik and Burgett 1992, pp. 31–34, and 1995, pp. 32–33, 35, 40–41, 43–45.

7

Localization: The Background

Anatomists having hitherto too readily formed Systems, and Moulded these soft parts in the manner that was most agreeable to each we cannot be surprised to find so little exactness in their Figures.

—Niels Stensen, *Discours de Monsieur Stenon sur l'anatomie du cerveau*, 1669

What were the "several reasons" Harlow had in 1868 for believing that the portion of Gage's brain traversed by the tamping iron was "the best fitted of any ... to sustain the injury"? Do we take Harlow to be offering his opinion of that year, or was he referring to what he had thought in 1848? On either or both occasions, was Harlow simply repeating the very old opinion that damage to the back of the head, or occiput, often caused the vital functions to fail? Or did he think the front or anterior part of the brain had few functions? Or even none at all? What sorts of observations supported Harlow's view? Clinical? Experimental? Teasing out the answers to these questions requires us to consider some aspects of the complicated way in which we have learned how the brain works. Even though it was not so, I shall deal with it here as if our knowledge of the functions of the brain accumulated gradually, in a relatively uncomplicated, linear way.

I start this history with our modern vision of the brain. Even with the naked eye we have as little difficulty in discerning the fissure separating the frontal and temporal lobes, or that separating the frontal from the parietal lobe, as we have in appreciating the irregular surface of the moon. It therefore comes as a surprise to learn that it was not until 1838 that the terms "frontal," "temporal," "parietal," and "occipital" were introduced for describing these lobes, or that the delimitation of the lobes themselves, begun by Gratiolet and completed by Turner, was accepted from only about the late 1860s. Exactly when the earlier and gross differentiation of the anterior or frontal parts (not lobes) from the posterior was first made, as distinct from the merely descriptive uses of those terms, is uncertain. Similarly, as the three illustrations of the brain in figure 7.1 show, the regularity we see in the convolutions of the brain evolved only gradually. The most modern of these, panel (c), is an 1866 "drawing from nature" made for Turner, panel (b) is from an etching prepared during 1810–1815 for Franz Josef Gall, and panel (a) is a woodcut prepared for the 1543 edition of Vesalius's *De Humani Corporis Fabrica*. The increased detail in the images closer to our era is not simply a function of how they were constructed: a well-made woodcut can reveal the details of the convolutions and fissures. What was perceived about the structure of the brain was influenced by what was conceived about its functions, and up to the first half of the nineteenth century, it was given very few functions.[1]

Early Clinical and Experimental Findings

Harlow's opinion about the lesser effects of anterior damage could have been drawing on the very old lore about the role of those parts of the nervous system lying between the spinal cord and the cerebral hemispheres or brain proper. Although it was not clear to the ancients just which of the functions of respiration, circulation, and movement these parts controlled, it was widely suspected they made a major contribution. The most common evidence was clinical, for example, that of Oribasius (c. A.D. 325–400), who observed that a death that followed from the back of the neck being stabbed was because breathing was arrested. Experiments by Galen (c. A.D. 129–c. 200) also showed that sectioning the cord above the first vertebra caused death immediately. Ancient theory similarly held that damage to the space in this part of the nervous system, as distinct from damage to the substance of the organs defining the space, was immediately fatal. Hence, whereas damage to the skull at the back and underside of the head often disturbed or even abolished the vital functions, damage elsewhere had less effect. If Harlow was referring implicitly to Gage's vital functions, he may have been drawing on this distinction.[2]

On the other hand, Harlow's opinion may have been based on clinical observations of damage to the cerebral hemispheres themselves. Coincident with the general attention given these parts of the nervous system by the mid-1700s, some attention also began to be given to the effects of

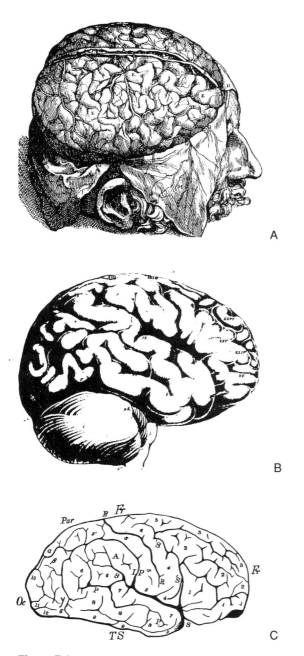

Figure 7.1
Illustrations of the convolutions of the brain: (a) Vesalius 1543, (b) Gall 1810–1815, (c) Turner 1866

I will not assert it to be a general fact, but as far as my own experience and observation go, I think that I have seen more patients get well, whose injuries have been in or under the frontal bone, than any other bones of the cranium. If this should be found to be generally true, may not the reason be worth inquiring into *?

* That this is true, has been proved by many instances. The cause is in great measure assigned, if we recollect that the cerebrum may be hurt with less danger than the cerebellum; and that the greater the distance of a wound from the cerebellum, the less danger there is of that part of the contents of the cranium being injured. It has been frequently demonstrated, that great part of the cerebrum may be taken away without destroying the animal, or even depriving it of its faculties; whereas the cerebellum will scarcely admit the smallest injury, without being followed by mortal symptoms.   E.

Figure 7.2
Facsimile of Pott on frontal damage and Earle's footnote on animal experiments From Pott 1790, p. 184. The footnote is 1790, but Pott's text here is the same as Pott 1768.

damage at different sites. In 1768 Percivall Pott (1713–1788), the English surgeon, in what may well be the first expression of a clinically based view about the effects of anterior damage to the brain, raised the possibility that injury "in or under the frontal bone" had less marked consequences than damage elsewhere. As we see from the facsimile quotation of Pott's work, Earle, his editor, indicated in his 1790 footnote that Pott's opinion was now "proved by many instances" and supported by the results of experiments on animals (figure 7.2). Pre-1800 experimental findings were thus consistent with Pott's clinically grounded possibility.[3]

By the second quarter of the nineteenth century, the opinion Pott expressed seems to have been reasonably widely accepted. Thus Tyrrell's comment on Rogers's case in 1827 is consistent with it, and the anonymous 1843 reviewer of Guthrie's On Injuries of the Head Affecting the Brain could take Guthrie to task for claiming that anterior brain wounds were more serious than those more posterior because it was a claim directly opposed to the opinion and practice of every practitioner with whose opinions we are acquainted, and is contrary to our own observation of the result of a considerable number of cases.

Consequently, if Harlow was drawing on recent clinical opinion in 1848, he was expressing what by then seems to have been the majority view. Hence in the choice between the anterior and posterior of Gage's brain, the frontal portion would best have resisted the damage done by the tamping iron.[4]

Some fifty years before Gage's accident, in 1792, Leny had drawn an important general theoretical conclusion from the fact that in his case of frontal damage, "Every function, both mental and corporeal, was unimpaired and indeed had always been so since the accident, except the short time he was delirious." Leny's patient was a boy of about fourteen who had suffered a right forehead fracture with an immediate loss of an amount of brain tissue "nearly the size of a hen's egg," and the subsequent loss of smaller quantities, apparently from the right frontal lobe. For understanding the role of the brain, Leny saw that

accidental injuries seem to bid fairest towards its elucidation; but even these, as a source of information, must be re-regarded as exceedingly uncertain. Sometimes, when to appearance small, their effects have been almost instantly fatal, while, at other times, when seemingly of much greater importance, they have been productive of little subsequent harm.

From these differential effects, Leny immediately drew the conclusion "that every part of the brain is not equally concerned in the execution of its functions." But with only the one case, the most he could have done would have been to see his case as illustrating Pott's thesis.[5]

Given that observations on the effects of injury to the brain go back thousands of years, we must ask why Leny's methodological pointer was not followed earlier, why it took so long to formulate a clinical opinion as simple as Pott's, and why the effect of anterior damage was still a matter of controversy until about the time of Gage's accident. A clue is found in a peculiarity of Home's 1814 attempt to relate different kinds of brain damage to changes in brain function. Possibly the first such series of cases to be published, and appearing only a few years after Earle had composed his footnote and Leny had drawn his conclusion, Home's introduction began with this plea:

The various attempts which have been made to procure accurate information respecting the functions that belong to the individual portions of the human brain,

having been attended with little success, it has occurred to me, that were all anatomical surgeons to collect in one view all the appearances they had met with, in
cases of injury to that organ, and the effects that such injuries produced upon its
functions, a body of evidence might be formed, that would materially advance
this highly important investigation.

Home's intention was to contribute to that advance by presenting his
own observations as "so many experiments made upon the brain." In a
sense, he was wanting to build on the same kinds of comparisons that
Leny had suggested.[6]

From our perspective, therefore, one might have expected Home to
have organized his cases according to the place or site of the damage.
Instead he classified them according to the nature of the agency causing
the damage (e.g., concussion, dilatation of the blood vessels, pressure
from tumor, pressure of water on the brain, etc.). Whatever clinical and
therapeutic significance Home's analysis may have had, his schema
required his readers to bring together for themselves the effects of damage at any particular site. For example, if one wanted to know the effect
of frontal damage, one had to search each of Home's ten agency categories. Home's scheme did not contribute to understanding the relation
between brain damage and brain function, and we must ask why he
failed to relate the damage to the site.

The answer is, I believe, the same as the answer to the questions of
why suggestions like Leny's were not followed, and why Pott had been
able to raise the anterior-posterior difference only as a possibility. For
hundreds of years the anatomy of the brain was studied by a method that
could not reveal the structures to which changes in function could be related. Even had those structures been identified, the few functions attributed to the brain were not conceptualized in ways that could be usefully
related to them.

Early Brain Anatomy

Not until about 1640, literally after hundreds of years of anatomical
studies, was the first of the brain's major anatomical landmarks first
described. It was then that Franciscus Sylvius identified the fissure now
named after him as the Sylvian fissure. Nearly 200 years more were to
pass before Luigi Rolando in 1829 described the second fissure, eventually also named after him. Why were these structures overlooked for so
long? I believe there were three reasons. First, a long tradition located

psychological functions like perceiving, thinking, and feeling in the heart, rather than in the head; second, there was a centuries-long method of dissection that revealed the spaces within the parts of the brain rather than of the substance of the brain itself; and third, there were technical difficulties in the methods for dissecting the brain.

Brain or Heart?

Until about 1500 the predominant view was that the heart, and not the brain, exercised psychological functions like perceiving, thinking, and feeling. Those who followed Aristotle and Avicenna—the majority—emphasized the heart; those who followed the Hippocratic writers and Galen—the minority—emphasized the brain. Because the brain won out only after the late 1500s, the positions taken before that time necessarily determined how injuries to the brain were construed.

The arguments for both orientations were as much speculative-philosophical as empirical. It was, of course, practically self-evident that life depended upon the heart: with the cessation of its movement, life itself ceased. Hence, Alfred pronounced "Cor igitur vitae domicilium pronuntio." Aristotle (384–322 B.C.), whom Clarke and O'Malley describe as the "most distinguished advocate" of the majority or cardiocentric view, in his *Parts of Animals* further pointed to the heart's movements being visible as soon as the embryo formed, to the lack of the brain's "continuity with the sensory parts," and to those sense organs near the brain being connected to it directly by vascular channels, as indicators that the faculties of sensation and motion were located in the heart. On general philosophical grounds, Aristotle also concluded that the nerves originated in the heart, that sensations were appreciated in it, and that the heart was the center for thought. Nature, having contrived the heart as the source of the blood vessels—the very containers of life—set it centrally in the body, in "the place of primacy and governance." The functions of the brain were designed only to balance the heat of the heart because, in his view, everything needed something to counterbalance it: "The brain, then, makes the heat and the boiling in the heart well blent and tempered."[7]

The importance given the brain by Hippocrates or the writers who made up the Hippocratic school (c. 430–350 B.C.) came from the role they gave it, in *The Sacred Disease*, as interpreter of "the phenomena caused by the air." The air conferred intelligence on the brain: "Eyes, ears, tongue, hands and feet act in accordance with the discernment of the brain." Therefore, they asserted, "the brain is the interpreter of consciousness.... Some people say the heart is the organ with which we think, and that it feels pain and anxiety. But it is not so." In the eloquent statement of this Hippocratic writer:

> Men ought to know that from the brain, and from the brain only, arise our pleasures, joy, laughter and jests, as well as our sorrows, pains, griefs, and tears. Through it, in particular, we think, see, hear, and distinguish the ugly from the beautiful, the bad from the good, the pleasant from the unpleasant.

Even though the members of the Hippocratic school so emphasized the role of the brain and provided, as Woollam put it in 1958, "a mine of wisdom and observation upon the diseases of the brain," their writings showed "but little evidence of any direct contact with the anatomy of the brain."

What do we make of this gap? It is relatively easy to understand how Aristotle's cardiocentrism could be responsible for his giving "a very scanty description of the anatomy of the brain," as Woollam also said, but this kind of explanation does not seem to apply to the Hippocratic deficiency. I believe the failure of the Hippocratic writers to question the humoral explanatory mechanisms they had proposed to be responsible. Humors provided the explanatory link between Hippocratic physiology and the psychology that went with it. If, as seems to have been the case, they were satisfied with that link, and if only a feeling of something's being wrong with an existing explanation drives the search for a new one, what would have required the Hippocratic school to give more consideration to the anatomy of the brain? The particular method of dissection they used told them what they needed to know; they had no need to modify anything.[8]

The Ventricles and Dissection

For centuries, the only method used for dissecting the brain sectioned it a limited number of times, probably not more than three, and then only in horizontal slices, or transversely. The technique readily revealed the ventricles, or spaces between the parts of the brain, and traced the connections between the ventricles and some of the immediately associated structures, but revealed little or nothing of structures making up the substance of the cerebral hemispheres themselves.

Herophilus (fl. c. 300 B.C.) is said to have been the first to observe the ventricles, and Clarke notes that from his time onward "in all descriptions of the brain the anatomist paid more attention to the ventricular system than to any other part because of its functional significance." The importance of these spaces derived from the fact that both physiological and psychological functions were located in them.

The first detailed account of the ventricles we possess is, according to Clarke and O'Malley, that of Galen from the second century B.C. Galen sectioned the brain transversely with the method that was to be used until the middle of the seventeenth century, that is, for the next 1,400 years. We have no illustrations of what Galen and others like him saw, but we get some sense of how the lateral ventricles dominated their vision from the earliest published, very crude illustrations of Lorenz Phyres or Fries, which appeared in 1518, and those of Berengario da Carpi and Johannes Dryander, published in 1523 and 1536, respectively.

In the much less crude illustrations with which Vesalius illustrated the steps of his dissection, published in 1543 (figure 7.3), we see the domination of the lateral ventricles especially clearly. Vesalius first removed the top of the skull and reflected the membranes to expose the two hemispheres and the corpus callosum. He then revealed the lateral ventricles

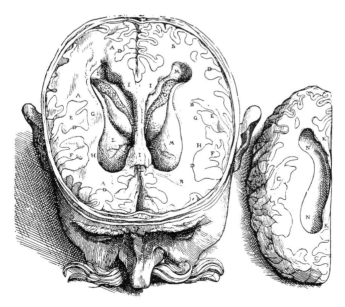

Figure 7.3
The lateral ventricles in Vesalius's dissection of the brain
From Saunders and O'Malley 1950, p. 191, plate 68.

by removing the upper portion of both hemispheres. In the remaining steps of his dissection, he explored, among other things, the relation of the two lateral ventricles to the third and fourth, and the connections of the hemispheres to the cerebellum and various of the cranial nerves. A small opening known as the interventricular foramen connected the third ventricle, the space lying under the hemispheres and above the midbrain and cerebellum, to the lateral ventricles. From the third ventricle, the cerebral aqueduct, or aqueduct of Sylvius, led to what was usually considered the fourth ventricle: the space between the medulla oblongata and the cerebellum (although in some versions of the theory the fourth ventricle included the cerebellum itself).

The first significant shift from this method of dissection was made known in 1573 when Varolio (1543–1575) published details of his novel and difficult method of removing the brain from the skull and dissecting it from below. Varolio's method allowed the connections between the brain stem and the brain to be traced more easily, and the *pons* (later the *pons Varolii*) to be identified. About 100 years later, the notable physician, physiologist, teacher, and anatomist, Franciscus de le Boë Sylvius, or Françoise de le Boë (1614–1672), introduced the second significant change, one that enabled some differentiation to be made *within* the cerebral hemispheres themselves. Some time before 1641, Sylvius uncovered the fissure now named after him by removing the right hemisphere entirely and pushing or rolling the left into the space previously occupied by it. Essentially, Sylvius's procedure separated what we now call the frontal and parietal regions from the temporal by moving the former upward and to one side.

The first published description of the fissure of Sylvius is a note signed "F. S." on page 262 of Caspar Bartholinus's 1641 *Institutiones anatomicae*, and the first illustration of the fissure is figure 5 of Bartholinus, reproduced here as figure 7.4(a). Sylvius may also have sectioned the brain in other directions that were also likely to have revealed the fissure. What is certain is that Stensen, one of Sylvius's most famous pupils, published what Clarke and Dewhurst describe as "the first reasonable drawing" of a coronal section in 1669. Reproduced here as figure 7.4(b), the Sylvian fissure is also very apparent.[9]

Difficulties with Methods of Dissection

In antiquity, human brains were so difficult to obtain that most early dissection was of animal brains. Although it may not be immediately

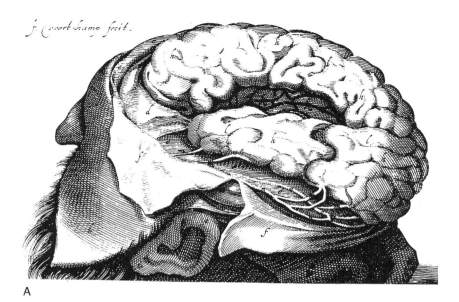

A

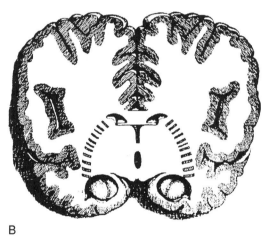

B

Figure 7.4
(a) Sylvius's dissection and (b) Stensen's coronal section
From (a) Bartholinus 1641, p. 261, fig. 5 and (b) Steno [1669] 1950, unnumbered appendix figure.

apparent from their writings, Galen and others based most of their conclusions about the human brain on studies of goats, sheep, pigs, and oxen. That the ungulate *rete mirabile*, an important circulatory structure below the brain, was attributed to the human brain, from which it is absent, was a not unsurprising consequence. Dissection of human bodies, mainly those of criminals, was not unknown, but it was not common. For example, according to Baker, Holy Roman Emperor Frederick II generously decreed in 1240 that "a cadaver should be dissected before assembled physicians and surgeons once every five years." Baker lists a number of European centers at which dissections were performed in the fourteenth and fifteenth centuries, usually at the rate of one or two per year. Not until the sixteenth century did the numbers grow; even then, as we know directly from Leonardo da Vinci and from Vesalius, some dissection had to be carried out hurriedly and in secret. The relative infrequency of dissection in general necessarily limited dissection of the human brain.

Early dissectionists generally did not fix or harden the brain before dissection, so that the anatomist could, as Niels Stensen (Steno) put it in his famous barb, mold the unhardened, soft, and plastic brain to accord with his preconceptions:

Every Anatomist who dissects the Brain demonstrates from experience what he advances. This soft and pliable Substance so readily yields to every motion of his Hand, that the Parts are imperceptibly formed in the same manner as he had conceived them before Dissection.

The lack of adequate methods of hardening also meant that anatomists worked under conditions that considerably limited what they could demonstrate. Consider, for example, Baldasar Heseler's detailed record of a public dissection carried out over fourteen days by Vesalius himself in Padua in 1540. The first of two of the bodies Vesalius used was "already stinking" by the second day and the homologous parts of freshly killed dogs had to be dissected to demonstrate his points. By the fifth day the body was "very much decayed," and was so dry and withered on the sixth and seventh that dogs had again to be used. To complete the demonstration, Vesalius commenced dissecting a second body on the ninth day and took another five days to complete his task. One can only imagine the condition of the brain when it was eventually dissected on the last day of work on each body, the eighth for the first and the sixth for the second. Except for the hotter summer weather causing him to hurry, Simon Paulii's dissections in Copenhagen in March and May of 1645 follow a similar sequence to that of Vesalius.

Finally, only macroscopic methods for examining the structures and the tissues of which they were constituted were available to Vesalius, Sylvius, and their contemporaries. Those methods changed only in the 1830s, when the compound achromatic microscope came into use. True, microscopes had been used from the middle of the seventeenth century, but the images they produced were of very poor quality, adequate in 1674 for Leeuwenhoek (1632–1723) to reject one of the major propositions of ventricular physiology, that peripheral nerve fibers and the spinal cord were hollow, but unable to resolve much more detail than that. That limitation, together with hardening the brain by boiling it in water or oil and the effects of tissue degeneration, probably contributed to the artifacts described by Malpighi (1628–1694) as minute glands and Leeuwenhoek as globules when they did examine the cells of the cortex in 1666 and 1684, respectively.

Methods for fixing brain tissue were developed at about the same time as reliable data from microscopic examination of cortical tissues became available. Reil first proposed the main hardening medium, alcohol mixed with an alkali, in the early 1800s; serial sectioning of frozen tissue came slightly later, in 1842; the use of paraffin and celloidin began in 1869 and 1882, respectively; and differential staining was introduced as late as 1858. Thus, only between 1830 and 1840, approximately, were the main histological methods for examining brain tissue established.

In the light of all these technical difficulties, how little was definitely established about brain structure prior to 1820 should surprise us less than how much.[10]

Ventricular Physiology and Clinical Observations

The ventricles gained their functional importance in ventricular physiology as the places in which "animal spirit" was manufactured and stored. Vesalius, for example, concluded that in the ventricles, the mixture of air inspired during breathing and the vital spirit transmitted from the heart were "altered by the power of the peculiar substance of the brain into animal spirit." From there the spirit was distributed via "the nerves to the organs of senses and of movement." How Vesalius thought the spirit caused movement and sensation is not clear. Unlike Galen, he did not believe the nerves were hollow, which the usual view of the transmission of animal spirit necessitated. If nerves were solid, by what means did spirit travel? How this problem of mechanism bedeviled ventricular physiology is evident in one of its most famous versions, that of René Descartes (1596–1650), who postulated the existence of threadlike structures that led from the sense organs to the ventricles. Sensations arrived there via the threads and caused pores in the interior of the ventricles to open, thus allowing animal spirit to be reflected to the muscles, where it caused movement. There was, of course, no more evidence for "threads" than for hollow nerves.

In all versions of this physiology, the only clinical observations relevant to the localization of function were those that could be related to the ventricles or the structures that subserved them. Pagel has observed that what "stands out as most characteristic" in the few accounts of cerebral localization up to the seventeenth century is that they are actually attempts at ventricular localization. However, ventricular physiology could not readily incorporate mechanisms or pathways of influence that explained the effects of damage to the brain, and the inability to connect symptoms with sites of damage in the few collections of clinical observations published prior to 1800 reflects this hiatus.[11]

Ventricular Physiology and Epilepsy
The Hippocratic explanation of epilepsy illustrates the inadequacies of the mechanisms postulated in ventricular physiology especially clearly. The Hippocratic *The Sacred Disease* contains very acute clinical descriptions of many epileptic symptoms—including the aura, the feelings of premonition, and the convulsive limb movements—as well as the seizure itself:

The patient becomes speechless and chokes; froth flows from the mouth; he gnashes his teeth and twists [contracts] his hands; the eyes roll and intelligence fails [he becomes insensible], and in some cases excrement is discharged.

Some manuscripts go further:

These symptoms manifest themselves sometimes on the left, sometimes on the right, sometimes on both sides.

No less an authority than Wilder Penfield said of these descriptions, "there is nothing in medical writing to compare with it until Hughlings Jackson."

Penfield's judgment sharpens the contrast between Hippocratic clinical acumen and the vagueness of Hippocratic explanation. The Hippocratic writers believed epilepsy was caused when phlegm, a humor that accumulated when the body failed to purge itself of impurities, blocked the movement of air to the brain and impeded its ability to interpret the phenomena detected by the senses. Halting the flow of air caused paralysis at the point where the flow was arrested, a mechanism proved by the feeling of numbness produced by pressing on a vein. Speech was lost because the passage of air to the brain, the ventricles, or the vena cava was checked. The hands were paralyzed and contracted because the blood was not moving, and the eyes rolled because the minor veins pulsated when they were shut off from the air, and so on. About 1,600 years after *The Sacred Disease*, Mondino de' Luzzi (c. 1270–1326) could do little better: if the ventricles alone were blocked the result was epilepsy, but if both ventricles and substance were obstructed, the result was apoplexy.[12]

We see a further difficulty for these ventricular explanations in the controversy over whether the convulsions and brain damage were on the same side of the body (ipsilateral) or on opposite sides (contralateral). As early as about 450 B.C., the Hippocratic writers had observed contralateral convulsions after wounds of the head:

And, for the most part, convulsions seize the other side of the body; for, if the wound be situated on the left side, the convulsions will seize the right side of the body; or if the wound be on the right side of the head, the convulsion attacks the left side of the body.

Similarly with the convulsions that might be produced by operations on the temple:

if the incision be on the left temple, the convulsions seize on the right side; and if the incision be on the right side, the convulsions take place on the left side.

But what ventricular structures or pathways linked the site of wound or incision on one side of the head with the muscles on the other side of the body?

Over the centuries the Hippocratic observation was so frequently confirmed it was repeated, according to Neuburger, as "a well-known fact." Yet, even in ancient times a minority of physicians disputed the observation. Thus Berengario da Carpi (c. A.D. 1460–1530) cited Avicenna (A.D. 980–1037) to the effect that after a head wound the paralysis was on the same side and the spasm on the opposite. According to Neuburger, this minority opinion created an uncertainty the resolution of which did not begin until about 1650. The first step in that resolution came when the vascular etiology of apoplexy began to be understood and some of the pathways by which that cause acted could be specified.

François Pourfour du Petit (1664–1741) then reconceptualized the pathways of nervous action in a way that should have removed the uncertainty, even though he retained animal spirit as the medium of nervous influence. Pourfour du Petit trephined the parietal bone in dogs, damaged the brain, and then removed the damaged matter. Movements were always weakened in the contralateral extremities, and complete paralysis was produced when the corpus striatum was also damaged. Through his anatomical studies, Pourfour du Petit then established that each hemisphere was linked to the muscles on the opposite side of the body by the crossing over of the pyramidal fibers. He therefore had "convincing proofs that the animal spirit changes from one side to the other," and he believed his anatomical studies showed how the crossing came about.

Neuburger summarized two of Pourfour du Petit's theses as follows: (1) the animal spirit that mediated limb movement issued from the cerebral hemisphere of the opposite side, and (2) the spirit passed through the corpora striata. That Pourfour du Petit retained animal spirit in his reconceptualization does not detract from the importance of his having exchanged the vagueness of the ventricular physiological explanations based on phlegm and venous obstruction for demonstrable pathways of influence. Not until late in the last century did studies using electrical stimulation confirm the functional connection of each hemisphere to the muscles on the opposite side of the body and vindicate Pourfour du Petit's explanation. And like the mixture of alcohol and alkali used for hardening brain tissue, the reconceptualization that made his achievement possible had been available to others well before 1710.[13]

Psychological Function and Ventricular Physiology

If ventricular physiology generated only limited explanations of physiological functions, the deficiencies in what was called "cell theory" limited the explanations of psychological functions even further. According to the various versions of cell theory, psychological functions were carried out in different spaces or "cells" within the brain. Perception, for example, took place in the space where the nerves of the five senses supposedly terminated. Constituted by the two lateral ventricles, this sensory terminus was known as the *sensus commune*. A second cell, usually constituted by the middle or third ventricle, was the locus of imagination and cognition and reasoning. Memory was located in the third cell or fourth ventricle. The placement of these mental functions in the ventricles meant that cell theory was really a ventricular psychology. It was also a particular version of faculty psychology that restricted the powers or faculties of the mind to those of perception, reasoning, imagination, and memory.

One sees immediately that, on its own terms, cell theory is unable to explain other than broadly conceived classes of psychological function. Thus a ventricular psychology could account for something like a generalized memory loss, but what of the very specific impairment of those many stroke victims whose understanding and use of language seems more or less intact but who are unable to name things correctly (nominal aphasia)? In other words, the very breadth of the faculties on which cell theory was based was responsible for its failure to generate useful explanations of the more specific and more common psychological abnormalities. Consequently, although some who adhered to ventricular physiology made very acute analyses of the symptoms that followed injury to the brain, they were unable to relate the symptoms to the damage. For example, Luzzatti and Whitaker showed that in the many case descriptions of language disorders Schneck and Wepfer published in 1584 and 1658, respectively, only in a minuscule number was reference made to the site of the damage. As described by Finger and Buckingham, Alexander Crichton's 1798 study of language disorders shows a similarly unsurprising lack of connection between damage and symptom.

Only in one of the many cases Schneck and Wepfer collected were the symptoms related to the site of damage. Ironically it was a negative instance. Theodoric reported that his Master, Hugo of Lucca, had successfully treated a man for a wound to the fourth ventricle. However, Theodoric went on:

Since it had been the cavity of memory, I saw that Master Hugo was greatly amazed by this; for the man had memory just as before; for he was a chairmaker and lost only his skilfulness.

Master Hugo's amazement is understandable. It would have been joined by the opposite kind of amazement of the many other physicians whose cases Schneck and Wepfer collected. In most cases, had post mortem investigations been conducted, they would have found no damage to the ventricles. Their only explanatory tools—ventricular physiology and psychology—could not have accounted for the disturbances in language function.[14]

Conclusion

Whatever Harlow's "several reasons" for believing that the frontal portion of Phineas Gage's brain was best fitted to sustain the injury from the iron, they were consistent with a clinical opinion that began to be formulated in the mid-1700s and an experimental consensus that began to emerge a little later. However vaguely localized, vital physiological functions were toward the rear of the brain. Consistent with Pott's surmise, Gage could sustain a frontal injury and live.

Ventricular physiology and ventricular psychology meant that by the end of the eighteenth century much more than that could not be said. Leny set out the level of ignorance of brain function very eloquently when he introduced his case:

Although the brain be not only the seat of those powers which distinguish animate from inanimate matter, but also of all those mental operations which dignify man above the inferior orders of animals, yet there is no part of the human body concerning which we possess so limited a knowledge. Its intricacy is great, and to that, our ignorance seems to bear proportion. We neither know the manner in which it performs its functions, nor the share which each of its parts have in their performance. The former is perhaps, for wise purposes, placed above human understanding; and the latter, though it appears more within our reach, has hitherto eluded the research of inquirers.

Yet at almost the same time as Leny expressed his pessimism, concepts were being developed that seemed to explain what had happened to Gage.[15]

At most there had been only slight damage to Gage's left lateral ventricle, and none of the changes in his behavior could be classed as impairments in sensation, reasoning, or memory (this latter at least not obviously). The faculties of cell theory were too broad to encompass these alterations and, had physical symptoms been present, ventricular physiology lacked concepts for explaining how the ventricular damage caused them. Only when physiologists and anatomists started to think that differentiation of function required differentiation of structures, and reciprocally, that differentiated structures implied differentiated functions, could what happened to Gage begin to be understood.

The most important contribution to this change in orientation came from the Viennese anatomist Franz Josef Gall (1758–1828), who decided that behavior had to be explained by faculties more specific than those proposed in cell theory. He believed he had found these faculties in the structures his new method of dissection had revealed in convolutions of the cortex, or outer layer of the cerebral hemispheres. Among his conclusions was that there was a faculty of Benevolence located on the median line at about the junction of the frontal and parietal bones. The primitive function of this organ was, in Gall's view, "to dispose man to conduct himself in a manner conformed to the maintenance of social order." From Benevolence developed the sense of morality and justice, and conscience was the affection or emotion that accompanied its action. Immediately behind Benevolence, Gall located an organ responsible for religious feeling. His colleague, Caspar Spurzheim, named it Veneration, and partly gave it the function of maintaining respect for one's fellows. The two faculties were also components of the moral sentiments that regulated the animal propensities located in the posterior areas of the brain.[16]

The *North Star* reported the injury to Gage's organ of Veneration. It was that which, together with the impairment of the adjacent organ of Benevolence and the manifestations of Gage's animal passions, was to be held responsible for the fact that Gage was "no longer Gage." In the next chapter I examine the basis of Gall's explanatory system, its fate, and the alternative to which it gave rise.

Notes

1. I have treated the topic of this chapter more generally in Macmillan 1994. For the delimitation and naming of the lobes, see Clarke and Dewhurst 1972, pp. 104, 107.

2. Ancient instances of injury from Neuburger [1897] 1981, pp. 93–96.

3. Pott 1790, p. 184. Earl's footnote is 1790 but, as can be seen in Pott 1768, the text he comments on is Pott's of 1768.

4. Rogers 1827 for his case, and "Review of Guthrie's," 1843 for the review of Guthrie.

5. Leny's case seems to have been published first as a pamphlet in Edinburgh in 1792, and was reprinted in a number of places without mentioning that fact. My source is Leny 1793.

6. Home 1814 for his plea.

7. Alfred's pronouncement is cited in Pagel 1958. Clarke and O'Malley 1968, p. 7, for their evaluation of Aristotle. In succession, Aristotle's "anatomical" arguments are from his *Parts of Animals*, sections III, iv; II, vii; II, x; II, i. The general philosophical arguments are in Sections III, iv, and II, vii.

8. Hippocrates (c. 460–379 B.C.) was real enough and did write a number of works attributed to him, but others are best attributed to a corpus of "Hippocratic writers." In order, the quotations are from Jones's (1923–31) translation of Hippocrates, *The Sacred Disease*, sections XIX, XX, and XVII. Woollam 1958 for his judgment.

9. Clarke 1968 for the opinion of Herophilus; Galen in Clarke and O'Malley 1968, p. 709; Phyres or Fries, da Carpi, and Dryander in Singer 1952, pp. 127, 128; Vesalius in Singer 1952 and in Saunders and O'Malley [1950] 1973, plates 67–72. Varolio's method is in Clarke and O'Malley 1968, p. 634; Bartholinus 1641, p. 261, for his method (see also Baker 1909; Clarke 1968; Clarke and Dewhurst 1972, p. 66 and fig. 90); Steno [1669] 1950, unnumbered Appendix Figure; and Clarke and Dewhurst 1972, p. 81 and fig. 103. Neither Sylvius, nor Stensen, nor Bartholin seems to have given reasons for the change to the method of brain dissection, and no authority I have consulted knows of any discussion of its introduction. Steno's figure of the coronal section may derive from Sylvius via Bartholin.

10. Emperor Frederick in Baker 1909; Steno [1669] 1950, p. 30, for the preconceptions of anatomists; and Heseler's account of Vesalius's dissection is in Eriksson 1959, pp. 107, 115–117, 147, 157, 177, 185, 201, 219–221, 287–291; and for Simon Paulii's dissections in Copenhagen in March and May of 1645, see Møller-Christensen 1958. Microscopic methods are in Clarke and O'Malley 1968, pp. 27–53, 415–420, and sectioning and staining in Bonin 1960, p. xii.

11. Vesalius 1543, cited by Clarke and O'Malley, 1968, p. 468, for animal spirit; the mechanism proposed by Descartes is in Riese 1958; and ventricular localization is in Pagel 1958.

12. The Hippocratic description of epilepsy is from Adams's (1849) translation of *The Sacred Disease*, sec. X; Penfield 1958 for his appreciation. Mondino de' Luzzi (1316) is cited by Clarke and O'Malley (1968, p. 23).

13. Hippocrates, *On Injuries of the Head*, secs. XIX and XIII for contralaterality in Adams's translation, and Neuburger [1897] 1981, pp. 53–59, for its general acceptance as well as the reservations. Pourfour du Petit's (1710) experiments are described by Neuburger [1897] 1981, pp. 59–63, his anatomical conclusions are quoted from Clarke and O'Malley 1968, p. 283, and his theses are summarized by Neuburger [1897] 1981, p. 61. Pourfour du Petit's error in attributing the inability of his dogs to see with the contralateral eye (homonymous hemianopia) to the animal spirit that made vision possible also passing through the lateral corpus striatum does not detract from the importance of his reconceptualization of the pathways of action as contralateral.

14. The lack of connection between symptoms and brain/ventricular damage in Luzzatti and Whitaker 1996 and Finger and Buckingham 1994; Theodoric [1267] 1955, vol. 1, p. 109, for Master Hugo's amazement.

15. Leny [1792] 1793.

16. Benevolence and Veneration in Gall [1822–1825] 1835, vol. 5, pp. 156–158 and 215–218 respectively. cf. Gall and Spurzheim 1810–1819, vol. 4, pp. 193–194 and 244–246.

8
Localization: The Beginnings

I, considering the organs of the brain to be near the base of the head ... usually begin the dissection from the ... base ...
—Varolio, *De Nervis Opticus Nonnullisque Alis*, 1573

One thing we seem to learn from the history of the attempts to localize functions in the brain is that there is a reciprocal link between the conception of the functions the brain exercises and the perception of its structures. When the brain is not perceived as having a differentiated structure, it seems not to be conceived of as having differentiated functions. Similarly, differences in function seem to be conceived only when differences in structure are perceived. When nineteenth-century thought began to displace that of the eighteenth, some physiologists explicitly used this relation between perception and conception as a general principle to guide their research. It was largely through it that the foundations of our modern views of brain function were laid.[1]

At the end of the eighteenth century the first systematic work on the brain to be guided by this reciprocal principle was begun by Franz Josef Gall, who argued for the localization of very specific functions in very specific parts of the brain. However, the experimental results of Marie-Jean-Pierre Flourens, published in the 1820s, seemed to deny Gall's theses completely. Nevertheless Gall's work contributed most to ending the domination of ventricular physiology and psychology, a rather surprising consequence given that the sensory-motor physiology that replaced the ventricular view owed much to Magendie and almost nothing to Gall.

The new sensory-motor physiology had disparate sources in the work of Charles Bell and Françoise Magendie on the functions of the roots of the spinal nerves, and that of Marshall Hall on the spinal reflex. The new way of thinking itself does not seem to have a single origin, although

Johannes Müller does seem to have strikingly foreshadowed it in the late 1820s and early 1830s. Its formulation was gradual, coming about only after much bitter debate, and was finally accepted only when its endorsement by notable dualists such as William Carpenter and Müller himself reassured the timid that there was still a place for a will that could work through a brain from which it stood apart. Hence although Müller's foreshadowing of a sensory-motor physiology appeared less than ten years after Flourens's, neither he nor those on whose work he drew made any real advance on the ventricular psychology that so irked Gall. In fact, the psychology the sensory-motor approach to localization spawned was little more than the old ventricular psychology.

I begin this necessarily complicated story with Gall and Flourens and contrast briefly the kinds of explanations of what happened to Gage that could be derived from their positions. After that I sketch the development of sensory-motor physiology that Müller put together from his own work and that of Magendie and Hall. I then point out the limitations of those aspects of it that were applied to Gage.

Functions for the Brain

We have already seen how knowledge of the brain's gross structures depended on particular methods of dissection, and especially how the transverse sectioning of the brain practiced since Galen's time had kept ventricular physiology and psychology alive. Gall and Spurzheim said that any method

> that prevents discovery of the parts that gradually bring the brain to perfection, that cuts the organs before their completion, or that begins ... by slicing and cutting them from above downwards, is contrary to nature and to the purpose of cerebral organisation.

They included the "wretched method of Vesalius" in this criticism. In the convolutions of the cerebral cortex, structures his method of dissection revealed clearly for the first time, Gall sited the psychological functions he thought important for explaining behavior.[2]

Gall: Localization and Fractionation

Franz Josef Gall (1758–1828) was regarded by many as the outstanding brain anatomist of his day and was the most important contemporaneous contributor to the doctrine that the brain was the organ of mind.

No less a person than Flourens, who was to become his great critic, granted that although that proposition had not originated with him,

the merit of Gall, and it is by no means a slender merit, consists in his having understood better than any of his predecessors the whole of its importance.... It existed in science before Gall appeared—it may be said to reign there ever since his appearance.

Gall based his identification of the brain's structures on a method of dissection that, like Varolio's, dissected the brain from below upward. Approached this way, the continuity of the cortical grey matter on the outside of the brain with the fibrous white matter underlying it, and that of the cerebral hemispheres themselves with the structures below it, was immediately apparent. In fact, it is said that Gall was the first to make the distinction between the grey and white matter and show the connection between them. Gall was also the first to insist that the convolutions of the cortex were not arranged randomly but had a regular structure. Flourens's recollection vividly conveys what Gall's method revealed: "I shall never forget the impression I received the first time I saw Gall dissect a brain. It seemed to me as if I had never seen this organ before."[3]

Gall rejected the general faculties of cell theory on the grounds that abstract, general faculties such as sensation, reasoning, and memory could not explain anything of interest about behavior. His aim was a psychology that would explain the differences between people in traits like foresight, stubbornness, compassion, and creativity and in the qualities that made man a social animal, and why people differed in sexual and other propensities. He also wanted to explain the differences between humans and animals and between the different classes of animals.[4]

Gall complained that none of his predecessors could explain such things as "the origin and exercise of the principle of propagation," or "the love of offspring," or "the instinct of attachment." How could such broad processes as sensation, attention, comparison, reasoning, or desire bring those kinds of behaviors into being? He therefore fractionated behavior differently from cell theory and postulated very specific functions located in the substance of the brain itself. The older cell psychology faculties merely accompanied behaviors; they necessarily belonged "to an object, to a particular talent, and are only attributes of it." The emotions ("affections") were conceived of similarly: pain, pleasure, joy, or fear, for instance, were generated when the abilities or faculties were affected in a particular manner. No place remained for the superordinate faculties of cell theory.[5]

Gall says he began thinking of discrete psychological functions as early as his school days. According to a frequently cited account of his own, the variation in the specific talents or abilities his fellow pupils possessed puzzled him. One such was rote learning, an ability that he himself lacked, but that a classmate who had large, bulging eyes possessed in marked degree. Observations of other good rote learners seemed to confirm this association so frequently that Gall took the bulges as an indicator of the size of a talent or ability for verbal memorizing. Even without preliminary knowledge, Gall said he could not avoid the inference that eyes so formed were a mark of an excellent memory. But

it was not until afterwards, that I said to myself, as I have already remarked in my introduction to my first volume, if memory manifests itself by an external character, why should not the other faculties have their characters outwardly visible?

This, he went on, "gave the first impulse to my researches, and which was the occasion of all my discoveries."[6]

Gall's systematic attempt to determine what these abilities or faculties were and where they were located began with his *Philosophische-Medizinsche* of 1791 and concluded with his better known *Functions of the Brain* of [1822–1825] 1835. A good illustration of Gall's method for investigating faculties comes from his account of how he identified what he called the instinct or faculty of self-defense and property, the disposition to quarrel, and courage (*Instinct de la défense de soi-même et de sa propriété, amour desrixes et des combats*). He collected together "a number of individuals of the lower classes of society ... such as coachmen, servants, &c," and, after gaining their confidence, and giving them beer, wine, and money, encouraged them to talk about each other's good and bad qualities, "in short, their striking characteristics." Their discussions soon narrowed to identifying those who were peaceable and those who provoked quarrels. Gall then tried to identify the features of the heads that differentiated the two groups:

I ranged the quarrelsome on one side and the peaceable on the other, and examined carefully the heads of both. I found that in all the former, the head, immediately behind and on a level with the top of the ears, was much broader than in the latter.

Observations of students expelled for dueling, of others who were especially quarrelsome or especially cowardly, and of a notable Viennese fighter of boars, bulls, and similar wild animals confirmed the importance of the skull peculiarity. The instinct of self-defense, known later as the organ of Combativeness, was clearly situated at the posterior-inferior angle of the parietal bone.[7]

As one can appreciate from Gall's example of his fellow pupil's bulging eyes, the language function had to be symmetrically distributed across the two cerebral hemispheres. In one sense, there was not one language function but two: both eyes bulged, ergo, the language function existed in the parts of the brain resting on each orbit. All the faculties were represented in both hemispheres. Consequently, unilateral brain damage or disease did not abolish a function. The undamaged side continued its work, but the overall behavior the affected faculty determined was enfeebled or weakened. In any case, Gall tended to place less emphasis on the effects of injuries to the brain than on malformations of the brain: what he called "natural" mutilations. This caution was partly because of uncertainty about the extent of damage, but it was partly because the other proofs were more important. As he put it:

It is true that I have rejected violent mutilations as a means of discovering the functions of a cerebral organ, or of any organ whatever.... Still, when, after the seat of an organ has been discovered by other means, and this discovery has been sufficiently proved, and this organ having been injured, there ensues any lesion of the faculty that is attributed to it, we may with the fullest assurance, regard this phenomenon as a new proof.

Gall illustrated his point with a case of "an inability to recollect names" caused by a bullet injuring that part of the frontal lobe resting on the orbit. This clinical observation gained its importance only because he had already established that the Faculty for Remembering Names was localized there. Another case in which the subject felt pain under the external angle of the eye when performing difficult calculations confirmed that the Faculty of the Relation of Numbers was located "on the most external lateral part of the orbitar plate." As Gall said, "no one will suppose, that it is bad reasoning, to regard these facts as so many new confirmations."[8]

From comparisons and analyses like these, Gall attempted to derive a limited number of independent, irreducible, and fundamental faculties for explaining behavior. His faculties were not material properties of the brain itself but were, as Hoff has insisted, nonmaterial "essences" that manifested or realized themselves in cortical tissue. The extent to which they did so was proportional to development: the more developed a given faculty, the larger the amount of tissue in the convolutions through which it was realized, and vice versa. Consequently, it seemed to follow that the size of the cranial prominence above a given organ betrayed its size. Gall eventually termed this new approach to studying the relation between brain and behavior "organology," rejecting "cranioscopy" and "craniology," the terms by which others referred to it, and the "phrenology" through which his one time colleague and disciple Spurzheim popularized it.[9]

Gall also located a faculty of Benevolence on the median line at about the junction of the frontal and parietal bones. The full list of French words in the heading with which he introduced his discussion of the organ well conveys its functions: "*Bonté, bienveillence, douceur; compassion, sensibilité, sens moral, conscience.*" Evidence for this faculty came in the first instance from three people known to Gall whose goodness, benevolence, and gentleness "was well acknowledged." He had casts made of their skulls and "examined them until I found the character common to these three heads, otherwise very differently formed." In each, "the superior anterior middle part of the forehead, or the middle anterior part of the frontal bone" projected in "a lengthened protuberance." Consequently, "the cerebral part" under the projection was "the organ whose energetic action constitutes goodness, benevolence, the gentle character." When Benevolence was active the emotion of conscience was felt, and from that feeling morality and justice developed. The primitive function of Benevolence was "to dispose man to conduct himself in a manner conformed to the maintenance of social order," that is, to conform to society's rules.

Immediately behind Benevolence, Gall located an organ for God and religion. The initial basis for this location was the configuration of the skull of one of his own brothers who was so much more religious than the other nine children that he "prayed to God and said Mass all day." Although Gall's father wanted this brother to become a merchant, his religious faculty was so developed that he "fled home and turned hermit." Five years later he joined a religious order, and until his death "lived in exercises of devotion and penance." Gall again studied many other individuals and confirmed the presence of a great elevation of the head "toward the crown," more particularly a "considerable projection" of "the posterior mean part of the superior half of the frontal," in those who were especially devout. Gall seems not to have given the organ a name, and Spurzheim seems to have named the organ "Veneration." He also broadened its scope to include the maintenance of respect for one's fellows, especially for those in authority.

Neither Gall nor Spurzheim described what happened when Benevolence or Veneration were injured. Presumably there were too few survivors. The pathological instances they cited were of cases of religious mania in which the organ of Veneration was inflamed. That is probably why they concentrated on the effects of a small organ of Benevolence or Veneration. Spinoza's atheism, for example, was indicated by his skull's being "flattened on the top" and was caused by Benevolence having "acquired only a very feeble development." Generally, though, when Benevolence or Veneration were small, other organs tended to become ascendant, and one discovered "mischievousness, a malicious, vindictive and ungrateful, character, and a spirit of detraction." In extreme cases, murderous and cruel impulses were released. Thus Gall implicated a depression of the skull in the area of Benevolence as the cause of what he referred to as the notable cruelty of Caribs and the murders committed by various "great criminals."

In the Scottish and American versions of Gall's doctrine at least, Benevolence and Veneration were also components of a system of "Moral Sentiments" that, together with nearby Conscientiousness, regulated the organs responsible for the instinct of propagation, love of offspring, social attachment, self-defense, and destructiveness (figure 8.1). Collectively these faculties were the animal propensities that Gall and Spurzheim located in the posterior areas of the brain.

As we have seen, in 1848 the *North Star* implied that Gage's organ of Veneration had been injured, but said nothing about any consequences. The writer of the 1851 *American Phrenological Journal* report, who implicated Benevolence as well as Veneration, clearly believed their injury was directly responsible for "his profanity, and want of respect and kindness." As weakened moral sentiments, they also gave "the animal propensities absolute control in the character."[10]

Flourens: Antilocalization and Antifractionation

The enthusiastic initial acceptance of Gall's system was matched by the violence of the criticism it also attracted. Nevertheless it survived pretty well unscathed until Marie-Jean-Pierre Flourens published the results of his experimentally based attack—the first—on it. Between the first publication of Gall's theory and Flourens's attack, physiology had been transformed from what can be fairly called a static discipline, founded on anatomy, into an experimental pursuit. In this context Flourens began his

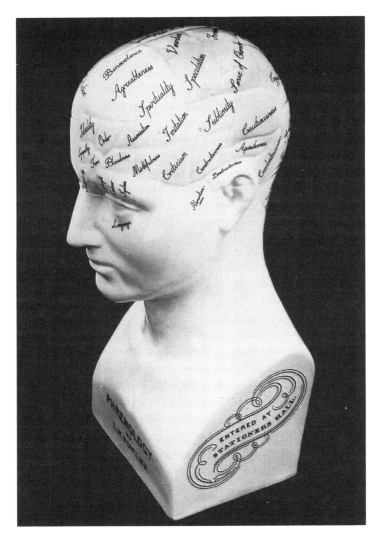

Figure 8.1
Phrenological head showing Veneration, Benevolence, and Relation of Numbers
Head by courtesy of Dr. Jason Mattingley, Melbourne.

work on the brain, and ironically, he was able to take advantage of the revolutionary contributions of Gall and Spurzheim to the brain's anatomy. Flourens's method was to identify particular parts of the cortex, remove them, and judge the effects on behavior. With this method of selective ablation, he seemed to establish that the changes depended upon the amount of cortical tissue removed rather than upon its location. The brain could not therefore be divided into the separate organs Gall's theory demanded. It functioned as a whole.

Despite his skill, Flourens's experiments were deficient in the way he removed tissue, in using birds and other species in which the hemispheres are relatively primitive, and in using crude behavioral changes for judging the operations' effects. Some of these criticisms were put forward at the time along with contrary experimental evidence, some collected by Gall himself, but Flourens's conclusion became widely accepted, especially among experimental physiologists. Not only did the ancients seem to have been correct in believing that mechanical injury did not affect the brain, they seemed to have been right to believe that the tissues of the cerebral hemispheres had nothing to do with the organism's behavior.[11]

Flourens did believe that the cerebral hemispheres were the seat of important processes. But they were the very general psychological processes of voluntary control, or will, perception (as distinct from sensation), and intelligence. How the will acted on the lower centers and how sensations reached the organ of perception and higher functions was something of a mystery, for Flourens was not at all consistent in describing the nature of their connection. To explain psychological changes Flourens could draw only on the abstract faculties of ventricular psychology. Had he known about the changes to Gage, he would have been quite unable to account for them, especially as there were no connections between any psychological processes, including "the will," and the frontal lobes.

But of course, Flourens could not have known about the changes to Gage. From Dalton's judgment of Gage, we can infer that Flourens would have been pleased at how well Gage fitted with his experimental results. Dalton, who appears to have been the first person to mention Gage in the literature on localization, sited his discussion of the case exactly between some opening remarks on the "insensibility" of the hemispheres to direct stimulation and a lengthy and positive appreciation of the ablation experiments Flourens pioneered. He concluded his discussion with an attack on phrenology.[12]

Functions in the Roots of the Spinal Nerves

Where the nerves from the muscles and senses like touch, temperature, or pain join the spinal cord, the fibers divide into anterior and posterior parts. These divided portions are known as roots, and each root joins the cord separately and independently. This anatomical fact had been known since antiquity, and although it had also long been known that the integrity of the roots was necessary for normal sensation and movement, their precise role was not. The attempt to understand that role led to the first localization of functions in the nervous system, and eventually to a sensory-motor physiology that replaced both Gall's organology and ventricular physiology.

By the time of Dalton's appreciation of Gage, the new sensory-motor physiology was well established. Based partly on the localization of distinct sensory and motor functions in distinct structures in the spinal cord, and evolving from a philosophy that stressed experiment as much as Magendie, it had had a good deal of success in explaining the regulation of many physiological functions and symptoms stroke and spinal injury caused. The sensory-motor psychology that accompanied it was a different matter. It was still so embryonic that its explanations of behavior had to fall back on the categories of ventricular psychology.

Charles Bell began the work on the functions of the spinal roots. He had a particular end in mind, one that caused him to see only a motor function for one of the roots. Free of Bell's particular preconception, and with better and more systematic experimental methods, Magendie established that each root had a different role. His work laid the foundations of the sensory-motor physiology that eventually dominated the approach to the localization of brain function.

Bell: Function by Analogy

Shortly after Gall began promulgating his organology, Charles Bell (1774–1842), also an anatomist, was seized with the conviction that the anterior and posterior parts of the brain must have different functions. It is known that he had absorbed a structure-function principle and had accepted the advice that he ought to study the brain by studying its connections with the spinal cord. Some time in about 1807 Bell seems to have arrived at the idea that the functions of the brain's different structures could be established by establishing the functions of the different classes of nerve to which they were connected.[13]

Bell based his central thesis on an analogy between the spinal nerves and the brain. His starting point was that "a distinct class of nerves" came to the brain from the sense organs and that from the brain went "all the common nerves of motion." He explained the analogy to his brother George in 1810 as follows:

It occurred to me that, as there were four grand divisions of the Brain, so were there four divisions of the spinal marrow: first a lateral division, then a division into the back and forepart. Next it occurred to me that all the spinal nerves had within the sheath of the spinal marrow two roots, one from the back part, another from before. Whenever this occurred to me I thought I had obtained a method of inquiring into the function of the parts of the Brain.

The two lateral parts of the brain to which he referred were the two cerebral hemispheres that together constituted the cerebrum. The anterior-posterior division of the brain was that between the cerebrum and the cerebellum, and the lateral and anterior-posterior divisions of the roots matched the divisions of the brain. The anterior root led to the front of the brain, that is, to the cerebral hemispheres, where sensation and movement were localized; the posterior root led to the back of the brain, that is, to the cerebellum, where the functions necessary to life were regulated.

Bell went on to tell George how touching the anterior root caused the muscles to convulse but that stimulating the posterior had no effect. In line with his preconception, he concluded that the anterior root carried the sensations that caused movement; it came "from the cerebrum." The posterior root was insensible and belonged "to the cerebellum." The following year Bell developed the point more formally in his privately printed *Idea of a New Anatomy of the Brain*. Bell's "new idea" was actually that of three years earlier. Each bundle of nerve fibers contained two sets of nerves: the anterior that led to and from the cerebrum and carried sensations to and movements from it, and the posterior that conveyed impressions vital to regulating life to and from the cerebellum. He again described his experiments and repeated the conclusions he had already conveyed to George. He had speculated that through the posterior portion of the spinal roots he might be able to touch the cerebellum "as it were," and seemed to have done that. As well, he had touched the cerebrum through the anterior roots.[14]

Magendie: Function by Experiment

Bell had begun his work with a particular end in mind, one that caused him to see a motor function for one of the roots. Free of Bell's particular preconception, and with better and more systematic experimental methods, Françoise Magendie (1783–1855) established the true role of both roots. His overcoming the limited significance of Bell's findings helped found the sensory-motor physiology that eventually dominated the approach to the localization of brain function. Magendie also believed there was a reciprocal relation between structure and function but was not committed to anything as specific as Bell's analogy. In fact, Magendie had a positive dislike of the way speculative theoretical ideas like Bell's intruded into physiology. His thinking is well-characterized by Foster's jibe that he thrust "his knife here and there to see what would come of it," and by Claude Bernard's saying that Magendie pushed "his empiricism to excess, even to the point of giving the raw results of experiments without disentangling the contradictory phenomena to which differing experimental conditions sometimes gave rise."

Largely through Magendie, physiological work was given an experimental direction. Before him, the most widely used three-volume physiological text of the time contained no contemporary experimental material and few case illustrations. To illustrate his dictum that "facts, and facts alone, are the foundation of science," Magendie packed his *Précis Élémentaire de Physiologie* (1816–1817) with experimentally established conclusions. In the Preface to the second edition of 1825, Magendie explained that he had published the *Précis* in order to align physiology with the other sciences. Its purpose had been

to contribute towards a change in the state of physiology, to reduce it entirely to experiment: in a word, to impart to that science the happy renovation which has taken place in the natural sciences.

In that spirit Magendie investigated the functions of the roots of the spinal nerves.

Bell's collaborator and brother-in-law, John Shaw, demonstrated some of Bell's experiments on the facial nerves, but not those on the spinal roots, to Magendie, who then went on to conduct his own experiments. He soon corrected Bell's findings on the functions of the roots. Magendie's two series of experiments were carried out in Paris, in 1821, in the presence of Spurzheim and Dupuy. Unlike the stunned or recently dead animals Bell used, the dogs he used were very much alive. In the first series, Magendie first cut the posterior root and stimulated the limb to which it led. Although sensibility was "entirely extinct," the limb moved. On the other hand, when only the anterior root was cut, the limb was completely immobile, even though the stimulation caused pain. Sensation was thus retained but movement was abolished. When both roots were sectioned, sensation and motion were lost completely.

Magendie concluded that

the anterior and posterior roots of the nerves that spring from the spinal cord have different functions, that the posterior appear to be particularly destined for sensation while the anterior seem to have a special connection with movement.

A few weeks later, in a slightly different series of experiments, Magendie observed that stimulation by pressure, touch, and galvanic electricity of that part of the anterior root still attached to the cord caused slight pain as well as movement. When the posterior root was similarly stimulated, there was some movement as well as pain. These mixed responses were difficult to explain, but did not really detract from the accuracy of Magendie's overall characterization of the posterior roots as sensory and the anterior as motor.

For the very first time, different functions had been localized in different structures of the nervous system. Whereas Bell had shown only the motor function, Magendie had demonstrated both. Many hailed his discovery as the most important in physiology since that by Harvey of the circulation of the blood. The functions were not in the brain, of course. Nevertheless they became the basis of the sensory-motor physiology that eventually dominated the search for functions in the brain. Although sensation and movement at the spinal level were also very far from the complex psychological functions of interest to Gall, they actually helped put paid to Gall's vision of a behaviorally relevant differential psychology. We see this foreshadowed in the psychological functions Magendie attributed to the brain: sensibility, memory, judgment, and desire or will. How these abstract faculties were related to the brain was a mystery. Magendie said, for example, that in all cases of the loss of memory for names, of number, or of language:

after death we observe more or less extensive lesions of the brain and medulla oblongata: but morbid anatomy has not yet succeeded in establishing any relation between the part injured and the species of memory abolished.

One deficiency that would have had more application to Gage was that of judgment, but it was no more explicable than a memory defect:

It is not known what part of the brain serves for the more immediate seat of the judgement: it was long thought to be in the hemispheres, but nothing proves it distinctly.

Neither Magendie's psychology nor his physiology could encompass anything in Gage's behavior. The more developed sensory-motor physiology was not much more useful.[15]

Sensory-Motor Physiology

The new sensory-motor physiology began to take shape once Müller aligned Magendie's distinction between the functions of the sensory and motor nerves with Marshall Hall's discovery of the spinal reflex. Sensory-motor psychology developed largely from the readiness with which this new physiology could be related to associationist psychology.

The first reflex movements physiologists studied were those initiated by external stimuli, such as those that set the limbs into action. Others were involved in maintaining aspects of the body's functions, for example, those of the lips and mouth in swallowing, or those of the muscles controlling facial expression. Reflexes were considered more or less invariant patterns of behavior elicited by the same stimulus. Spinal reflexes depended on the integrity of the nervous pathways in the spinal cord, where nervous impulses from the sense organs were reflected back to the muscles. They did not depend on the brain or seem to require the participation of the will or even to be under its control. Müller's sensory-motor physiology began with the spinal reflex Marshall Hall described.

Hall: Spinal Reflex Function

When the leg of a decapitated frog is stimulated, the leg moves despite the absence of any connection with the brain. In 1832 Marshall Hall (1790–1857) showed that whether movement occurred or not depended on the state of the spinal marrow. When the marrow was intact, movement was normal; when it was destroyed, there was no movement. Hall interpreted this observation to mean there was a distinct system of "excito-motory nerves" that linked the sense organs directly with the muscles through the grey matter of the spinal cord or spinal marrow. This connection was distinct from Magendie's sensory-motor nerves that communicated with the brain *via* the columns of the spinal cord.

Hall also studied reflexes in animals rendered unconscious and tetanic by opium, a drug that he believed simultaneously abolished the "will" and enhanced sensibility. Because volition or willing was due to the mind playing upon the brain in response to the sensations transmitted to it, and because the mind's willed acts traveled down the marrow to the muscles via the motor nerves, and because movement still occurred when the will was abolished, "these experiments ... establish a property or function of the nervous system—of the sentient and motor nerves,—*distinct from sensation and voluntary or instinctive motion.*" Five years later the title of his second memoir, *On the True Spinal Marrow and the Excito-Motory System of Nerves,* utilized the name he had given the new nerves. Hall also identified a number of other reflexes as components of his supposed excito-motory system and was careful to maintain the maximum differentiation between this "True Spinal System" and what he called the "Cerebral System." Nothing about the reflex was conscious. It belonged completely to the spinal system.

Hall was especially anxious to dissociate himself from Magendie's discovery. Like many other physiologists of the time, Magendie believed that the impulses carried by the sensory nerves were conscious. "Sensation" was practically synonymous with "consciousness." For Hall the spinal reflex occurred entirely without consciousness, and he would not grant sensation a role in its production. Primarily for that reason Hall would also not grant any resemblance between his True Spinal System of reflexes and Magendie's sensory-motor nerves. He was not even prepared to consider that the two systems might have pathways in common. So anxious was he to distance himself from the Magendie distinction that he insisted on his own term, "incident," for the incoming nerves of sensation and refused to use the term "sensory."

The functions Hall did allow the cerebral system were sensation, perception, judgment, volition, and voluntary movement. He stressed that "all these functions are strictly *psychical.* They imply consciousness," and that his ideas were close to those of Flourens. Six years later Hall dedicated his *New Memoirs on the Nervous System* to Flourens. Despite his differences with Magendie, Hall was content with the same pre-Gall faculties that he as well as Flourens had retained from cell psychology.[16]

Müller: Sensation, Movement, and Associations

Hall and his work on reflexes generated enormous controversy, partly on experimental and partly on conceptual grounds. In his two-volume *Handbüch der Physiologie* [1833–1842] (1833–1840), Müller confirmed the experimental observations of both Hall and Magendie, at the same time doing away with Hall's hypothesis of a separate system of excito-motory nerves. This integration provided the main foundation of a sensory-motor physiology that eventually extended from the spinal cord to the brain and made a sensory-motor psychology possible. This end-point was unlikely to have been Müller's aim because he made sure his physiology did not conflict with the dualist philosophy that he shared with most investigators of that period. What he retained, however, was something Hall and Magendie had in common: a maximal differentiation between the nervous system's cerebral and spinal functions.

Müller did localize in the medulla oblongata a center for controlling movements more complex than those regulated by the spinal reflexes Hall described. Sensations led to this center and movements issued from it, and here rather than in the brain proper voluntary movements were generated in response to incoming sensation. Consequently the medulla was the seat of the will's action. For a complete theory of the will, Müller required a connection between the brain and the medulla. His well-known metaphor clearly sums up the problems of his conceptualization:

> The fibres of all the motor, cerebral, and spinal nerves may be imagined as spread out in the medulla oblongata and exposed to the influence of the will like the keys of a piano-forte. The will acts only on this part of the nervous system, but the influence is communicated along the fibres by their action.

Müller's stopping short of allowing sensory-motor representation in the brain itself was an integral part of the way he maintained the traditional dualism between mental and neural processes.

From our point of view, Müller's great achievement was to synthesize associationism with sensory-motor physiology, because that step marked the beginning of sensory-motor psychology. Associationism, the well-established philosophical trend that went back to antiquity, was best known in the early nineteenth century through the versions of it pro-mulgated by Hobbes, Locke, and Mills. The central notion was that repeated experience of simultaneous, successive, or contrasting ideas caused those ideas to become associated with one another. Repetition of the association could strengthen the link so that the recurrence of one of the ideas would cause the others to be revived. In sensory-motor physi-ology it was most often used to explain the connection between incoming sensation and outward movement. Müller took this doctrine further to explain willed actions.[17]

Müller and the Will

For Müller, the basis of volition was what he called the "voluntary" movements of the fetus. The fetus first moved its limbs "not for the attainment of any object, but solely *because it can move them*" (emphasis added). Müller went on:

Since, however, on this supposition, there can be no particular reason for the movement of any one part, and the foetus would have equal cause to move all its muscles at the same time, *there must be something* which determines *this or that* voluntary motion to be performed, *which incites* the retraction, first of this foot or arm, and then of the other. (emphasis added)

Once it had come into being, however, this "voluntary" excitation

gives rise to motions, changes of posture, and consequent sensations. *Thus a connexion is established in the yet void mind between sensations and certain motions.* When subsequently a sensation is excited from without, in any one part of the body, the mind will be already aware that the voluntary motion, which is in consequence executed, will manifest itself in the limb which was the seat of sensation; the foetus in utero will move the limb that is pressed upon, and not all the limbs simultaneously. (emphasis added)

What Müller called "the nervous principle" in the medulla oblongata was in such "a state of extraordinary tension, or proneness to action" that "every mental impulse to motion" caused "a discharge of nervous influence" to "a certain number of fibres in the nervous motor apparatus."

What the piano player in the brain composed and played on the keys in the medulla was the "particular reason" for a specific action. Müller's integration of sensory-motor physiology with associationist psychology thus did not conflict with his dualism. The movements the fetus produced were associated with the sensations that accompanied them and strengthened by repetition. The deliberate control of movement became possible when the will selected one rather than another of the associations on which to play.

Müller was vague about where the associations were formed. He rejected the phrenological conception of faculties: ideas, thoughts, and emotions were modes of consciousness rather than powers of the mind. The hemispheres played their part because it was in them that

the sensorial impressions are not merely perceived, but are converted into ideas ... in them resides the power of directing the mind to particular sensorial impressions—the faculty of attention.

Attention, clearly a mental power the brain possessed, was the means by which a starting point was created for associating ideas and movements. The behavioral hiatus between brain and mind was thus as wide as ever even though the physiological gap between brain and cord was slightly reduced.

Müller did recognize that lesions of the brain sometimes caused quite specific defects, especially of memory, but basically he was antilocalization. Prepared to grant that there might be "a certain part or element" of the brain that enabled ideas to acquire an affective quality, he also argued "the existence of such a part or element cannot be proved, nor its locality demonstrated." Although the cerebral hemispheres were insensible to injury and unresponsive to direct stimulation, they had to be "the seat of the mental faculties." Obvious effects such as losses of consciousness produced by mechanical pressure on the brain meant that the hemispheres had to be "the seat of the mental faculties."[18]

Nothing Müller proposed could have been applied to understanding the effects of the damage to Gage's brain. Alexander Bain soon provided a much more advanced psychology that could.

Bain's Sensory-Motor Psychology

Alexander Bain (1818–1903) is not as well known these days as he was in the last century, and some account of his background is in order. Born in Aberdeen, Scotland, he was the second child and one of the five surviving children (of eight) of a poor Scottish weaver of narrow religious views. Largely self-educated, he had mastered several of the branches of mathematics, knew a good deal of astronomy and natural philosophy (i.e., science), had begun to teach himself Latin by comparing Newton's *Principia* with an English translation, and was reading metaphysics by the time he was seventeen. He was then admitted on a small bursary to Marischal College, now one of the constituent colleges of the University of Aberdeen, from which he was graduated in 1840, at the age of twenty-two, equal top in his year in an examination covering Classics, mathematics, science, and philosophy. As a result of his upbringing and his self-education, Bain became an agnostic, and this lack of belief prevented him from obtaining a suitable university position. He therefore moved to London, where he held various government positions and wrote many papers on philosophical topics. In 1860 he was appointed to the Chair of Logic and English at the University of Aberdeen, where he founded the philosophical journal *Mind* in 1876, and from which he retired in 1880, because of ill health, at the age of 62. He died on 18 September 1903 and is buried in Aberdeen.[19]

A Sensory-Motor Will

Bain began the study of anatomy and physiology in Aberdeen, attending practical classes with medical students and later teaching those subjects to them. After arriving in London he attended the lectures and demonstrations of anatomists and physiologists like Richard Quain and William Sharpey and became friendly with William Benjamin Carpenter, the physiologist. In London, his philosophical empiricism and political liberalism led to his becoming friendly and working with John Stuart Mill. His own philosophy is usually regarded as a development of James Mill's doctrine of association.[20]

Bain's associationism and physiology are often treated as if they were separate aspects of his work, whereas they were really two sides of the one process, a unity that becomes very apparent in the first of his major psychological works, *The Senses and the Intellect*. What he wanted to do in his "full and systematic account of the Science of the Mind" was to give "a recognised place" to "many of the striking discoveries of Physiologists relative to the nervous system." In fact he began by pointing out the similarity of his analysis of mental phenomena to the physiological one made by Sharpey in Quain's *Anatomy* and set out his arguments for the brain's being the organ of the mind. He then quoted Sharpey's version of the new sensory-motor physiology: the nervous system consisted of ganglia to which afferent nerves conducted impressions and from which efferent nerves imparted stimuli to the muscles. Although Bain knew transmission was not electrical, he sometimes used words like "current" and "conduction" to refer to the process. The circle of nervous action was the reflex that completed the transmission inward that produced feeling (sensation) with the transmission outward that caused movement.

Drawing largely on accounts by Todd and Bowman and by Carpenter of experimental work on reflexes, Bain concluded it was beyond doubt that (1) the spinal cord was able to complete "a circle of nervous action" in isolation from the brain, and that (2) the medulla oblongata and the grey matter of the cord possessed "the property of sending out motor power." He therefore concluded that

the nerve centres of the spine have in them a constant charge of nervous energy, which flows out at all times, a force originating there *independently of outward impressions*, and merely yielding itself in greater abundance under such outward stimulus. (emphasis added)

The movements caused by this internally generated energy were the basis of Bain's concept of the will.[21]

Physiology and Volition
When he began to discuss "Movement, Senses, and Intellect," Bain provided more physiology, this time of the muscular system. Quoting extensively from one of the Sharpey editions of Quain's *Anatomy* on the distinction between voluntary and involuntary muscle fibers and their nervous regulation, Bain included the feelings of pleasure and pain that arose from movement and exercise as muscular sensibility, and classed emotions and willing as mental stimuli capable of causing muscle contractions. After listing eight "proofs" of spontaneous nervous system activity, he tried to explain the growth of volition by drawing extensively and explicitly on Müller. What Müller had called "voluntary" movements in the fetus, but which Bain termed "spontaneous," were the basis of the will. As Ribot later attested, this starting point was an entirely novel one. Bain first endorsed Müller's belief that the balance of tension of "the nervous principle" in the medulla oblongata was so extreme that it readily excited "fibres in the nervous motor apparatus" to action, and began looking for an incitement that provided the "particular reason" for a specific action.

Bain's proposal was that the germ or rudiment of volition lay in the way that infantile feelings, especially painful ones, impelled action. In infancy no channel existed to direct the stimulus into appropriate action. For example, an active stimulus undoubtedly impelled a child whose foot was pricked by a needle but in the absence of a link between the irritation in the foot and the movement of the hand toward the part affected, its movements were in vain. It could do nothing but drown the pain in an outburst of pure emotion. Hence:

It is the property of almost every feeling of pain to stimulate *some action* for the extinction or abatement of that pain; it is likewise the property of many emotions of pleasure to stimulate an action for the continuance and increase of the pleasure; but the primitive impulse does not in either case determine *which action*.

How was action like this acquired?[22]

Bain assumed that when the occurrence of a spontaneous movement alleviated pain, a "volitional impulse belonging to the feeling" that sustained the movement arose in the brain. Feeling itself did not initiate appropriate action but once the act of avoiding pain began, the effects of that avoidance sustained and prolonged the action. Bain illustrated his thesis with an example of an infant lying in bed experiencing the painful sensation of cold. The cold produced "the usual emotional display, namely, movements, and perhaps cries and tears." But this *"latent spur to volition"* (emphasis added) had "nothing to lay hold of." However, if the child's spontaneity was "awake," to use Bain's quaint term, "the pained condition" irritated "the spontaneous centres" and

in the course of a variety of spontaneous movements of arms, legs, and body, there occurs an action that brings the child in contact with the nurse lying beside it; instantly warmth is felt, and this alleviation of the painful feeling becomes immediately the stimulus to sustain the movement going on at that moment. That movement, when discovered, is kept up in preference to the others occurring in the course of the random spontaneity.

Associations important to willing were acquired when

the movement and the feeling become so linked together that the feeling can at times awaken the movement out of dormancy: *this is the state of matters in the maturity of volition.* The infant of twelve months, under the stimulus of cold, can hitch nearer the side of the nurse, although no spontaneous movements to that effect happen at the moment; past repetition has established a connexion ... whereby the feeling and action have become linked as cause and effect. *A full-grown volition is now manifested.* (emphasis added)

Bain had placed considerable emphasis on the physiological distinctions between sensory and motor nerves, between voluntary and involuntary muscle, on the sensibility of muscle, and on centrally arising spontaneous activity in the nervous system.

These distinctions allowed him to separate sensation from action and voluntary from involuntary movement, to have sensations produced by movements of the muscles experienced directly, and to allow for action that arose independently of external stimulation. These were the aspects of physiology useful to understanding the will. He now had only to account for the formation of associations.[23]

Forming and Reviving Associations

Bain believed that most associations formed in accord with the Law of Contiguity, that is, when mental events occurred simultaneously or successively. In his version of the Law:

Actions, Sensations, and States of Feeling, occurring together or in close succession, tend to grow together, or cohere in such a way that when any one of them is afterwards presented to the mind, the others are apt to be brought up in idea.

Repetition was the most important of the factors influencing this cohesion, coherence, or "adhesive growth."

Although Bain did not know what adhesive growth was, physiologically or mentally, it seemed clear to him that it took place in the brain:

A stream of conscious nervous energy, no matter how stimulated, causes a muscular contraction, a second stream plays on another muscle; and the fact that these currents flow together through the brain is sufficient to make a partial fusion of the two, which in time becomes a total fusion, so that one cannot be commenced without the other commencing also.

Adhesiveness linked movements together in trains, the feeling of the effect produced by one movement could become the link in a transition to the next, and complex trains could result.[24]

Thinking

Bain began his analysis of thinking by considering what happened when the sensation or feeling of a movement was continued or revived without the movement itself being made. He explicitly rejected the "cerebral closet" conceptualization of ventricular psychology by saying that the brain could not be

a sort of receptacle of the impressions of sense, where they lie stored up in a chamber quite apart from the recipient apparatus, to be manifested again to the mind when occasion calls.

The persistence of a sensation or feeling could be due only to "a continuance of the same diffusive currents" that had caused the initial sensation and nerve currents that passed through the brain and out to the muscles. Hence the renewed feeling "occupies the very same parts and in the same manner as the original." When one recalled an energetic action, it was difficult to prevent oneself from repeating the movements because the "rush of feeling has gone on to the old tracks, and seizes the same muscles, and would go the length of actually stimulating them to a repetition." Consequently:

The truth can only be that the train of feeling is re-instated on the same parts as first vibrated to the original stimulus, and that recollection is merely a repetition which does not usually go to the same length; which stops short of actual execution. No better example could be furnished than the vocal recollections. When we recal [*sic*] the impression of a word or a sentence, if we do not speak it out, we feel the twitter of the organs just about to come to that point.

Bain cited Müller's similar view of revived sensations in support of his own thesis.

During the recollection of a visual image the same thing happened. "A visible picture is in fact a train of rapid movements of the eyes, hither and thither, over luminous points, lines, and surfaces," and the "inward operations for holding a remembered ... picture in the view" were "the very same as the actual examination of the original." In the perception of the material world, the difference between what was real and the idea of it, what Bain termed the "ideal picture," could be assessed through movement:

A mere picture or *idea* remains the same whatever be our bodily position or bodily exertions; the sensation we call the *actual* is entirely at the mercy of our movements, shifting in every possible way according to the varieties of action we go through.

For Bain, therefore, one of the important criteria of the sense of reality was the effect that a movement had on a sensation or perception.

Bain outlined the role of volition in controlling which of a set of recollections or ideas would be selected or followed and which of its parts would be focused upon. Because the mental eye was "still the bodily one," the same will that ruled "the bodily eye" also ruled "the mental." The will operated "through the power of directing and fixing attention on any of the objects present to the mind at the time, to the exclusion of others."[25]

The Will and Attention in Thinking

Bain's second major psychological work, *The Emotions and the Will* (1859), explored the relation between willing and thinking in more detail. One of his main theses was that the will operated on the voluntary muscles and fixed the attention through its effects on them. The argument faced a problem, because it was not at all obvious that the voluntary muscles retained an idea in the mind. Bain therefore asked, "Which moving organ is put in force when I am cogitating a circle, or keeping my attention wedded to my recollection of St. Paul's?" He derived his reply from his earlier thesis that a remembered idea occupied "the same place in the brain and other parts of the system, as the original sensation." The idea of a circle was, therefore,

a restoration of those currents that would prompt a sweep of the eyes round a real circle; the difference lies in the last stage, or in the stopping short of the actual movement performed by the organ.

This "muscular element" of the recollected idea also differentiated it from the real:

> I know of no other distinction between the remembered and the original, except this stoppage or shortcoming of the current of nervous power.... We can direct the currents necessary for keeping an imagined circle in the view, by the same kind of impetus as is required to look at a diagram in Euclid.

Attending to the relevant element of a recollection required the inhibition of other competing but irrelevant elements. That, in turn, required the inhibition of other competing but irrelevant movements.[26]

Although Phineas Gage's lack of deference to his fellow men and his inability to plan some action and carry it through could be thought of as resulting from deficits of will and/or attention, Bain had nothing with which to link those deficits to frontal lobe damage. For Bain, willing was based on inhibiting particular actions, but he did not base the will or attention on any specific physiological mechanism. Nor did he localize the will in any specific part of the brain.

Bain's conception of nervous action was reflex in nature, but he does not seem to have adopted the view that the brain itself functioned in a reflex manner. Yet if by the mid-1850s, the notion that reflex functions could be extended to the brain was not the conventional view, it was a fairly widely accepted one. Despite Bain's wanting to give "a recognised place" in his psychology to "the striking discoveries" about the nervous system, and despite having taken sensory-motor psychology well beyond Müller, a physiology that separated the functions of the brain from the rest of the nervous system limited his explanations of willing and attention. In this Bain remained true to Carpenter and to Quain. It was his pupil, David Ferrier, who, basing his experimental work on a reflex conceptualization of the brain, localized an inhibitory mechanism in the frontal lobes that seemed to explain the changes in Gage.

Conclusion

During Gage's recovery in 1848, Harlow noted that Gage's sensorial powers were unimpaired, but in 1868 Harlow reported that a partial paralysis of the left side of the face had been evident then. Nevertheless, there was no substantial sensory or motor impairment. We also know that in 1848 Harlow alluded to some reduction in Gage's ability to judge the monetary worth of things (valuing the pebbles and not being particular about the prices he had to pay), and possibly to a difficulty in his recalling the names of those who had visited him during recovery. J. B. S. Jackson also recorded that Gage's family believed his memory had been affected. During the recovery period, Harlow did mention the problems of controlling Gage's behavior in passing and foreshadowed a future communication on the "mental manifestations." It did not appear until twenty years later.

We do not know why Harlow delayed telling anyone other than the phrenologists about the manifestations. He had Gall's faculties of the Relation of Numbers, Remembering Names, Benevolence, Veneration, and the Animal Propensities on which to base an explanation. Not that Gall's explanatory concepts were without problems. Even if the faculties were as Gall described, their independence from one another prevented the generation of adequate explanations of behavior involving (1) variations in their manifestations and (2) how they interacted in the same behavior. Gall's problem is illustrated in his own story of a thief with a large organ of Acquisitiveness who also had large but somewhat smaller organs of Murder and Compassion. After robbing a woman he later returned to untie the cord with which he had strangled her (Gall [1822–1825] 1835, vol. 6, p. 302). Harlow may have had the first of Gall's difficulties in accounting for the difference between Gage's overvaluing of the pebbles and the accuracy with which he made his purchases from the local store.

On the other hand, for Bigelow the absence of sensory or motor symptoms meant there were really no symptoms at all. Barker (1995) has also pointed out that Bigelow's virtual denial of the changes in 1850 was consistent with his antiphrenological stance.

During the first few years after Gage's injury, few outside of New England seem to have been aware of the changes to his personality. That there was no substantial sensory-motor damage was understandable—at the time those functions were localized well below the level of the hemispheres—and that there may have been, at most, some weakening of the intellectual powers further illustrated the correctness of the remnants of the cell psychology the pioneers of sensory-motor physiology left to the hemispheres.

Twenty years later, in 1868, when Harlow did report the changes in Gage, a variety of factors conspired to prevent the news from reaching either a wide medical or general public. One was the hold that sensory-motor physiology had by then achieved. For many, especially for the antilocalizationists, sensory-motor physiology excluded what they called "the higher mental functions" from consideration altogether. They therefore tended to describe an unchanged Gage. On the other hand, the defeat of phrenology was almost complete by then, and those who accepted that Gage's personality had been fundamentally altered had only the psychology spawned by sensory-motor physiology with which to explain what had happened. As we shall see in the next chapter, that psychology was just as inadequate as cell psychology.

Notes

1. Leys (1990, p. 388 and n. 127) cites Carpenter's explicit 1840s formulation of functions being inconceivable apart from structure as one of the early statements of the principle. So common are the premonitions of this view that it is difficult to know when it was first formulated. For example, Gall stated his belief in a version of it some forty years earlier than Carpenter when he led into his introductory remarks on the proofs of the plurality of the organs of the brain with the heading, "In all Organized Beings, Different Phenomena Suppose Different Apparatus; Consequently, the Various Functions of the Brain Likewise Suppose Different Organs." He also said it was unquestionable that "the functions of the brain are as diverse as the five senses, and, consequently, that they have a necessity as imperative for different organs" (Gall [1822–1825] 1835, vol. 2, pp. 254–255). Although the thought of the first French edition is similar, it is not exactly the same (Gall and Spurzheim 1810–1819, vol. 2, p. 266. cf. pp. 247–252). Bell's slightly later spatial analogy (c. 1810) was clearly based on the same principle. In one sense, though, only one side of the principle appears in Bell and Gall, rather than the reciprocal one.

2. Dissection in Gall and Spurzheim 1810–1819, vol. 1, p. 174, cited by Clarke and O'Malley 1968, p. 826. This particular paragraph is not included in Gall [1822–1825] 1835, although the other paragraphs that surround it are.

3. Flourens [1842] 1846, p. 27, for his praise of Gall. Flourens on Gall's dissection in Critchley 1979, p. 247. There are differences in the estimates of Gall's "discoveries." For an apparently authoritative list, see Critchley 1979, p. 246. Temkin [1953] 1975 shows the relation between Gall's crainoscopical presuppositions and his (and Spurzheim's) anatomical conceptualizations especially clearly.

4. The scope of Gall's mature program requires us, as Robert Young (1970) has so persuasively argued, to regard Gall as the first empirical psychologist, the first with a program that had the potential to establish the differential and comparative psychologies that were not in fact founded until almost a century later.

5. My discussion of the orientation of Gall's work is from Gall [1822–1825] 1835, vol. 3, pp. 82–85. The more diffuse version of the original is in Gall and Spurzheim 1810–1819, vol. 2, section 2.

6. Gall [1822–1825] 1835, vol. 5, pp. 7–8. cf. Gall and Spurzheim 1810–1819, vol. 4, p. 48. As Gall makes clear, he was then reasoning about a fairly primitive physical marker of a fairly primitive *psychological* faculty, and not about anything in the brain.

7. Gall [1822–1825] 1835, vol. 4, pp. 14–15 on so establishing the validity of the organs (cf. Gall and Spurzheim, 1810–1819, vol. 3, pp. 129–130). Present-day psychologists use the method and term it "criterion validity."

8. We see that Gall's position on the importance of evidence from brain damage is certainly not a simple one of dismissing it, as I once thought and is commonly believed. My examples of his more complex arguments about case material are from Gall [1822–1825] 1835, vol. 3, pp. 128–129. cf. Gall and Spurzheim 1810–1819, vol. 3, p. 55. Much case material is reported in the Scots and U.S. phrenological literature (e.g., A. Combe 1823; Fowler 1873, 1877; Boardman 1851; Capen 1881; Drayton and McNeil 1892; Hood in Whitaker 1998).

9. Hoff (1991) discusses the nonmaterial nature of Gall's faculties and clears up the confusion about what Gall meant by "function." I agree with Hoff's assessment that this conceptualization is the basis for Gall's dismissing the charge that his doctrine was a materialist one likely to lead to the spread of antireligious sentiment. Gall's own reply to the charge of materialism is in Gall [1804] 1838. Hildebrandt (1991) takes up another aspect of Gall's concept of function in critically evaluating the alleged similarity in the independence of his faculties with modern views of the modules constituting the mind. A convenient source and summary of significant parts of Gall's argument is his letter to Joseph Retzer. Here Gall describes the inner senses as "the inner organs of the actions of the soul" and then draws an analogy between the external and internal senses, for example, the eye and the parts of the brain responsible for vision. It is not, he then says, the eye or the brain that sees but the soul that sees through them (Gall [1798] 1994). For untranslated examples of the various names Gall used to describe his new doctrine, see Gall [1798] 1994 and Gall and Spurzheim 1810–1819, vol. 3, p. 57, and vol. 4, pp. 190–191, 198, 206.

10. The quotations for Benevolence, Veneration, and Conscientiousness and their relation to the "animal propensities" are in Gall [1822–1825] 1835, vol. 5, pp. 156–157, 167, 183, 216–218, 235–236. cf. Gall and Spurzheim 1810–1819, vol. 4, pp. 137–162, 172–194, 244–246, 263–264. The *American Phrenological Journal* report is "A most remarkable case" (1851).

11. The context and Flourens from Neuburger [1897] 1981, pp. 269–271, 276, 277; Krech 1963 for the deficiencies of Flourens's methods.

12. Flourens and will in Young 1970, p. 74; Leys 1990, pp. 109–111, and n. 67 on pp. 458–459, n. 68 on pp. 319–320, and n. 188 on p. 504. Dalton 1859, pp. 359–363.

13. Bell's acquisition of the structure-function principle during his training is in Keith 1911, and his brother John's advice is cited by Flourens (1858, reprinted in Cranefield 1974).

14. Charles's letters to George Joseph Bell of 5 December 1807 and 2 March 1810 in Shaw 1869, pp. 151, 152 and the experiments in Bell 1811, pp. 20–22, 26, both reprinted in Cranefield 1974.

15. Foster (1899) and Bernard (1867) are both reprinted in Cranefield 1974; the nonexperimental nature of the physiology of the era is in Olmsted 1944. Magendie 1816–1817 and [1825] 1829, pp. xv, xvii, for his *Précis*. Shaw's account of his visit to Paris contains the vague phrase that he also presented Magendie with "a short account of [Bell's] system (as it still stands)." This has led some to infer that Magendie obtained knowledge of Bell's spinal root experiments from Shaw. The complexities of this aspect of the priority dispute are discussed in Cranefield 1974, pp. 8–9. Magendie's two sets of experiments in Magendie [1822] 1974a, [1822] 1974b; their explication is in Cranefield 1974, pp. 51–53; the comparison with Harvey in Olmsted 1944 and Müller [1833–1842] 1833–1840, vol. I, pp. 192–193; Magendie 1829, pp. 113–114, for his cell psychology and views on localization.

16. Hall's first paper is Hall 1832; the various *Memoirs* are Hall [1833] 1837a, 1839, 1843. I have especially drawn on sections II, V, VI, and VII of the first paper; the excito-motory system is in Hall [1833] 1837a. For the complex story of Hall's findings, his interpretations of them, and the battles over their acceptance, see Leys 1990, especially her Introduction, chapters 4 and 5, and Conclusion.

17. Müller [1833–1840] 1833–1842, p. 836. For reconciling Müller publication date discrepancies, see Boring 1950, p. 46, and Clarke and Jacyna 1987, pp. 470–471.

18. Fetal movements: Müller [1833–1840] 1833–1842, vol. 2, pp. 935–937; will as pianist: Müller [1833–1840] 1833–1842, p. 934; will and attention: Müller [1833–1840] 1833–1842, p. 836; localization: Müller [1833–1840] 1833–1842, p. 836.

19. Bain's life is in Bain 1904; Davidson 1904; Hooper 1920; and Hearnshaw 1964.

20. Bain provided extensive annotations to the second edition of James Mill's *The Analysis of the Phenomena of the Human Mind* (1869), amplifying and correcting many of Mill's points, and also wrote biographies of both Mills (Bain 1882a, 1882b). John Stuart Mill granted the superiority of Bain's analysis of voluntary action as involving willing and association over that of his father (Mill 1869, p. 379, n. 67). Bain became so knowledgeable about associationism that John Stuart Mill deferred to him as the authority on the subject, and he mastered physiology well enough for him to be regarded as the first physiological psychologist (Boring 1950; Cardno 1955; Hearnshaw 1964; Warren 1912).

21. Bain 1855, Preface and pp. 1–13, 38, 46–47, 52–53, 58–59. Bain several times gives either the fourth or fifth editions of what seems to have been Jones Quain's *Elements of Descriptive and Practical Anatomy for the Use of Students* as sources of his anatomical knowledge, but the fourth, published in 1837, would have been out of date by 1855. He probably drew on the two-volume fifth edition edited by Richard Quain (Jones's brother) and William Sharpey (1848). Todd

and Bowman (1845) and Carpenter (probably the fourth edition of 1851); Todd and Bowman do not specifically mention Hall, probably because they did not get on well with him. I have not been able to compare Bain's quotations from these various works with the originals.

22. Bain 1855, pp. 68–80, 293–298; cf. especially pp. 289–291 and Müller [1833–1840] 1833–1842, vol. 2, pp. 935–937; Ribot 1874, p. 209. In view of Bain's explicit acknowledgment of Müller as the source of the physiological basis of his theses, it may seem odd that Boring (1950, p. 238) could write that "it was probable [Bain] did not know Müller's psychological physiology" and Hearnshaw (1964, p. 12) could claim Bain "was handicapped by his imperfect knowledge of German and of the great German physiologists of the time." Clearly, however, although he was quite knowledgable about contemporary German physiological work, Bain was not primarily interested in one of the main aspects of the physiological psychology of the day, that relating to psychophysics. He required a basis for "spontaneous" activity and an associationism in which muscular activity featured prominently. The physiology he used, especially that supplied by Müller, gave him almost everything he needed.

23. Bain 1855, pp. 295–296.

24. Bain 1855, pp. 318, 325. Successive acts were similar. Thus if the brain stimulated a movement for articulating one syllable that was followed by a second, a continuity was established "between the two, *a sort of highway made*, and a bent given to pass from the one act to the other" (Bain 1855, p. 325, emphasis added). My emphasis here is meant to point to the similarity of Bain's term to the German *bahnung*, which Exner later used to refer to the same process.

25. Bain 1855: recall of movement is pp. 332–335; visual recall is pp. 350, 357, 373; and will and attention are pp. 560–561.

26. Bain 1859, p. 410, for his "stoppage" thesis.

9

Localization in the Brain

There are but two ways at coming at the knowledge of a Machine, either to be taught the whole Contrivance by the Maker, or to take it to pieces, and to examine each Piece by itself, and as it stands in relation to the rest ... but the generality of Inquirers have thought they had better guess at it than be at pains to examine it thoroughly.

—Niels Stensen, *Discours de Monsieur Stenon sur l'anatomie du cerveau*, 1669

We have seen how functions localized by experiment and conceptualized in sensory-motor terms crept up to the level of the medulla oblongata by the 1840s. Theoretical considerations moved some of them a little higher over the next twenty years or so, but they did not invade the hemispheres proper. Suddenly two independent and parallel developments between about 1860 and 1880 accelerated the upward movement. One development came from studies of the effects of stimulating the exposed brain, the other from clinical studies of the language disorder that became known as aphasia.

Laycock's 1840s theoretical proposition that the brain was a reflex organ and the clinical work of Hughlings Jackson in the 1860s based on it pointed to experiments on the effects of stimulating the brain. The experiments themselves, begun in 1870 by Fritsch and Hitzig and taken up by Ferrier in 1873, seemed to show that sensory-motor functions were localized very precisely in the cortex. The second development began in the 1820s with the work of Bouillaud and passed through a tangle of observations made by (among others) Dax in the 1830s and Broca in the 1860s. Again by the 1870s, it seemed that quite specific language functions were also localized in the brain.

After setting out these two developments separately, I bring them together by showing how the Gage case was used in the criticisms made of

Ferrier's findings and Broca's inferences. Central to these criticisms is the assessment of the changes in Gage's behavior and the site and amount of damage to his brain. I conclude my analysis of the small but important role the Gage case played in these controversies by making the ironic point that the main limitation of Ferrier's explanation of the effects of Gage's brain damage derived from its sensory-motor nature.

Sensory-Motor Processes in the Brain

Prior to 1870 many attempts had been made to stimulate the brain directly, but all had failed to produce observable effects. In that year, Fritsch and Hitzig showed that electrical stimulation of a dog's brain caused movements of the limbs on the opposite side. Soon after, David Ferrier used a variant of their method and demonstrated how extensive and precise the localizations were. Laycock's thesis that the brain functioned like any other reflex organ provided one part of the context in which he conducted his work; another came from Hughlings Jackson's clinical inference that the nervous processes for movement were localized in the brain. Ferrier found that the frontal lobes of the monkey were unresponsive to stimulation and that ablating them produced no sensory or motor changes. Basing himself partly on Bain, Ferrier then argued they were the locale of an inhibitory-motor function. I begin this section with Laycock's arguments for extending reflex function to the brain.

Laycock's Theory of Brain Reflexes

Thomas Laycock (1812–1876), born at Wetherby, in the West Riding of Yorkshire about 20 kilometers west southwest of York, began his training in medicine at the age of fifteen by way of an apprenticeship to a local physician, expanded on it in London by passing the examinations for membership of the Royal College of Surgeons and the London Society of Apothecaries in 1835, and completed it with an M.D. from Göttingen in 1839. In 1842 Laycock became physician to the York Dispensary and, in 1846, Lecturer in Clinical Medicine at the York School of Medicine. Ten years later, in 1856, he was a controversial appointee to the Chair of the Practice of Physic at Edinburgh University.[1]

Laycock founded the doctrine that the brain itself was as much subject to the laws of reflex functioning as the lower parts of the nervous system. He first set out part of this view in various papers on hysteria that he began to publish in 1838, and consolidated it two years later in *A Trea-*

tise on the Nervous Diseases of Women. His address "On the Reflex Function of the Brain," to the British Association for the Advancement of Science meeting held in York in 1844, set out the doctrine in its final form. He began his address by stating that the brain was the organ of mind and that there were now a "multitude and variety of facts" from which its laws and mode of action could be induced. He found these facts in comparative physiology, where it had been shown that "the structure and functions of the nervous system of all animals are subject to the same laws of development and action." He then made a novel appeal to the reciprocal relation between structure and function:

The brain, although the organ of consciousness, was subject to the laws of reflex action, and that in this respect it did not differ from the other ganglia of the nervous system. I was led to this opinion by the general principle, that the ganglia within the cranium being a continuation of the spinal cord, must necessarily be regulated as to their reaction on external agencies by laws identical with those governing the functions of the spinal ganglia and their analogues in lower animals.

Laycock felt obliged to apologize to Marshall Hall for locating reflexes in the very organ of consciousness itself.

The facts Laycock drew on in his address were of two main kinds. First were those movements that seemed to be involuntary but were accompanied by sensation, like the jerking of the legs during tickling. They apparently contradicted Hall's view that reflex action had to be without conscious sensation. Second, just as causes within the spinal cord could produce reflexes, so causes within the brain could excite the central part of the connection of the cerebral nerves of sight, olfaction, and audition with the muscles. Thus the reflex convulsions in hydrophobia, ordinarily caused by peripheral stimulation of Hall's excito-motory system by splashing water on the face, could also be produced by the idea of water, which, of course, arose centrally. Consequently Laycock concluded:

The cerebral nerves being analogous to the posterior spinal nerves, and the encephalic ganglia analogous to the spinal ganglia, the spectrum of the cup of water [in the hydrophobic example] will traverse the optic nerves, and enter the analogue of the posterior gray matter in the brain causing changes, (ideagenous changes), corresponding to the idea of water; thence the series of excited changes will pass over to the analogue of the anterior gray matter exciting another series ... by which the necessary muscles are combined in action.

The correspondence of the white and gray matter of the brain with that of the cord, and the purposeful and combined action of muscles that took place without volition in the spinal cord, forced the question, "How can we deny the same qualities to the … cerebral hemispheres and their connexions?" Laycock's positive answer marked the invasion of the hemispheres proper by sensory-motor physiology.

Laycock had previously remarked that stimulation of an afferent nerve caused an instantaneous change in the gray matter of the ganglion where it terminated, a change that was then propagated to the roots of the muscular nerves. But that was not all:

A change passes also along the twigs of the sympathetic nerve connected with the ganglion, and so the secreting as well as muscular and sensory structures have an influence communicated to them. In short, a change is effected in *all* the fibrils entering into the composition of the ganglion.

And there was more:

Like the association of movements, the true explanation of the association of ideas is to be found in the doctrine of the reflex functions of the brain. The mode of action of the sensory gray matter is strictly analogous to that of the motor gray matter, both with reference to its substrata and the diffusion of afferent impulses through it.

Laycock's doctrine thus included an associationist sensory-motor psychology that could have moved into the brain at about the same time as the physiology.[2]

A sensory-motor psychology was many years away, however. Several interrelated factors seem to have impeded its development. Aspects of the complex debate over the nature of reflexes continued for some time, especially whether consciousness was necessary to them, and it was also a long time before the anatomical and physiological connections among the roots of the spinal nerves, the spinal cord, and the brain itself were established. Complex philosophical and religious factors also played a role. Laycock allowed no place in his reflex theory for a will that stood apart from the nervous system. As he said in 1871:

Under the guidance of text-books you will too often meet with useless metaphysics. You will read of "palsy of the will" … that "the mind plays" upon the nerves like a performer on the keys of a piano; and therefore you will be led into fallacies in observation and practice.

For Laycock, reflexes in the brain only *seemed* to turn humans into automata: the neatness of the way reflexes were adapted to circumstances that evoked them was what the Creator of the Design himself had intended. Old-fashioned dualists like Müller and Carpenter, on the other hand, avoided the automata criticism by having the sensory-motor processes driven by ideas that somehow existed separately from the brain. As Danziger has pointed out, many who joined the debate seem to have had difficulty in evaluating the similarities and differences between the two conceptualizations.[3]

Even allowing for such powerful factors, I suspect that a major part of the delay was due to gaps in Laycock's evidence. Ingenious as Laycock's arguments were, they were after all very general, and his evidence was sparse. Few clinical observations had been made on sensation and reflexes in those whose spinal cords had been severed, and there were almost no experimental findings. Laycock did criticize Flourens because the kinds of stimulation he had used were not appropriate to the "proper endowments" of the gray matter, but had nothing to suggest other than that skilful applications of strychnine (an excitant) and narcotics to the motor and sensory tracks in the brain (not then identifiable, of course) "might lead to important results." The push of sensory-motor physiology and psychology into the brain waited on clinical deductions and experiments like those of Hughlings Jackson and David Ferrier, respectively. Both had worked with Laycock.[4]

Hughlings Jackson's Clinical Inferences

John Hughlings Jackson (1835–1911) was, like Laycock, also born near York, but about 18 kilometers to the west northwest in Green Hammerton. He also began his medical career as an apprentice to a local physician, this time in York itself. He attended the York Medical School between 1852 and 1855 when Laycock was lecturing there, and it is likely that he became interested in the nervous system and its diseases through Laycock. In 1856 Jackson gained his memberships of the Royal College of Surgeons and the London Society of Apothecaries in London. He then took up an appointment as house surgeon at the York Dispensary, where Laycock had been physician until he had left for Edinburgh in 1855. Jackson says reasonably frequently that Laycock's reflex conceptualization of the brain's functions influenced him greatly, but there are not many specific instances of his use of it in his papers. It seems most likely that Laycock had provided him with a framework that most influenced him in his general thinking rather than in particular ways.[5]

During the three years following Jackson's completing his M.D. externally at St. Andrews in 1860, he was appointed to the London Hospital and the then new National Hospital for the Paralysed and Epileptic at

Queen Square, also in London. Within a year of being graduated Jackson initiated work on what was to become one of his main clinical interests: a particular kind of epileptic convulsion, first described by Bravais in 1824, and most often a consequence of syphilitic affections of the nervous system. The seizures were intermittent, and were sometimes accompanied with only a limited loss of consciousness, or even none at all; they involved only one side of the body, and were followed by a temporary or permanent hemiplegia. Most frequently localized tremors in the extremities (for example, a twitching in the foot and leg) preceded the seizures before gradually extending to involve the rest of the body (for example, the side of the body, the arm, and the side of the face) and developing into something less than a full-scale convulsion. Most physicians thought the seizures unimportant on the grounds that they did not result from genuine epilepsy.

Cases of unilateral epilepsy that came to autopsy usually showed clear traces of the effects of syphilis on the bones of the skull, on the dura mater, and/or on the brain itself. Structural changes like these were permanent, whereas the seizures and hemiplegias were not. In his paper of 1861 Jackson therefore aligned himself with authorities like Todd who had concluded that the seizures were probably initiated by a discharge through what Jackson came to call the "eccentric irritation" of "a persistent lesion of some part of the nervous system" on the side opposite the convulsion. In his earliest paper, Jackson also hinted that the first movement seen in the seizure gave a clue about the locale of the lesion, and the sequence in which it spread through the body gave clues about the way the discharge spread through the brain.

In 1869 Jackson said the lesion did not cause epilepsy, but that changes "in a particular region of the nervous system led to convulsions, in which the spasm began in the right hand, spread to the arm, attacked next the face, then the leg, &c." By 1873 he made explicit his conviction that

cases of paralysis and convulsion may be looked upon as the results of experiments made by disease on particular parts of the nervous system of man. The study of palsies and convulsions from this point of view is ... just what the physiologist does in experimenting on animals; to ascertain the exact distribution of a nerve, he destroys it, and also stimulates it.

Jackson also believed he could discover

the particular parts of the nervous system where particular groups of movements are most represented (anatomical localisation), but, what is of equal importance, we shall also learn the order of action (physiological localisation) in which these movements are therein represented.

As if to indicate his indebtedness to Laycock in working along these lines, Jackson introduced a 1875 reprinting of this paper with Laycock's statement from his 1845 Address that the brain necessarily functioned in a reflex way.

Hughlings Jackson's method rested on the assumption that there was a relation between the site of the lesion and the innervation of the motor nerves. If so, it followed that the order in which the different parts of the body joined in the convulsion (the "march of the fit," as Jackson called it) allowed inferences about the separate and specific parts of the brain where the movements of those body parts were localized. Where was the evidence about the location of the lesion, about its heightened tendency for discharge, and that its irritation provoked the seizure? Post mortem examination often revealed tumors or deposits in or near the corpus striatum, a structure lying in the white matter between the cortex and the ventricles. Brain hemorrhage often left clots there that that caused permanent hemiplegias, and direct stimulation of the structure in animals caused movements. Jackson felt justified in assuming that the lesion and the nervous processes representing movements were located in the corpus striatum.

But what of those cases in which there was no change anywhere in the brain? Jackson's answer revealed a decided gap: "the very fact that the convulsion has been one-sided or has begun on one side warrants the inference that there *is* in such cases a local lesion, although we are unable to detect it." Granting his freedom to infer the presence of such lesions, Jackson still had the problem of demonstrating directly that they had a heightened tendency to discharge, and that the movements seen in the seizure were the motor components of processes located near it. Before 1870 there were no such demonstrations but, in that year, Fritsch and Hitzig provided the first, and in 1873 David Ferrier many more.[6]

The Experiments of Ferrier and Fritsch and Hitzig
In the fifteen years after Laycock announced his reflex thesis, no method of stimulating the brain appropriate to what Laycock called its "proper endowments" was found. Then in 1870, Fritsch and Hitzig showed that the cortex or outer surface of the dog's brain did respond to electrical stimulation. It is often said that Fritsch and Hitzig began this animal work *after* similar experiments on soldiers with head injuries, but I have not found any published evidence that that was the case. The possibility has been canvased that their work may have originated in similar observations. Kuntz says:

According to Percival Bailey [the American neurologist], the legend goes that Fritsch discovered in dressing a wound of the brain during the Prussian-Danish war in 1864 that irritation of the brain causes twitching of the opposite side of the body.

Plausible though this more prosaic story may be, it also seems unlikely. Over the many years during which physicians and surgeons had treated the injured and exposed human brain, such movements were certainly not commonly reported. Nothing is said of this incident in Fritsch and Hitzig's first report of their work.

Hitzig does say quite explicitly that some time previously he had observed that galvanic stimulation of the posterior and temporal regions of a man's *head* reliably elicited eye movements. He seems to have been led to these experiments by using what was then a fashionable treatment for nervous disorders: applying galvanic stimulation externally to various parts of the body, including the head. In Fritsch and Hitzig's later experiment, in contrast, they stimulated the surface of the exposed brain of a dog by direct current from a galvanic pile (a type of battery) applied through blunted electrodes to various areas on the cortex. Initially they found only five points from which responses could be elicited: one for extension and another for contraction of the forelimb, and others for movements of the hindleg, the neck, and the face. Stimulation elicited movements on the side of the body opposite the side of the brain being stimulated. Increasing the intensity of the current caused convulsions that commenced in the same parts of the body as had moved at lower intensities. Limited as these findings now seem, and even though Hughlings Jackson does not seem to have become aware of them immediately, they were just what he needed. They also began a completely new approach to studying the localization of functions.[7]

Soon after Fritsch and Hitzig's results were published, David Ferrier (1843–1928) followed the path they had opened up. As a friend of Jackson, he especially wanted "to put to experimental proof the views entertained by Dr. Hughlings Jackson on the pathology of Epilepsy, Chorea, and Hemiplegia...." Ferrier was born at Woodside near Aberdeen, Scotland, and attended the University of Aberdeen, from which he was graduated in 1863 with double first-class Honours in Classics and Philosophy. Alexander Bain had so influenced him as an undergraduate that he went to Heidelberg in 1864 to study psychology. There, "more or less as an afterthought," he also began to study anatomy, physiology, and chemistry. The following year he returned to Edinburgh where, in

1868, after winning most of the university medals in the subjects he studied, he was graduated as Bachelor of Medicine with First-class Honours.

Ferrier's first appointment was as assistant to Thomas Laycock, then in Edinburgh. His duties included giving a weekly lecture summarizing Laycock's lectures for the previous week and teaching the practical classes for Laycock's students. He soon resigned the position to become an assistant to Dr. Image, a Suffolk general practitioner, who encouraged him to work on the comparative anatomy of the corpora quadrigemina. Ferrier was awarded the Gold Medal of the University when he submitted that work as his M.D. thesis in 1870. After commencing a private practice in London and holding a lectureship in physiology at Middlesex Hospital for a year, Ferrier resigned to become Demonstrator in Practical Physiology at King's College, London, in 1871. The next year, at the age of thirty, he was made Professor of Forensic Medicine at King's.[8]

Ferrier conducted his experiments at the new Pathological Laboratory at the West Riding Lunatic Asylum at Wakefield, Yorkshire, directed by his friend and fellow Edinburgh graduate, J. Crichton Browne, because facilities for experimental physiological work throughout Britain, including those at King's, were then almost nonexistent. He aimed to show that the nervous processes for movement were represented in the brain, and that their excessive discharge would produce seizures like those Jackson had described. He aimed to place Jackson's clinical conclusions on a firmer basis.[9]

At the beginning of March 1873, scarcely two months after commencing his experiments, and using faradic stimulation rather than galvanic, Ferrier had mastered the method's very considerable technical difficulties. Using more than thirty animals, he identified areas in what we now know as the motor cortex of the brain of the cat, the dog, the guinea pig, and the rabbit where stimulation caused movements on the opposite side of the body. Stimulation at higher intensities also produced facsimiles of Jackson's convulsive patterns. Within another five weeks, by mid-June, Ferrier had also mapped out these motor centers in the monkey.

Like Fritsch and Hitzig, Ferrier found that stimulation of any one center caused well-defined movements of the muscles on the side of the body opposite the stimulation. However, as can be seen from his diagrams, he located more centers than they (figure 9.1). He also elicited a greater range of movements, a large number of which were very precise.

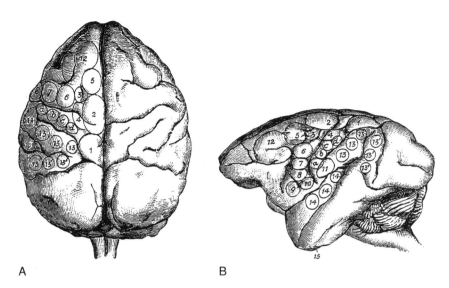

Figure 9.1
Ferrier's monkey localizations: (a) upper surface, (b) left lateral surface
From Ferrier 1876, p. 142, figs. 28 and 29.

For example, stimulation of areas *a*, *b*, *c*, and *d* in figure 9.1(b) provoked various movements of the fingers and wrist and 4 and 5 caused backward and forward movements of the arm. Excessive stimulation caused seizures that followed the sequence of movements observed by Jackson.[10]

On the basis of the homologies of structure, Ferrier was then emboldened to extrapolate his monkey localization map directly to man. What is most striking about Ferrier's monkey and hypothetical human localizations is the absence of functions in the frontal areas. Except for one monkey in whom irregular movements of the eyeballs were produced, electrical stimulation of the frontal lobes produced little response. Further, almost complete removal of these lobes in three monkeys caused, as he said when summing up the first two to three years of his work in *The Functions of the Brain* in 1876, "no symptoms indicative of affection or impairment of the sensory or motor faculties." Nevertheless, *something* had changed:

Notwithstanding this apparent absence of physiological symptoms, I could perceive a very decided alteration in the animal's character and behaviour, though it is difficult to state in precise terms the nature of the change. The animals operated on were selected on account of their intelligent character. After the operation, though they might seem to one who had not compared their present with their past, fairly up to the average of monkey intelligence, they had undergone a considerable psychological alteration. Instead of, as before, being actively interested in their surroundings, and curiously prying into all that came within the field of their observation, they remained apathetic, or dull, or dozed off to sleep, responding only to the sensations or impressions of the moment, or varying their listlessness with restless and purposeless wanderings to and fro. While not actually deprived of intelligence, they had lost, to all appearance, the faculty of attentive and intelligent observation.

Ferrier concluded:

What the psychological function of the frontal lobes may be is, therefore, not clearly indicated, either by the method of excitation or by the method of destruction. That the removal of the frontal part of the hemispheres in dogs causes no positive symptoms, in the domain of sensation or voluntary motion, is also proved by the experiments of Hitzig.

Having said this, Ferrier immediately cited Gage for a second time:

And that extensive disease may occur in the frontal lobes in man, without any manifest symptoms in life, is likewise illustrated by numerous pathological cases, among which may be reckoned the celebrated "American crow-bar case" already alluded to.

The allusion was to his earlier placement of Gage in the conventional context as an instance of those cases "in which extensive disorganization of the brain substance has co-existed with little or no apparent symptoms during life."[11]

Ferrier's Inhibitory Function

Clearly the changes in Ferrier's monkeys were profound; just as clearly they were not disturbances of sensation or movement. Ferrier saw the problem posed by what had happened and reached for a solution that stretched the sensory-motor framework more than a little. He granted that "until further light is thrown upon it experimentally," any explanation of the relation between the frontal areas and movement had to remain "more or less hypothetical." And because the phenomena following ablation had "more of a psychological than a physiological character," he postponed considering them until he took up "the subjective or psychological aspect of brain functioning" at the end of *Functions*. When he did so, Ferrier drew heavily on Bain's 1873 analyses of psychological processes. Bain had adopted the philosophical view that physiological and psychological processes formed a "double-faced unity," a view that Ferrier knew Hughlings Jackson had endorsed, and took (probably incorrectly) to be equivalent to Laycock's psychophysical parallelism. Ferrier asserted that it followed from this view "that mental operations in the last analysis must be merely the subjective side of sensory and motor substrata."

Ferrier's main argument was based on Bain's proposition that intelligent and reflective thought required the retrieval of previous ideas and selecting the most relevant from among them by fixing attention on them. That attention required the inhibition of movement:

During the time we are engaged in attentive ideation we suppress actual movements, but keep up in a state of greater or less tension the centres of the movement or movements with which the various sensory factors of ideation cohere.

Inhibiting the motor reaction directed the excitatory force inward and caused the other ideas with which the idea/motor center was currently connected to enter consciousness:

This inhibited excitation of a motor centre may be compared to a tugging at a plant with branching roots. The tension causes a vibratile thrill to the remotest radicle. So the tension of the motor centre keeps in a state of conscious thrill the ideational centres organically coherent therewith.

Inhibitory centers formed "the chief factor in the control of consciousness and the control of ideation."

Educating the centers of inhibition caused acts of will to become less impulsive and more deliberate. Current impulses or feelings no longer excited action automatically, as in the infant, but simultaneously stimulated the inhibitory centers. Action was therefore suspended until "the associations engendered by past experience between actions and their pleasurable or painful consequences, near and remote, have arisen in consciousness," and the deliberate mature act of will set in action. But what evidence was there for inhibitory centers? Here Ferrier stretched the sensory-motor framework to the breaking point:

It has already been shown that electrical irritation of the antero-frontal lobes causes *no motor* manifestations, a *fact* which, though a *negative* one, is *consistent* with the view that, though *not actually motor*, they are *inhibitory-motor*, and expend their energy in inducing internal changes in the centres of actual motor execution. (emphasis added)

In other words, the motor-inhibitory function supposedly exercised by the faculty of attention was localized in the frontal areas *precisely because no other function could be found there* (figure 9.2).

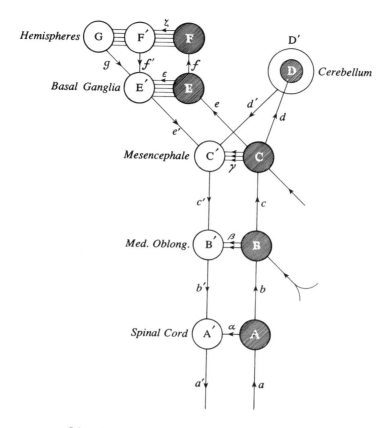

Schematic Diagram of the Cerebro-spinal Nerve-centres.
The further explanation of the diagram is given in the text.

The Cerebral Hemispheres.

§ 111. The sensory regions of the hemispheres are represented in the diagram by
(F), and the motor by (F), while ζ indicates the associating fibres between the
sensory and motor centres. By (G) are indicated the frontal regions, the centres,
as has been argued (XI., § 104), of inhibition, or inhibitory-motor centres.

The respective communications between these centres and the basal ganglia are
represented by the arrows f, f', g, the direction of the arrow indicating the centri-
petal or centrifugal direction.

Figure 9.2

Ferrier's diagram of the inhibitory centers in the frontal lobes
From Ferrier 1876, p. 290, fig. 58. Lower text added from p. 294.

Despite the logical problem, Ferrier believed he could now explain the behavioral changes following frontal lobe damage:

The removal of the frontal lobes causes no motor paralysis, or other evident physiological effects, but causes a form of mental degradation, which may be reduced in ultimate analysis to the loss of the faculty of attention.

We have seen that at the time of formulating this thesis Ferrier did not apply it to Gage or any other specific case. In fact he averred that Gage had not manifested "any special symptoms which could be attributed to such a serious injury of the brain."

Now it is dangerous to conclude, as I once did, that Ferrier simply disregarded the behavioral changes, and meant by "symptoms" only that there had been no changes in Gage's sensory or motor functions. He may have meant that, but it seems more likely that he was drawing on one of the many summaries of Harlow's 1868 address that contained nothing on the psychological changes. Ferrier clearly knew something of this report of Harlow's, because he said that Gage "lived for thirteen years afterwards," but we shall see that he did not learn of the changes until 1877. The following year, in his *Gulstonian Lectures*, he used his inhibitory thesis to explain the effects of disease and injury of the frontal lobes. Gage was then the most notable of his instances.[12]

What provoked Ferrier to so use Gage was Dupuy's citing the case as negative evidence in an attack on the whole doctrine of localization. Dupuy made two criticisms. First, there was no impairment of Gage's motor functions, and second, his language was not affected. To understand why Dupuy included language in his attack, we have to take up the second line of development, that which came from attempts to localize a language function.

Language and the Brain

Although Gall's inferences from the analysis of cranial prominences about faculties were faulty, he had actually made some quite sound inferences about the effects of brain injury on language. Indeed, no less an authority than Henry Head credits Gall with "the first complete description of aphasia due to a wound of the brain." As we have seen, Gall claimed to have localized a faculty responsible for the memory of words in the brain's anterior lobes. One line of evidence that worked against Gall and those who persevered with his doctrine or some form of it was the many cases in which frontal injury seemed unaccompanied by language impairment.[13]

Gall and Broca's Aphasia

The main clinical evidence broadly consistent with Gall's thesis was collected independently but at about the same time by Jean Baptiste Bouillaud and Marc Dax. Beginning in 1825, Bouillaud, a founding member of the *Société Phrénologique* in Paris, devoted a series of papers and lectures to the proposition that loss of speech was always associated with lesions of the frontal lobes. Bouillaud argued that loss of speech was due either to the destruction there of "the organ for the memory of words" or to the "alteration of the nervous principle which presided over the movements of speech." By 1848, coincidentally the year of Gage's accident, Bouillaud was confident enough to offer a prize of 500 francs for anyone who could produce a case of severe frontal lobe lesion without loss of speech.

Working in Montpellier, Marc Dax quite independently demonstrated a somewhat different relation between language and the brain. He began his studies with the case of a cavalry officer wounded by a saber blow on the left parietal bone. Although he suffered "a major impairment in his memory for words," his memory for things was intact. Because Gall's system differentiated between the two types of memory, Dax first sought an explanation in it, but had to reject it because the wound was not above the orbit. Gradually he accumulated other cases until he had "more than forty" of his own, together with an unspecified number others had reported in the literature. In each the loss of speech was associated with damage to the left hemisphere and was not due to paralysis of the vocal apparatus.

Marc Dax is said to have reported his conclusions in Montpellier in 1836, although the paper was not published until 1865. Speech was localized in just one hemisphere, the left, and not necessarily above the orbit. However, although some injuries he reported were obviously left-sided, others were less so, and post mortem data were few. Moreover, in cases where there was only a right hemiplegia and loss of language, Dax seems to have *assumed* the lesion was on the left. Yet as we have seen, whether brain lesions caused paralyses on the same or the opposite side of the body was then still a matter of controversy. Dax, however, regarded it as "a general law."[14]

When Bouillaud's challenge began to be met it was without anyone's knowledge of Dax's work. Localization began to be debated again in

1860, this time at the *Société d'Anthropologie de Paris,* a society founded by Paul Broca, who also served as its secretary. At the February 1861 meeting of the *Société*, Pierre Gratiolet, an outstanding brain anatomist who agreed with Flourens "in a general manner," raised the question of the relation between intelligence and brain size. Auburtin, Bouillaud's son-in-law, replied that the total volume was less important than knowledge of the functions of its different parts. Broca himself apparently said very little, and it was left to Gratiolet to allow that "certain faculties of the mind stand in special relation, although not exclusively, with certain cerebral regions."

Broca continued the brain volume discussion at the March meeting of the *Société* but also discussed whether the brain acted as a whole or as a group of coordinated organs. After paying tribute to Gall's anatomical work and praising his principle of localization, he announced his own belief in localization, although not in Gall's particular doctrine. At the 4 April meeting Auburtin argued for the precedence of clinical over experimental evidence in determining the relation between speech and the frontal lobes. He cited much case material in support and virtually repeated Bouillaud's challenge in nonmonetary terms: he would abandon his belief in cerebral localization if there were cases of speech loss without lesion of the anterior lobes. Gratiolet countered, of course, but the issue was left unresolved.

A few days later, Broca asked Auburtin to judge whether a hemiplegic patient who had recently been admitted to his surgical wards had a language defect of the kind that would persuade Auburtin to accept him as a test case. The patient, a M. Leborgne ("Tan"), could answer simple questions with signs and communicate with gestures but could utter only the sounds "Tan, tan" when he tried to speak. If he became angry he would sometimes utter "Sacré nom de Dieu," a phrase he could not produce voluntarily and that functioned as a swear word. After examining the patient, Auburtin agreed that a frontal lesion ought to be present. M. Leborgne had a serious leg infection and was in such a weak condition that he died on 17 April, six days later. Broca's post mortem demonstrated a complex of changes in the brain, including "the most extensive lesions, the most advanced, and the oldest" in the middle part of Tan's left frontal lobe.

The following day, at a meeting of the *Société d'Anthropologie*, Broca presented his results. Although it was patently obvious that the lesion was on the left, he made no mention of that fact, concluding only that "the lesion of the frontal lobe was the cause of the loss of speech." According to Head and Critchley, Broca's audience displayed little interest. Later that year, in August, Broca gave a much more complete account of Leborgne's case to the *Société Anatomique de Paris*. He set out his arguments in much more detail, but he again failed to give the left hemisphere a specific role.

Then, in November of the same year, Broca found a similar change in the brain of another patient whose language was impaired. M. Lelong, an eighty-four-year-old laborer, died after suffering a stroke some eighteen months earlier. He had seemed to be able to understand "all that was said to him" but had been left with only an abbreviation of his name, "Lelo," that he used correctly, and four words: "Yes" and "No," also used correctly, "three," which he used for all numerical concepts, and "always," an utterance having no fixed meaning. The lesion was very obvious, "incomparably more circumscribed" than Tan's, and occupied "the left frontal lobe immediately below the anterior end of the fissure of Sylvius." Even though the center of the area of M. Lelong's lesion was "identically the same" as M. Leborgne's, Broca again emphasized only its frontal locale. M. Lelong's aphasia was the result of a lesion "of the second and third frontal convolutions."

Broca's analysis differentiated between a "general faculty of language" responsible for establishing the relation between an idea and a sign and "a special faculty of articulate language" that could be abolished without having effects on the muscles responsible for speech. Destruction of the general faculty made language impossible, whether by sign, sound, or gesture. The loss of the special faculty had afflicted MM. Lelong and Leborgne. Broca termed the condition "aphemia," but it later became known as "aphasia." As to where the faculty was localized, Broca wanted "more confirmation" of what the brains of Leborgne and Lelong seemed to tell him. Until he obtained it, he was prepared to say only that "the integrity of the third frontal convolution (and perhaps of the second) appears indispensable for articulated speech." Broca's emphasis was still on the frontal lobes rather than on the left hemisphere.

Of course, the evidence from Leborgne's case was not as compelling as some writers seem to believe, even now. Of the two, Lelong's profound aphasia with the obvious, accurately circumscribed lesion of the posterior third of the second and third frontal convolutions, was really the more important. But as Broca pointed out, two cases were not enough from which to generalize. And he placed no special importance on the left-sidedness of the lesions. Nonetheless, according to Head, by the end of 1861 Broca's communications were producing "the greatest excitement in the medical world of Paris," an excitement indexed, for example, by being specially commented on by the secretary of the *Société Anatomique* in his annual report for that year.[15]

In April 1863 Broca announced he had found left frontal damage in each of eight cases of aphasia. By 1864 he said he knew of more than twenty-five cases with the same left frontal involvement and only one in which there was not a left-sided lesion. It was then that he came to place as much significance on the left hemisphere as on the frontal lobes. The evidence previously collected by Dax was consistent with this new emphasis. By March 1863, Gustav Dax, Marc Dax's son, had presented his father's paper to the *Académie Impériale de Médicine* (with additional data of his own) for assessment of his father's priority in demonstrating the role of left hemisphere lesions. Even though it was supposedly being examined there in confidence, Broca could easily have known what their data showed. Dax had stated his conclusion in the title of his paper, and that title was published when the *Académie* reported on 24 March that it had been deposited for assessment. The conclusion had also been made public in the same way on the paper's simultaneous submission to the *Académie des Sciences* the day before.

Despite the possibility of Dax's conclusions so influencing Broca, he actually seems to have started leaning to the left some time before Dax's paper was deposited for assessment. Broca had made the left-right distinction in an annotated bibliography clearly prepared before the end of March 1863 that appeared, coincidentally, in the same number of the journal as the announcement of the deposition of Dax's paper with the *Académie de Médicine*. Certainly Broca knew before December 1864 about Dax's conclusion. By then it had been commented on in public (the previous August) and Lélut had reported his unfavorable opinion to the *Académie de Médicine*.[16]

In April 1865 Bouillaud attacked Lélut's report on the two Dax papers. Although a member of the examining committee, he had evidently not helped to prepare the report. He praised Gall and Broca in extravagant terms and accepted Broca as one of his own, even though he believed Broca's doctrine was not sufficiently proven. He also seemed to dissociate himself from the Drs. Dax. The protracted debate spread over the next three months of the regular weekly *Académie de Médicine* discussions. On 23 May, as the debate was drawing to a close, Velpeau claimed the 500 franc prize. After what Schiller calls a long and heated discussion, it was concluded that the evidence was against Bouillaud, and he had to pay. However, a few weeks later, at a meeting of the *Société d'Anthropologie*, some of the apparently exceptional cases began to be understood. Broca publicly announced his view that in most people the left hemisphere was specialized for language, a dominance that explained the common association of aphasia with right hemiplegia. The exceptional cases were left-handed people whose right hemispheres carried the language function. Bouillaud's loss was more a symbol of the complexity of what aphasia was beginning to reveal about localization than a real defeat.

Support for Broca's thesis grew very gradually. Many years elapsed before it was accepted even in the modified form in which it is held today. First, there was the admixed opposition to localization on political, religious, and philosophical grounds, partly characterized by Head and strikingly illustrated by Dupuy's virtual denial as late as 1877 of the proposition that the brain was the organ of mind. Second was the argument discussed in the 1860s, for example, by Bateman, Flint, and Maudsley that the two hemispheres were so much alike in structure that the one could not have a function not possessed by the other. So central was this view of brain symmetry that it caused even Broca to hesitate to move left. As another example, Brown-Sequard tried to show in the late 1870s that physicians since the time of Aretaeus had been wrong in attributing hemiplegias to contralateral lesions. Third, and with this, it was some time before a role was given to hemispheric dominance, and a number of the exceptions in those cases of aphasia with frontal lesions in the right hemisphere aligned with the left-handedness that could be taken to indicate that the right hemisphere was dominant. Fourth, much confusion surrounded clinical matters in the early literature. According to Hughlings Jackson, Bateman, and Flint, for example, there were simple-minded confusions about whether "aphasia" covered speech losses due to the very muscle paralysis that Bouillaud and Broca had ruled out! There was also uncertainty about what language was (cf. Seguin, Maudsley, and Broadbent), what was to count as its loss (cf. Hammond and Head), what constituted a lesion of a convolution (Foulis), and how the sites of lesions were to be determined (Maudsley).

Over and above these arguments were the negative instances: the cases of anterior damage without language being affected. In this context Gage appears, for the second time, in the localization literature.[17]

Gage and the Localization of Language

In 1868, the very year of Harlow's final report on Gage, Eduardo Seguin considered the bearing of all the cases reported until that time on the various propositions of Gall, Dax, Bouillaud, and Broca of language localization. He counted 514 cases in favor of and only thirteen against the Gall-Bouillaud view that the localization was somewhere in the anterior lobes. But the contra total, he went on,

includes four (such remarkable) instances of injury to the brain without loss of language, as to require quotation at length. Professor Bigelow of Boston has reported a case which occurred in the practice of Dr. Harlow of Cavendish.

Seguin also counted Gage against Dax's view that language was localized in only the left anterior lobe, and also against Broca's more specific nomination of the third left frontal convolution. In fact Seguin cited five cases and in his summary devoted slightly more space to Gage than to the other four combined. The difference seems to evidence the importance he placed on it among the cases that "at once settle the question in the negative."

Hammond, the American neurologist and author of the first English-language text on nervous and mental diseases, echoed Seguin, but with some ambivalence. In his chapter on aphasia, Hammond lamented the lack of experimental literature bearing on the localization of language, before saying:

But unintentional experiments have been performed upon the human subject, which tend to show that, though the faculty of language may be located on one or both anterior lobes, either may be seriously injured without the faculty of language suffering to any appreciable extent. Two of them have happened in this country, and, although referred to in connection with aphasia by Seguin and Harris, I take satisfaction in bringing them forward on account of their great importance to the question under consideration.
The first is related by Dr. Harlow of Vermont.

Hammond based his description of the accident and the damage to Gage's brain and skull on Harlow's 1848 paper (wrongly dated as 1849) and J. B. S. Jackson's description in the *Catalogue* of the Warren Anatomical Museum:

From this account it will be seen that the left anterior lobe of the brain suffered severely by this injury, and yet it is not stated that the subject had ever shown any difficulties in speech. If the faculty resides in the whole of the lobe, such an immunity should scarcely have existed.

Broca's thesis was by then, of course, precisely that the faculty did not reside in the whole of the lobe. Then, as if ambiguously acknowledging that fact, Hammond went on to remark that "the photograph of the cranium establishes the fact that the third frontal convolution and the island of Reil escaped all injury." His ambiguity then got worse:

Another interesting circumstance is the addiction to profanity after the accident. A like phenomenon has been noticed in cases of aphasia.

Hammond was therefore citing Gage against the Gall-Bouillaud view while simultaneously using him in favor of and against Broca!

The French neurologist Dupuy was much more definite than Hammond in his use of Gage. Also basing himself on the description in J. B. S. Jackson's *Catalogue*, Dupuy concluded that there was no aphasia despite the complete destruction of the left frontal lobe. Four years later, by then resident in New York and having examined Gage's skull at the Museum, Dupuy again called on Gage. In a long article critically reviewing the localization data, he subjected Ferrier's work to special scrutiny. As soon as he came to consider Ferrier's remarks about aphasia, Dupuy introduced Gage as a negative instance:

The first and most striking case of destruction of the so-called speech-centre without consequent aphasia is the celebrated American crowbar case. I believe I was the first to report that extraordinary case in France [presumably in Dupuy 1873]. Dr. Ferrier, in commenting on it, lays it down that only the anterior portion of the frontal lobe was destroyed by the accident.... The tamping iron ... passed, according to measurement which I have made, through the brain on the left side, in such a manner as not only to destroy the left Sylvian artery, which sends a special branch to Broca's convolution, but it actually destroyed the greater part of the island of Reil. A great quantity of brain-matter was discharged for several days after the accident, in consequence of sloughing. I had an opportunity of seeing that cranium in Boston last winter, and also the iron bar. That man (Gage) was never aphasic, nor paralysed.

Why did Dupuy link Gage's lack of aphasia with the absence of paralysis? The answer comes from some of the details and implications of Ferrier's localization of motor processes in the monkey.[18]

Sensory-Motor Processes and the Localization of Language

Figure 9.3 shows Ferrier's extrapolation of his findings from monkeys to humans. If the extensions were accurate, stimulating the areas indicated by the same numbers and letters in the two species should produce the

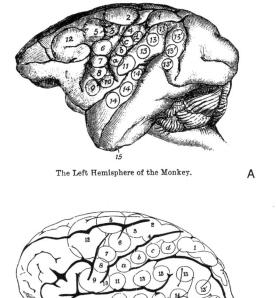

The Left Hemisphere of the Monkey.   A

B

Figure 9.3
Ferrier's left localizations in (a) the real monkey and (b) the hypothetical human
From Ferrier 1876, p. 142, fig. 29 and p. 304, fig. 63.

same responses. Thus if stimulating areas 9 and 10 in the monkey caused its mouth to open and the tongue to be protruded and retracted respectively, stimulating those areas in humans should do the same. Similarly, leg movements in the human should result from stimulating area 1, arm, finger, and wrist movements from 3, 4, and 6 together with the set of *a*, *b*, *c*, and *d* respectively. Now, areas 9 and 10 are within or close to where Broca found the lesions that caused aphasia. Areas 1, 3, 4, and so on correspond to the areas Hughlings Jackson considered to be the site of those discharging lesions in unilateral epilepsies in which the fingers, arm, and leg joined in the seizure. Dupuy believed that Gage's tamping iron had damaged both sets of areas. Consequently, Gage should have been aphasic and paralyzed.[19]

Dupuy's critical review appeared on 7 July 1877 and Ferrier's reply on 15 March 1878. Given the times, it was quite a quick reponse. It was also important, and in a curious way, decisive.

Ferrier and Gage

On 12 October 1877 Ferrier wrote from London to Henry Pickering Bowditch, Professor of Physiology at Harvard, asking "a little favour" over Gage. His choice of correspondent was ironic. Only three years before, Bowditch himself had opened a review article largely devoted to a critical examination of the localization literature, including the work of Ferrier and Hughlings Jackson, by citing Gage as a negative case:

> The phenomena of aphasia were at one time regarded by most physiologists as affording satisfactory evidence that at least *one* mental faculty has its seat in a definite, circumscribed portion of the brain. The accumulation, however, of recorded cases in which the disease has been observed without the lesion, and of those in which the lesion has been found without the disease (among which may be mentioned the celebrated "crow-bar case"), has gradually led to the abandonment of this view, as being, at best, only a partial expression of the truth.

The favor Ferrier asked was for Bowditch to examine Gage's skull and help him determine the exact site of the lesion.

Ferrier's letter pointed to what seemed to be a contradiction between Dupuy and Bigelow:

> From the account given by Dr. Bigelow in the American Journal of the Medical Sciences, July 1850 and the drawing which he there gives of his experiments on a skull with the object of determining the exact seat of the lesion I came to the conclusion that the injury was confined to the region in advance of the coronal suture. Dr. Dupuy has lately been writing in the Medical Times & Gazette that he can prove conclusively that it destroyed the Island of Reil and what not.
>
> Now I should be very much obliged to you if you would examine the skull carefully & tell me exactly the line of entrance and exit of the iron bar & the appearance presented. Better still if you could furnish me with a sketch of the preparation.

Bowditch evidently agreed to the request because, on 27 December, Ferrier received what he described as "magnificent photographs" from Bowditch.[20]

Ferrier's examination of the photographs raised questions about the accuracy of Bigelow's reconstruction. He asked Bowditch

if you agree with me in thinking that Bigelow has represented the track of the bar
a little too much towards the middle line & beyond it & also somewhat nearer
the coronal suture than was actually the case. It seems to me from the opening at
the left-side of the middle line that the bar did not cross the middle line at all, &
that it emerged more in front raising the flap of bone hanging on the line of
fracture on the right side of the frontal. In which case the left anterior lobe alone
was injured.
Bigelow also represents the hole in the base of the skull a little further outwards
from the middle than the photograph warrants.

Ferrier's reasons for believing that the flap of frontal bone was raised
from the left and that the flap was hinged on the right line of fracture
perhaps drew on his knowledge and experience as Professor of Forensic
Medicine at King's (see figure 6.5).

Ferrier's asking if there was "any further account of the case with post-
mortem etc. beyond that given by Bigelow," tells us that until then he
had relied mainly or solely on Bigelow. That he "had an idea" there was
a later account, but could not find the reference, together with his saying
in *Functions of the Brain* that Gage had survived unchanged for thirteen
years, also tells us that Ferrier very probably knew of Harlow's 1868
address only through one of the secondary reports that had failed to
summarize the changes. On 10 February 1878 Ferrier acknowledged
receipt of what must have been the booklet form of Harlow's address, and
immediately sent a telegram asking if Bowditch could obtain the woodcuts
from Harlow. We know he did, because Ferrier specifically acknowledges
Harlow's lending them in the *Gulstonian Lectures*. In the actual lectures
he used slides made from Bowditch's photographs, but the illustrations in
the printed lectures were made from cliches of Harlow's woodcuts.

As the illustrations themselves indicate, Ferrier made the case an
absolutely dominating feature of the first of his *Gulstonian Lectures* on
15 March 1878. From his figures, he told his audience, they would
clearly see that

the whole lesion is situated anterior to the coronal suture. If you will now compare the track of the bar through the skull and brain with [Turner's diagram of
the brain in situ] showing the relations between the skull and the brain you will,
I think, have no doubt in convincing yourselves that the whole track is included
within that region of the brain which I have described as the prefrontal region,
and that, therefore, the absence of paralysis in this case is quite in harmony with
the results of experimental physiology.

Ferrier did not give an account of his own of Gage's subsequent history
but presented Harlow's account of the changes in its entirety.[21]

When the lectures were over, Ferrier thanked Bowditch for his help, and added:

The case has excited very considerable interest here, & your photographs created quite a sensation at the College of Physicians—as they brought the facts home in such a telling manner.

Those abstracts or reviews of the *Lectures* that mentioned Gage substantiate Ferrier's description of the effect of his presentation. Relatively lengthy summaries of Gage or mentions of the impact of the illustrations were frequent.[22]

Dupuy's point had been decisively rebutted. Curiously, Ferrier represented Dupuy as appealing to the Gage case only as "showing that lesions of the so-called motor region may occur without paralysis," and said nothing about Dupuy's claim that Gage was "never aphasic." For Dupuy, the damage was posterior enough to produce both symptoms. Whether Ferrier was responsible for the shift in opinion or not, after his arguments for a more frontal site, no one seems to have referred to Gage in the aphasia literature as a negative instance again. Indeed, in a comprehensive review paper appearing soon after Ferrier's reply to Dupuy, Dodds cited the Gage case in relation to the role of the third frontal convolution and the island of Reil only to practically dismiss it. First, he accepted Hammond's view over Dupuy's that both structures had escaped injury. As a case it was therefore "of very inferior significance to many of those previously given." It was important only because "it showed a coincidence between escape of certain convolutions and the survival of speech."[23]

In the face of the publicity Ferrier gave Gage's case, it is surprising that some writers continued to maintain that Gage had not changed in any way. For example, in reporting Ferrier's *Lectures*, the *London Medical Record* and the *Dublin Journal of Medical Science* left Gage out of their comparison of the monkeys and the human cases. Then, when the *Medical Record* (New York) reviewed the American edition of the *Lectures*, it failed to mention Gage, and *Lancet* managed to say almost nothing about the *Lectures* at all. For all these, Gage was therefore unchanged. One can only speculate about the reasons for this contemporaneous silence, but for omissions that were made much later the situation is a little clearer. As their references showed, these later denials were generally based on ignorance of what Harlow reported in 1868, or they were made by unrepentant protagonists of the antilocalization position Flourens advocated.

Conclusion

Under Ferrier the sensory-motor physiology that Magendie had unknowingly founded, that Hall had unwittingly extended, that Laycock had encouraged, and that Hughlings Jackson had used to such remarkable effect spread from where Müller had left it at the medulla oblongata to the posterior border of the frontal lobes. There it stopped. Extensions of the localization doctrine had followed what may be termed a cordocephalic progression. Beginning with the sensory-motor distinction in the spinal roots, progressively higher levels of the nervous system were made the locale of more and more complex sensory-motor functions. But for Ferrier, the sensory-motor systems ceased at the rear of the frontal lobes. This had two consequences. First, despite its success, the sensory-motor approach had not routed Descartes's dualism in a decisive way. "Ideas" localized above the sensory-motor processes could still initiate their activity in much the same way as did Müller's piano player suspended above the medulla. Second, rather like the pre-1850 inability to demonstrate what functions the whole brain might have, the apparent absence of functions in the frontal lobes left the door open for Ferrier to attribute inhibitory functions to them. Others assigned almost anything to them, a consequence that was to have considerable impact on how the functions of the frontal lobes were conceptualized, especially in the consideration given to the Gage case in the development of brain surgery and psychosurgery.

Notes

1. Details about Laycock from Seccombe 1921–1922, pp. 744–745; Barfoot 1995; and a personal letter of 18 July 1998 from Dr. Frederick James, whose Ph. D. dissertation at the University of London was on Laycock.

2. Laycock's British Association address is Laycock 1845, and the *Treatise* is Laycock 1841. For the psychology, see Laycock 1854, 1855, 1860.

3. Laycock 1871; Danziger 1982.

4. Laycock 1845 on Flourens. The issue of Hall's priority in the discovery of the reflex may also have played a role. It was not really resolved until well after Laycock's translations of the works of Unzer ([1771] 1851) and Prochaska ([1784] 1851).

5. Details about Hughlings Jackson from Taylor 1920; Greenblatt 1965, 1977; Harris 1993; Critchley and Critchley 1998. I have to thank Dr. Greenblatt for a copy of Jackson's (1863) speculative attempt to relate specific vertebra to specific

kinds of disease, and I agree with him that it draws on Laycock's reflex thesis, even though his name is not mentioned.

6. My setting out of Hughlings Jackson's theses is based on Jackson 1861, 1869, 1873, 1874a, 1874b. The problem over the three components of what he needed to demonstrate (lesion, discharge tendency, movement representation) remained when he shifted the locus of the nervous processes representing movements, first from the corpus striatum to the convolutions near it, and finally to the cortex itself. Young (1970) and Greenblatt (1977) discuss the shift.

7. Bailey's story is in Kuntz 1970; Thomas and Young 1993 discuss some aspects of the early work of Fritsch and Hitzig but it is Finger (1994, p. 38) who identifies the role of Hitzig's (1870) therapeutic use of electricity; Bowditch (1874) includes a description of the effects of the stimulation, mainly the subjective ones; Arndt (1892a, 1892b) and Stainbrook (1948) give details about how it was used in treating various "insanities." Translations of Fritsch and Hitzig's papers appear in Fritsch and Hitzig [1870] 1960, [1870] 1963. For various methodological issues in the study of localization, including stimulation and ablation, see Walker 1957a, 1957b.

8. Details about Ferrier from Sherrington 1937 and Woolsey 1951. Dr. Frederick James drew my attention to the mentions of Laycock, Jackson, and Ferrier in Ashworth 1986.

9. Ferrier described his aim slightly differently in different places. I have followed his 1876 formulation (Ferrier 1876; cf. 1873, 1880). For the extraordinarily backward state of experimental physiology and the other sciences in Britain at the time, see Geison 1972. This backwardness was the main factor that took Ferrier to the West Riding Lunatic Asylum.

10. Ferrier's lack of success in eliciting responses from the brains of birds throws additional doubt on some of the conclusions Flourens drew.

11. Ferrier 1876, pp. 231–232, for the frontal changes and pp. 125–126, 232, for Gage.

12. Ferrier quotes Bain from *Mind and Body* (1873, p. 131). My quotations from Ferrier come from *The Functions of the Brain* (1876, pp. 125–126, 231–233, 255–257, 286–289) and are here in the order in which they occur in Ferrier.

13. Gall's cases are discussed in Brown 1991 and Head 1926, pp. 9–11; the latter also sets out Bouillaud's 1825 theses on pp. 15–16. Broca's papers are translated in Broca (1861a 1861b, 1861c, [1865] 1986). See note 16 for Dax's paper.

14. My version of the 1861 discussions comes from various sources, principally Head 1926, pp. 13–29, Stookey 1954, and Schiller 1979. It has also been influenced by the sociology of science analysis made by Woodill and LeNormand 1991. I recognize that these authors and the authorities they quote do not always tell the same story, and my reconciliation is based on what I have found in such original documents as exist. I have not set out my reasons for preferring the fragments cited by any one author. One fact that seems to me to be most harshly

treated is the failure of many authors, for example, Head 1926, Stookey 1954, and Krech 1963, to make Bouillaud's phrenological leanings explicit or even to hide them. A contemporary description of him is "a zealous phrenologist" (Browne 1833) and there are several quotations from him in Schiller 1979. Later descriptions include an "enthusiastic phrenologist" (Castiglioni 1958, p. 700), his "fervent championship ... of Gall" (Critchley 1979), and a "follower of Gall" (Ackerknecht 1982, p. 187).

The failure of Gall's followers to point out the very common connection between right hemiplegia and aphasia is worth noting. Dax took it that a language function localized only on the left contradicted Gall's thesis, but the more orthodox of Gall's followers do not seem to have done so. Dunn (1845, 1850), for example, explained those language functions that survived, like an otherwise speechless patient's being able to read, by the right hemisphere's "centre of intellectual action" not being affected but the corpora striata, where the will connected thought with action, being damaged.

15. Leborgne's brain showed changes in other than the frontal convolutions that, at the time and subsequently, were held by many to vitiate or at least to qualify Broca's conclusion (Broca 1861a, 1861b, 1861c; Maudsley 1868; Dodds 1877–1878; Marie 1906a). Broca did consider the nature and likely history of these other changes very carefully before ruling them out as causes of Leborgne's aphasia, and although a modern CT scan of his brain shows some damage to other areas, the main damage was where Broca's analysis placed it: in the third left frontal convolution. Hence, "Broca was right" (Signoret et al. 1984; cf. Castaigne et al. 1980). One notes also that the critics seem to have overlooked the evidence from Lelong's case, which even Marie accepted.

16. Broca [1865] 1986 for his extended findings. The relation between them and those of Marc and Gustav Dax is too complex to go into here. Joynt and Benton (1964) have translated what was presented by Gustav as his father's original report (M. Dax 1865). Finger and Roe (1996) have translated the paper by Gustav himself, reporting evidence from 146 cases and including his "claim" to Marc Dax's priority (G. Dax 1865), together with Lélut's (1864) report to the *Académie de Médicine*. Gustav Dax adduced 87 cases in which loss of language followed left hemisphere lesion, 53 of right hemisphere lesion without loss, and 6 that seemed to contradict his thesis. A further 225 were put aside because there was not precise enough information on them. Each group of the translators of these papers comments to varying degrees on (1) the chronology and significance of the three publications, especially in relation to Broca's; (2) the quality of Marc Dax's data; (3) the reaction to Lélut's report, especially Bouillaud's; and (4) the search for Dax's 1836 paper and/or a record of its presentation. Stookey (1954, p. 576) provides an informative footnote on the two Drs. Dax but Schiller (1979) and Critchley (1979) provide most of the detail. The two most useful discussions I have found on Broca's alleged use of the data in the papers by Marc and Gustav Dax before their findings were made public are by Schiller (1979, pp. 192–197) and Finger and Roe (1996). The *Académie des Sciences* does not seem to have evaluated the claim.

17. Head's oft-cited characterization, which I am not sure can be documented, is in Head 1926, p. 25, and Dupuy's virtual denial of the role of the brain is in Dupuy 1877a. Samples of the argument from anatomical similarity are in Bateman 1865, Flint 1866, and Maudsley 1868. Brown-Sequard is cited by Ferrier (1878a, 1878b; cf. Dupuy 1873, 1877b, and Ballance 1922, pp. 57–58). Samples of clinical confusions are discussed by Hughlings Jackson (1864), Bateman (1865), and Flint (1866); those of language and loss are in Seguin 1868, Maudsley 1868, Broadbent 1878–1879, Hammond 1871, and Head 1926; and those about lesions and loss are in Foulis 1879 and Maudsley 1868.

18. Seguin 1868; Hammond 1871, pp. 174, 179–180; J. B. S. Jackson 1870; and Dupuy 1873, pp. 31–33, and 1877. Maudsley's (1868) negative-instance argument may be based implicitly on Gage. Hammond is very difficult to follow in two respects. Harlow frequently quoted verbatim from Gage's conversation what seem to be whole phrases and sentences having completely normal communicative significance. Nothing he or Bigelow recorded even hinted that Gage's language consisted of the remnants of speech usually in the form of the obscene words or phrases sometimes left to the aphasic. Nor is it clear what the case is to which Hammond says Harris refers. Under the various *aphasia* headings for the period, the *Index Catalogue of the Surgeon-General's Library* lists no one of that name, and no publications are listed on aphasia under any of the *Harris* names. Although it is possible that someone called Harris discussed the issue of aphasia without publishing his remarks, that thesis suffers from the fact that it would then have to have been a Harris whose reputation was high enough for Hammond to take him seriously but who seems not to have published anything on aphasia. Finally, the next of Hammond's negative instances is Jewett's (1868) case of Joel Lenn, who actually did have some aphasic symptoms!

19. Critchley (1979, p. 247) gives an amusing table correlating some of Ferrier's areas with the locale of Gall's faculties. Thus Gustativeness was located at areas 9 and 10 and Hope was in the area from which tailwagging in the dog could be elicited.

20. Bowditch 1874 is the review. Ferrier's letters to Bowditch are reproduced in Appendix D by the kind permission of Richard Wolfe of the Countway Library. The transcriptions, in which I have not altered any of the spelling or punctuation, are mine. However, in this opening quotation I have made one alteration and used "line" where Ferrier wrote "lines" when he asked for Bowditch's opinion. A "line" was once a commonly used anatomical measure that varied with place and time and equaled either one-tenth or one-twelfth of an inch. Ferrier could have been asking for the distances that the entry and exit points were from known skull landmarks, expressed in this unit. That does not seem to me to make as much sense as his question's being about the general direction of the iron.

Unfortunately I have been unable to locate Bowditch's actual replies or any correspondence between Harlow and Ferrier. What I say about them is largely construction (not, of course, in the modern ahistorical sense of that term) from the sequence of ideas in the letters themselves and from Ferrier's references to Bowditch and Harlow in the two different printings of his *Gulstonian Lectures.*

My construction of the sources of the illustrations Ferrier used in the *Lectures* draws additionally on the two printings: Ferrier 1878a, p. 445, in the main text under his fig. 2, and the footnotes marked * and † in the right-hand column; and 1878b, p. 26, and footnote 2, and the Prefatory Note. My guess is that Bowditch sent him copies of photographs of the skull held by the Warren.

21. Ferrier's *Gulstonian Lectures* first appeared in successive numbers of the *British Medical Journal* almost as soon as they were delivered. Later that year they appeared in book form. Gage is discussed in Lecture I (Ferrier 1878a, 1878b, pp. 29–30, 37). The illustrations are most striking in the journal version. Spillane (1981) rather oddly cites Ferrier's *Gulstonian Lectures* as showing that "Ferrier did not apparently know that the patient … did suffer from epilepsy and altered personality."

22. *The Practitioner* (London), 1879, vol. 23, pp. 120–122; the *Medical Times* (London), 1878, no. i, pp. 299, 327, 355, 385, 455, 472, 499; the *Edinburgh Medical Journal*, 1878–1879, vol. 24, pp. 1116–1119; *Brain* 1878, 1, 132–133, and Ferrier to Bowditch, 10 February 1878 and 15 January 1879; *Lancet*, 1879, no. i, p. 339; the *Medical Record* (New York), 1879, vol. 15, p. 280; the *London Medical Record*, 1879, vol. 7, pp. 171–173; *The Dublin Journal of Medical Science*, 1879, vol. 67, pp. 53–58. These reviews and abstracts almost certainly underrepresent the extent to which Gage appeared in the literature, because reviews and abstracts were not always indexed. For example, as far as I can determine, neither the *New York Medical Journal* nor the *Medico-Chirurgical Transactions* contained an abstract or review.

23. Dodds (1877–1878, p. 470) does not mention Gage by name, but his citation of the details of the damage from Hammond's textbook provides unmistakable identification. Nor does he otherwise refer to Gage in his extensive discussion of Dupuy's antilocalization arguments and Ferrier's replies to them.

10

Gage and Surgery for the Brain

"Awful?" said Ferrier, "the operation was performed perfectly."
"Yes," replied Jackson, "but he opened a Scotsman's head and failed to put a joke in it."
—J. D. Spillane's version of a story from the first operation for an intracranial tumor, 1981

Phineas Gage's case made a small but significant contribution to the development of brain surgery, although that fact is much less often remarked than his supposed contribution to the development of psychosurgery. I explore and reestablish the contribution of his case to brain surgery in this chapter before showing in chapter 11 that what is said about its contribution to psychosurgery is almost completely erroneous.

I begin this chapter by mentioning briefly five important early cases of brain surgery, each of which was the first or among the first in which surgery was planned or conducted on the basis of what was then known about localization. I then discuss them in the context of the particular aspect of the localization debate to which they were related, the first two in relation to aphasia, the third to sensory-motor processes, and the last two to frontal lobe damage. Diagnostic rules derived from cases of frontal damage, of which Gage was the most important, had some vogue until about 1890. Criticism of these rules became sharper at about that time and their use fell into abeyance.

The five early cases are:

1. On 27 June 1871, a thirty-eight-year-old man was admitted to Broca's Service at L'Hôpital Pitié with a 6–7 cm cut to the left side of the head. After an initial healing, the cut became infected, suffered a hemorrhage, and finally there were signs of an intracranial abscess. To all questions asked of him at this latter stage, the patient could reply only, "It is not

going badly." From this and some motor symptoms, Broca concluded that the abscess was affecting the third left frontal convolution.

2. A young man was admitted to the Royal Infirmary, Glasgow, in July 1876 with convulsions and symptoms of brain abscess. William Macewen, his physician, noticed that for about two hours after a convulsion he was able to utter only the word "No" in response to questions. Macewen diagnosed an abscess "in the immediate vicinity of Broca's lobe."

3. Nearly nine and a half years later, on 3 November 1885, a twenty-five-year-old man, paralyzed in the left hand and arm, was admitted to the Hospital for Epilepsy and Paralysis, Regent's Park, London. He had had left-sided attacks of twitching that culminated in left-sided "fits" and a generalized convulsion. His physician, Alexander Hughes Bennett, diagnosed a right-sided tumor "situated at the middle part of the fissure of Rolando."

4. Three years after Macewen's first case, on 22 July 1879, a girl of fourteen was admitted to the Glasgow Royal Infirmary, again under his care. She had a pain in the head, a permanently contracted left pupil and "mental" symptoms. In Macewen's view, the mental symptoms pointed "to the probability of a lesion in the left frontal lobe."

5. On 14 January, 1893, American neurologist M. Allen Starr examined a forty-year-old farmer who had been admitted to the Nervous Department of the Vanderbilt Clinic in New York. His main complaints were also of what Starr called "mental symptoms." Largely from them, Starr diagnosed a brain tumor in the left frontal lobe, occupying "the posterior part of the second frontal convolution, just anterior to its junction with the anterior central convolution."

What made these diagnoses and the planned surgery possible was knowledge of how the functions that had been disturbed were localized.

In the first two cases, there was an obvious application of what seemed to follow from Broca's contention about the function of articulate language being localized in the third left frontal convolution. Second, in all five cases, but especially in case 3, the first conducted for removal of a brain tumor, there was an equally obvious application of Ferrier's and Hughlings Jackson's conclusions. Third, although it is not at all obvious, especially to the modern reader, the diagnosis in the first of the two earliest operations for the removal of a frontal tumor, case 4, probably drew on Phineas Gage, and the second, case 5, certainly did. The second and third of these uses constitute the beginning of Phineas Gage's contribution to brain surgery. I now consider the cases and their contexts in order.[1]

Aphasia, Localization, and Brain Surgery

Knowledge of brain function was not the only necessary precursor to brain surgery. As Macewen himself pointed out many years later, in 1888, there had actually been two formidable barriers to surgery in the region of the brain:

first, the fact that the majority of intra-cranial operations were attended by inflammatory action, which so often proved fatal as to cause surgeons to shun active interference; and, secondly, the brain was a dark continent, in which they could descry neither path nor guide capable of leading them to a particular diseased area.

Lister's pioneering work on aseptic surgery, conducted on the very wards where Macewen worked, had overcome the first barrier. The second began to fall, Macewen noted, when "Broca, in 1861, from observation on human pathology, isolated a particular limited area as the faculty of articulate language."[2]

Beginning with Broca's case 1 and Macewen's case 2, in which the symptoms included aphasia, I now consider the diagnostic use of findings from studies of localization in more detail.

Broca's Craniotomy (Case 1)

According to what Broca wrote in 1876, his 1871 diagnosis of M. Pierre Baron's abscess had been "based on the knowledge of the site of the faculty of articulate language." He also took into account a paralysis "of the right extremities" that developed when the patient's condition became much worse. He believed that the abscess was above the dura mater and that it was pressing on the third left frontal convolution. Broca therefore decided to drain the abscess, and after locating it where he thought it would be, successfully did so. However, the gravity of the symptoms convinced him that "there must exist further alterations, deeper," which he unsuccessfully searched for after the patient's condition again deteriorated. Eventually M. Baron died, and post mortem examination found the abscess where Broca had expected it to be. There were, as well, signs of inflammation of the brain itself in and around the third left frontal convolution.

Macewen and Broca's Thesis (Case 2)

According to Macewen's 1888 account, it was primarily the aphasia that led him to locate the abscess "in the immediate vicinity of Broca's lobe." He planned an operation "to open the abscess aseptically by exposing Broca's lobe" but the boy's parents denied permission, and the boy died. The post mortem examination was then carried out as if it were the planned operation. It showed Macewen's localization to have been accurate: an abscess, "about the size of a pigeon's egg, was situated in the white matter of the basis [*sic*] of the second and third frontal convolutions" (figure 10.1a).

Phenomena other than the transitory aphasia also helped Macewen to recognize the seat of the abscess:

A convulsion accompanied by loss of consciousness commenced on the right side, and gradually involved the whole body. On its cessation absolute hemiplegia of the right side was present, and remained for two hours, during which the patient was aphasic.

These additional phenomena have significance, of course, only because of the work of Hughlings Jackson and Ferrier. In fact, after pointing out that Broca's observations "on human pathology" had isolated a particular limited area as the faculty of articulate language, Macewen went on to say:

This very important investigation foreshadowed the localisation of function in other cortical centres ... [and] the question arose, how many other centres with specialised functions might there be?

We have seen that much of the answer to this more general question was provided by Jackson and by Ferrier's extrapolation of his monkey findings to humans.[3]

Sensory-Motor Physiology and Brain Surgery

Although Broca had shown the way, it was through Ferrier's confirmation of Hughlings Jackson's theses about the representation of motor functions that, as Macewen put it, "the mind of the physiological world was fairly awakened." But more direct confirmation of Ferrier's

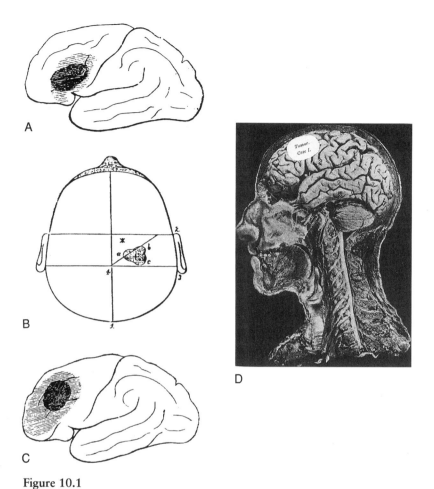

Figure 10.1
(a) Case 2 (Macewen), (b) Case 3 (Bennett and Godlee), (c) Case 4 (Macewen), (d) Case 5 (McBurney and Starr)
From (a) Macewen 1888, fig. 1; (b) Bennett and Godlee 1885b, fig. 1; (c) Macewen 1888, fig. 3; (d) McBurney and Starr 1893, fig. 2.

extrapolation was really needed. The case of the unfortunate Mary Rafferty provided such confirmation, in 1874, almost immediately after Ferrier had published his preliminary results. Rafferty's brain being exposed because of an incurable ulcerating disease of the skull, Roberts Bartholow, her physician, asked her to make it available for investigation by electrical stimulation. Mary, close to death and described by Bartholow as "rather feebleminded," agreed. Depending on the site of stimulation, Bartholow produced contralateral movements of the palpebral opening, dilation of the pupils, and sensations and movements in the limbs. On the third day of experimentation, however, convulsions resulted and Mary Rafferty died.[4]

Bartholow's investigation of the motor functions of the human brain was probably the earliest attempt to confirm Ferrier's conclusions on a human subject, and it was certainly the saddest in its consequences. On the other hand, in the same period that Ferrier's and Jackson's findings made the first operation for the removal of a brain tumor possible, Victor Horsley seems to have pioneered the use of Ferrier's stimulation method for identifying dysfunctional brain tissue more accurately. His first use of the method was to determine the function of a portion of brain protruding from a congenitally incomplete occipital bone ("occipital encephalocele") in a six-week-old infant. He then seems to have used it to determine the sites of suspect lesions prior to their removal. The technique had two special virtues. It gave the surgeon something more than poorly viewed anatomical landmarks to decide exactly where particular "centres" were situated. It also enabled the surgeon to determine the place and extent of excision when there were no gross signs of disease. The method was soon widely adopted, at least experimentally.[5]

Bennett and Godlee's Localization (Case 3)

The first operation for the removal of a tumor from the brain was that carried out on a twenty-five-year-old Scotsman, a Mr. Henderson from Dumfries, on 25 November 1884, eleven years after Ferrier began his work. He was our case 3 and, although faradic stimulation was not employed as a preliminary to his surgery, it is easy to assess the contribution of localization to the diagnosis. Henderson had originally suffered from left-sided epileptic attacks beginning in the face and tongue, with occasional losses of consciousness. Over a three-year period, his left hand and arm had also become involved, forcing him to give up work at the beginning of November. By the time he was admitted to the hospital there were also severe pressure symptoms: paroxysmal headache and vomiting, and papilloedema with hemorrhages. Bennett, his physician, diagnosed "an encephalic growth, probably of limited size, involving the cortex of the brain, and situated at the middle part of the fissure of Rolando."

Bennett planned the operation and persuaded Rickman Godlee to carry it out. Godlee was a nephew of Lister, who had made his own appreciation of asepsis by visiting Glasgow some eleven years earlier. On Godlee's operating, a tumor was indeed found, directly under the opening that had been made in the skull, and a little smaller than it. The tumor was removed, immediately relieving all the symptoms completely except for a slight increase in the hemiplegia. There were no mental effects, but an infection set in leading to Henderson's death from meningitis four weeks later (figure 10.1b).

Bennett and Godlee's achievement is well recognized. As Trotter put it, they had

proved for the first time that without the least external abnormality of the skull to point the way, a focal lesion of brain substance could be found and could be removed by operation leaving the general functions of the brain unimpaired.

Ferrier was present during the operation, and he and Hughlings Jackson were the first to contribute to the discussion that followed it. By relating Mr. Henderson's symptoms to areas 3, 4, 6, and 7 on figure 9.3, it can be seen how their work made it possible.[6]

Ferrier, Frontal Localization, and Gage

In now turning to cases 4 and 5 to examine the diagnostic use to which the Phineas Gage case was put in cases of frontal tumor, the first thing we should notice is that Ferrier's confirmation of Hughlings Jackson's theses did not awaken the whole of "the mind of the physiological world" as Macewen had put it. It will be recalled that the most striking thing about Ferrier's monkey and hypothetical human localizations is the absence of sensory-motor functions in the frontal areas. Frontal ablation in the monkey produced behavioral changes that Ferrier came to consider as being exemplified by Gage and that could be explained by the loss of a frontally localized inhibitory-motor function. The loss of that function caused "a form of mental degradation, which may be reduced in ultimate analysis to the loss of the faculty of attention."

After describing the changes in Gage in his first *Gulstonian Lecture*, Ferrier concluded that it could not be said that "the 'American Crowbar Case' is in opposition to the experimental facts which I have adduced as to the effects of lesions of the frontal lobes" in the monkey. At the end of the *Lecture* he directed his listeners attention to four other cases with "similar" characteristics (Baraduc's, Selwyn's, Lepine's, and Davidson's). His premier placement of Phineas Gage in this series makes it possible to class the operations on cases 4 and 5 as the first of Gage's contributions to brain surgery.

Macewen and Frontal Localization (Case 4)
According to Macewen's 1888 account, when he made his diagnosis in case 4 in 1879 he drew on a thesis that some kinds of psychological functions were localized frontally. The symptoms in his fourteen-year-old girl patient included "obscuration of intelligence, slowness of comprehension, [and] want of mental vigour" as well as the stability of the left pupil and pain in the head. Although Macewen seems to have taken the mental symptoms alone as pointing to the frontal condition, he was cautious enough to have her admitted to the hospital for observation. A few days afterward a series of convulsions commenced. His 1881 description was that

while sitting at the bedside, she uttered a cry, and immediately the muscles of the right side of the face began to twitch, the right arm was violently flexed, and violently twitched. The twitchings lasted for two or three minutes, and were entirely confined to the right side. An interval of ten minutes elapsed, when the spasms re-appeared in the right side of the face and on the right arm, lasting for about fifteen minutes. Two minutes after a third attack ensued, this time involving the whole of the right side of the body.

As the attacks became prolonged, the intervals between shortened, until they were continuous, and the convulsions became more general until consciousness was lost.

Macewen said in 1888 that he had construed the convulsive phenomena

as indicating extension of the irritation to the lower and middle portions of the ascending convolutions; and when this was considered along with the former evidence, it was concluded that an irritative lesion existed in the left frontal lobe.

On operation, a tumor of the dura mater spreading "all over the anterior two-thirds of the frontal lobe" was found and removed, leading to complete recovery (figure 10.1c).[7]

Macewen does not say so explicitly but I am almost certain that the importance he placed on the mental symptoms derived from Ferrier's theses about the psychological functions of the frontal lobes. By 1879 no one but Ferrier had proposed them. His monkey experiments had been published in various scientific periodicals prior to their consolidated appearance in *Functions of the Brain* in 1876, but they were specifically reiterated in relation to Gage in the *Gulstonian Lectures* of 1878, delivered just one year before Macewen's operation.

Starr's Recommendations for Frontal Surgery

If there is doubt about the contribution of the Gage case to Macewen's diagnosis, there can be none at all about it concerning the patient on whom McBurney and Starr operated in 1893, sixteen years later (case 5). To appreciate that fact we need to return to 1884, when the first modern comparison of the effects of different kinds of lesions and tumors was published. In it, the changes in Gage were very much in the forefront.

Data had been reported on the effects of lesions and tumors of the brain earlier in the century, of course, but they were not analyzed in a systematic way; they tended to be about individual subjects, rather than about groups; and it was not often that data about damage to the frontal areas were included. In any case, the reports said little about the behavioral and psychological consequences of lesions and tumors. Further, where systematic attempts had been made to evaluate even these limited data, as with the early series reported by Home that I mentioned in chapter 6, the investigator's limited physiological framework and narrow clinical-therapeutic aims restricted the conclusions even more.

There were some exceptions to the kinds of comparisons made by Home, for example, the series of Charcot, Charcot and Pitres, Pitres, and Lewis, but the numbers of cases were usually small and even when that was not true, as in Bernhardt's series, little or no attention was paid to frontal lesions. Starr's 1884 study was virtually the first of its kind and was quite different from all those conducted before. First, it was extremely comprehensive, being based on *all* of the nearly 500 cases of cerebral lesions reported in the American medical literature over the previous twenty-five years. Second, Starr restricted his analysis to the ninety-nine reports meeting Nothnagel's criteria of the damage's apparently being due to "a single lesion of small extent, accurately located, and of considerable duration." Third, Starr included the first large series of frontal lesions cases, twenty-three in all.[8]

Starr's comparisons began with the frontal lobes and actually used Gage as a standard:

Lesions affecting the three frontal convolutions may be classed together. Ever since the occurrence of the famous American crowbar case it has been known that destruction of these lobes does not necessarily give rise to any symptoms. That case is given in order to compare others with it.

He gave Bigelow's 1850 paper and J. B. S. Jackson's 1870 account in the Warren Museum catalogue as the sources of his information about Gage. Although he had observed that Gage had no motor symptoms, Starr summarized the psychological change as "his disposition was altered, and ... he was irritable, easily excitable, and emotional."

Starr's other cases of damage caused by foreign bodies included Lewis Avery and three in which bullets had lodged in the brain. According to Starr, in one-half of the cases of frontal lesion there was "decided mental instability." Any kind of damage could cause this instability, but it occurred only when the damage was frontal, never elsewhere. The change, he said, "did not conform to any one type of insanity. It is rather to be described as a loss of self control, and a consequent change of character."

Starr was familiar with Ferrier's experimental and clinical findings, listing the *Gulstonian Lectures* among his references. Although he did not mention Ferrier by name, Starr clearly drew on a similar inhibitory thesis:

The mind exercises a constant inhibitory influence upon all action, physical or mental; from the simple restraint upon the lower reflexes, such as the action of the sphincters, to the higher control over the complex reflexes, such as emotional impulses and their manifestation in speech and expression. This action of control implies a recognition of the import of an act in connection with other acts; in a word, it involves judgment and reason, the highest mental qualities. By inhibiting all but one set of impulses it enables one to fix attention upon a subject, and hold it there.

Just as Ferrier had done, Starr then argued that because the size of the frontal lobes separated man from the animals and the normally intelligent from the intellectually handicapped, it was "probable" that judgment and reason had their physical basis there. If that was the case, he said, one of the first manifestations of partial destruction of the frontal lobes would have to be some "striking" change in judgment and reason. What he had in mind was the lack of that self-control, which is the constant accompaniment of mental action, and which would be shown by an inability to fix the attention, to follow a continuous train of thought, or to conduct intellectual processes.

So characteristic did Starr judge this mental change to be that he recommended examining the patient's reason, judgment, and character or behavior whenever frontal lobe lesions were suspected. About eight years later he followed those recommendations in planning the operation on his farmer patient.[9]

McBurney and Starr's Frontal Tumor (Case 5)

Case 5 was, according to McBurney and Starr, the seventh operation on the frontal lobes. They said there had been six such operations, out of a total of seventy-four of all types, up to 1893. But the patient on whom McBurney operated following Starr's diagnosis of his left frontal tumor was, Starr claimed, "the first case ... in which operative interference has been so *directly dictated by the existence of mental symptoms*" (emphasis added). The illness of their farmer patient had been heralded by an attack of dizziness and distress in which his head was forcibly turned to the right. There had then been a convulsion followed by a two-and-one-half-hour period of unconsciousness. After the attack he was left with a slight right-sided weakness and a difficulty in talking, which passed off after about two weeks.

The patient had no subsequent similar attack but, over the next year, suffered from headache, nausea, and a gradual loss of vision. He also noticed

a progressive dullness of thought, general hebetude, an aversion to work which was unnatural to him, and a slowness of mental activity which he described as increasing stupidity; and an increasing difficulty in the use of language, so that it took him longer to express his ideas, there being, however, no difficulty in articulation and no lack of words.

These self-reported changes constituted what Starr called his mental symptoms. On examination, Starr found a slight right hemiplegia and an optic neuritis, more marked in the left eye than the right, which had caused a partial blindness. There was also a spot about three inches in diameter on the top of the head, tender to percussion, that corresponded to the location of his headaches. Starr also observed the behavioral symptoms that the patient had himself reported on, adding that "it was not easy for him to hold his attention to any subject continuously for any length of time."

Localizing the tumor was not easy. The hemiplegia indicated that the motor zone was involved, but the history indicated that the tumor had not begun there, and the absence of sensory symptoms, including sensory aphasia, ruled out the parietal lobe. The mental changes pointed to a left frontal location. In discussing their significance, Starr reproduced his 1884 description, the one that included Gage, and cited other cases as confirmation, most notably the series Welt analyzed. McBurney and he decided the lesion occupied "the posterior part of the second frontal convolution, just anterior to its junction with the anterior central convolution" (figure 10.1d).

During the operation, on 23 June 1893, McBurney and Starr found an ovoid-shaped sarcoma measuring $2.5 \times 2 \times 1.75$ inches, weighing 4 grams, and 50 cc in volume. It corresponded "very accurately to the diagnosis made before operation but the size of the mass was much greater than had been anticipated." So large was the tumor, so great the cavity, and so profuse the bleeding, that the patient survived the operation by only eight hours. There was no opportunity to observe any changes the removal of the tumor might have caused.[10]

Elder and Miles's Use of Mental Symptoms
About nine years after the operation by McBurney and Starr, Elder and Miles also followed Starr's recommendation. Their patient's main physical symptoms were pain and swelling in the left frontal region and a partial right-sided paralysis of the arm and lower facial muscles. However, the patient is particularly worth noting because some of his mental changes resemble those in Gage. His friends were annoyed "that he seemed to lose all sense of decency and shame and exposed his person unduly and needlessly." His attention could not be sustained and his memory seemed to be affected in that he would forget "in a few moments what he had been saying." He had also become very emotional, weeping at the sight of his friends, and had recently had an episode of depression.

On operation, a tumor (a syphiloma) was found where Elder and Miles expected it to be; it was successfully removed, and the patient recovered completely within a month. Nothing untoward took place except that for a few days after the operation the patient resembled "a man slightly intoxicated and began to use bad language, and became emotional." Comparing the importance of the mental with the physical symptoms, Elder and Miles asserted:

His mental or psychical symptoms were, however, not only confirmatory, *but if they had been taken alone* would have been sufficient to have justified an operation over the left frontal region. These symptoms may all be considered as a loss or depression of the inhibitory power of the individual. (emphasis added)

They cited the whole of Starr's description of "the mental instability," explicitly endorsed the practical diagnostic point he had made about it, and explicitly related these mental symptoms to Ferrier's and Starr's inhibitory theses. Perhaps their patient was fortunate in the accuracy of their localization, and the success of the surgery, because the problems of localizing frontal lesions had already come under critical scrutiny.[11]

The Criticisms of Frontal Localization

As early as 1885, only four years after Starr's recommendation and in the very year of the original Bennett and Godlee operation, Gowers had said of frontal lesions that while the "mental change is rather more frequent than in other situations," sometimes taking "the form of chronic insanity," "these symptoms are neither characteristic nor invariable." Then in major addresses to a symposium on "Cerebral Localisation in its Practical Relations," held on 19 September 1888 as part of the First Triennial Congress of American Physicians and Surgeons, C. K. Mills and Ferrier made similar points.

Mills's comprehensive review of almost all the clinical and experimental findings on localization was published as a 105-page Critical Digest in *Brain*. He concentrated especially on the practical value of localization rules in guiding the surgeon. He made it very clear how strikingly brain surgery had advanced since 1885 and that it was an advance that continued to be linked to knowledge of localization. At the beginning there had been virtually only Ferrier's extrapolation from his monkey studies and Hughlings Jackson's inferences from his clinical material. Now even the faradic stimulation Ferrier pioneered for use in the laboratory had been adapted by Horsley for use on the exposed human brain.

Mills particularly noted how

more and more has that region been narrowed which cannot be reached by the venturesome surgical explorer.... Absolutely inviolable ... are only the middle region of the base, and its bordering convolutions, the corpora quadrigemina, and the pons oblongata.

He concluded that in the accessible areas there were

(1) regions in which an absolute localisation can be made by positive symptoms; and (2) regions in which a close approximate localisation can be made by positive symptoms, combined with methods of exclusion and differentiation. Under the first head, come the motor, visual, and motor speech areas and tracts; under the second, the cerebellum, the pre-frontal, and the temporal lobes, with their more or less positively determined functions.

Mills was explicit about how much of this advance the field owed to Ferrier. All that had been necessary since Ferrier was "to modify and enlarge" on Ferrier's findings.

Without specifically mentioning Starr's proposal, Mills drew attention to some of the problems in using mental alterations in diagnosis. He felt diagnostic guides to lesions of the prefrontal lobe were only gradually "becoming more definite." More definite guidance might be obtained by combining "the few positive localising symptoms" with general symptoms of a brain tumor, such as headache and changes in the optic discs, and the exclusion of lesions of or associated with the motor, speech, and visual and auditory areas. The "distinctive manifestations" shown "in a large percentage of the carefully studied cases" were

mental disturbances of a peculiar character ... such as mental slowness and uncertainty, want of attention and control, and impairment of judgement and reason; closely studied, the inhibitory influence of the brain both on psychical and physical action is found to be diminished. Memory is not seriously affected although a continuous train of thought cannot well be followed, and complex intellectual processes cannot be thoroughly performed.

Although psychical phenomena could not "be studied with accuracy in animals below man," Ferrier's and others' ablation of the frontal lobes of animals showed behavioral changes that were "difficult precisely to describe." Therefore the phenomena

did not measure in usefulness for the average diagnostician with such positive objective manifestations as hemianopsia or Jacksonian spasm, but they should be valuable aids in the hands of close observers.

In his invited address to the same conference, Ferrier also drew attention to the difficulty.

For Ferrier, the characteristic history of unilateral spasm followed by monoplegia and the successive monoplegiae resulting in general hemiplegia made lesions of the Rolandic or motor zone the "most easily determined." In contrast, lesions of the prefrontal region cannot with certainty be diagnosed from the symptoms of the lesion as such. The irritable dementia not unfrequently observed in connection with such lesions cannot with certainty be distinguished from the general effects of other cerebral diseases, such as tumour, abscess, and the like.

Ferrier's seeming endorsement of the opinion of Mills, and of the one quoted earlier from Gowers, shows how the tide had turned by the very end of the last century against the strict use of localizing signs in general, and not just for frontal diagnosis. Some critics completely rejected the value of localization to brain surgery. For example, although John W. Robertson, Professor of Nervous and Mental Disease at the University of California, San Francisco, agreed that if "the strict localisation" views were correct a vast area of surgery did open up, he took the (mainly animal) evidence to show "that very little" had been "irrefutably demonstrated" about localization and concluded that brain surgery based on it was neither justified nor likely to be of benefit. Only in "exceptional cases," he later offered, was localization "of material assistance to the surgeon."[12]

Starr's Cases Reconsidered

Enthusiastic as he was over localization's usefulness, C. K. Mills was also to point to another aspect of the problem, one that seemed to be purely practical: "The symptoms are largely psychical, and unfortunately the physician is not usually well trained to study such phenomena." Among the psychical symptoms of frontal damage and disease, Mills included slowness and uncertainty, lack of attention and control, impaired judgment and reason, diminished inhibitory influence, and the inability to perform complex intellectual processes thoroughly. Memory was not affected. These symptoms posed the difficulty, and animal experiments were not very helpful "because psychical phenomena cannot be studied with animals lower than man."

Although it is true that phrases like "mental instability," "progressive dullness of thought," "mental degradation," "irritable dementia," "defect of attention," or even "loss of self-control" may be the not very precise descriptions to be expected of not "well-trained" physicians, the real difficulties come from trying to fit these kinds of behaviors into the sensory-motor framework. The point is clearer when we examine Starr's descriptions of what he believed the loss of the inhibitory function caused.[13]

In three of the first five of Starr's frontal cases, "foreign bodies entered and destroyed portions of the brain" and resulted in no change, including the case of Lewis Avery (Starr's case II) (see figure 10.2). That all three cases were as unproblematic as Avery's may be illustrated by this one:

Case III Corporal G[eorge] W[ashington] S[tone], of the 12th. Massachusetts Volunteers, a 28 year-old farmer from Roxbury, Massachusetts, lost the sight of his right eye on December 13th. 1862, at the battle of Fredericksburg. During his regiment's unsupported action against Stonewall Jackson's flank, a conoidal ball penetrated his right orbit, and unknown to him or the army surgeons at the Baltimore hospital to which he was taken, the ball came to rest outside the dura mater and on the inside of the left tempero-sphenoidal bone. He appeared to recover completely, showing no symptoms or changes in his behaviour until two days before his death from the effects of a late-developing left frontal lobe abscess on 15th. February, 1863.[14]

More problematic about Starrs' cases are those in which there was change, such as this one:

Case IV. Charles Burklin was a heavy drinker who, after making an unsuccessful attempt to kill his wife, attempted suicide on 9th. March, 1872, by shooting himself through the left forehead. After an intermittent fever that was serious enough to have him admitted to hospital on 6th. January, 1873, his condition gradually became much worse, and he died on 13th. February that year, nearly eleven months after the shooting. Post-mortem examination revealed a sac filled with 6 ounces of pus lying on the underside of the left frontal lobe and reaching from its beginning almost to the fissure of Sylvius. The bullet lay incysted in front of the sac.

Starr summarized the change in Burklin with the phrase that he had become "stupid and listless." But what Prewitt originally reported in 1873 was:

He [Burklin] was rather morose, seemed indisposed to talk, and not altogether rational. His answers to questions, however, were always relevant, both upon admission and afterwards ... the patient at no time show[ed] any marked sign of delirium, although it was evident that his mind was not just right. He did not seem to appreciate his position, expressed frequently a wish to go home, mani-fested no anxiety about his own fate, though when told that his wound might, and probably would prove fatal, he expressed a hope that it would kill him quick. He asked repeatedly about his wife, manifested a good deal of anxiety about her condition, said he did not know why he had shot her, that he must have been crazy, and at one time when insisting on being permitted to go home, and upon being told he would be thrown into prison if released from the hospital, he said they could not hurt him for it—referring to the shooting of his wife—that he was crazy when he did it.

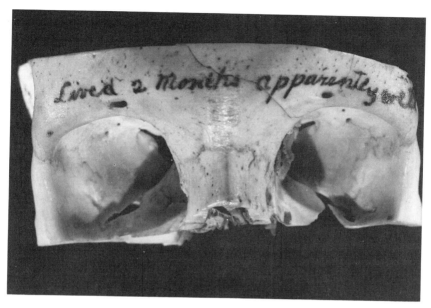

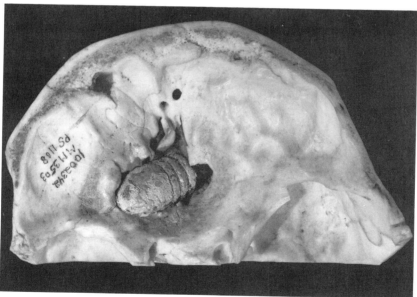

Figure 10.2
Corporal Stone's skull with conoidal ball lodged in it
Photograph of AFIP specimen 1108 by courtesy Paul Sledzik, Armed Forces
Institute of Pathology, Washington, D.C.

If Starr had already been less than true to Harlow's original in using words like "irritable," "easily excitable," and "emotional" to describe the changes in Gage, he now compounded the inaccuracy by jointly summarizing the "mental symptoms" of Gage and Burklin by saying both showed "a deficiency of self-control."

As Starr outlined them, the changes in the three of the seven cases of softening or abscess were actually just as varied:

Case VII had "no cerebral symptoms at any time but it was noticed that the patient was querulous, complaining, and timid, and a little slow of speech";
Case X became "sulky and morose instead of cheerful as formerly";
Case XII was "much more talkative than before the injury."

Starr summarized these cases as showing "an undue excitability and a lack of self-restraint."

Mental symptoms in the eleven cases of tumor were similarly varied:

Case XVI "became incoherent," possibly not long before his death;
Case XVIII showed "mental hebetude and uncertainty with a tendency to hallucinations." About a month before he died "he was too stupid to be tested accurately [for sensory capacity]. His intellect was much impaired. Formerly he had been intelligent and energetic, now he was slow and seemed to have difficulty in receiving mental impressions and in directing voluntary movements. The faculty of attention was almost gone, and his attention was only to be fixed by vehement command." When answering questions "he seemed unable to retain the same idea or follow a line of thought. He would not wander, but would stop speaking. He was very emotional. He would at times have outbursts of speech, saying a few sentences very loud and then stop suddenly. Exclamations of this kind would be repeated every few minutes for several hours";
Case XX showed the faculty of "attention was wanting, and continuous thought was impossible. He was very emotional and cried often";
Case XXI was "very sad, he never smiled, and never conversed except to answer inquiries. The expression was neither one of pain nor of idiocy, but was very pathetic. If questioned he answered correctly in a clear low tone and very distinctly. His memory of past events was good, but of recent occurrences was poor. 'His intellection was retarded, but not absent nor irrational.'"

Starr gave no separate summary of the mental symptoms in these cases of tumor but went on to include them in the overall summary I have already quoted, which stressed the lack of self-control, "the constant accompaniment of mental action," shown in "an inability to fix the attention, to follow a continuous train of thought, or to conduct intellectual processes." If Starr's interpretations seem cavalier, what of Ferrier's use of Gage as exemplar?[15]

Gage as Exemplar

After Ferrier presented Harlow's account of the changes in Gage to the audience at his 1878 *Gulstonian Lecture*, he went on to mention briefly four other cases of frontal damage "without sensory or motor affection" in which there had also been marked changes in behaviour. Even though he was unable to specify "the symptoms directly indicating disease of the prefrontal lobes," experimental physiology "had brought into prominence certain facts" to which attention would have to be paid in the future. The facts? The apathetic, dull, restless, and purposeless behavior of his monkeys. Ferrier continued:

I have elsewhere attempted some explanation of the faculty of attention—the basis of the higher intellectual operations—and its relation to the anatomical substrata of the prefrontal lobes; but I will not enter further on these speculations at present. I would, however, call your attention to the psychical characters in some of the cases of disease and injury to the frontal lobes to which I have referred ... as in many respects similar to those seen in monkeys after removal of the prefrontal lobes.

Ferrier placed considerable importance on Gage as an example of the loss of inhibitory function. Not only did he use Harlow's illustrations, but he devoted approximately twice as much text to Gage as to the other four cases together.

Although Gage was impatient and obviously suffered from a lack of social inhibition, how does his obstinacy, capriciousness, and vacillation relate to that symptom? How apt were Ferrier's descriptions of these other cases in relation to Gage?

1. Baraduc had described his patient as being in a "state of complete dementia, marching about restlessly the whole day, picking up whatever came in his way, mute, and quite oblivious of all the wants of nature, and requiring to be tended like a child."

2. Selwyn said his patient had a very defective memory and was "incapable of applying to any pursuit requiring mental activity. His disposition is irritable, especially after indulging in liquor, or after any unusual stimulus."

3. Lépine pictured his patient as "in a state of hebetude. He seemed to comprehend what was said but could scarcely be got to utter a word. He would sit down when he was told to do so, and when taken up could walk a few steps with assistance."

4. Davidson's patient seemed to understand everything but "every action he performed left the impression on the mind of the observer that it was purely automatic."

At the very least, these behaviors differ markedly from one another.

How well do these descriptions match Harlow's of Gage? Can the behaviors be encompassed as "a form of mental degradation, which may be reduced in ultimate analysis to the loss of the faculty of attention"? Recall now that Ferrier's evidence for localizing an inhibitory-motor function in the frontal areas and linking it with attention was peculiarly negative. The failure of electrical stimulation and ablation to have an effect was literally a "negative fact," and Ferrier's evidence for attention being involved was no stronger. Hence, essentially the same combination of negative findings and subjective reasoning that had led Müller to localize attention in the whole of the hemispheres now led Ferrier to localize it in the frontal lobes.[16]

If Ferrier's cases are not closely considered, it is as easy to be seduced by his summaries as by Starr's. The difficulty is that "symptoms" other than the sensory-motor, especially complex behavioral symptoms, posed problems in principle for both sensory-motor physiology and psychology. They continued to do so well into the twentieth century. Consider, for example, Dandy's 1933 comments on the seemingly minimal effects of the removal of whole lobes from the brain. He granted that he had not gathered his behavioral and psychological data in a standardised or systematic way and was prepared to concede that his tests might not have revealed what he called the "little peculiarities of mental origin, such as those in the famous crow-bar case" that might "be obvious to those who are thrown in frequent contact." To imply that the changes in Gage were "little peculiarities" confirms how difficult it was to describe complex behaviors within the sensory-motor framework.

The criticisms made at the end of the century thus anticipated part of what Dandy was to say forty years later. There were, Dandy stressed in 1933, "very good reasons" why attempts to localize cerebral functions through the effects of tumors and degenerative processes had led to contradictory results. First, a tumor's effects were not restricted to the immediate region of the brain the tumor occupied, and, second, the absence of signs or symptoms appropriate to an area did not mean a tumor was not present in it. Without knowing it, Dandy went on to echo Leny in an almost uncanny way:

The net result of tumor analyses furnishes a seeming paradox, for some tumors in a given region produce no obvious loss of function, whereas others of the same size and in precisely the same location cause the most widespread and profound alterations in their workings.

In the light of these judgments we can say that Macewen, Bennett and Godlee, McBurney and Starr, and Elder and Miles had all been very fortunate that their use of localizing signs that were sometimes misleading and at other times vague had directed them to areas of the brain affected by reasonably circumscribed lesions. Many of those who came later found things to be more complicated.[17]

Conclusion

The emergence of brain surgery depended on the development of surgical techniques in the narrower sense (e.g., anesthesias, asepsis, operative procedures) and on knowledge of how the brain's functions were localized. Phineas Gage's two contributions to brain surgery can be specified within the context of those developments. First, Gage's survival probably encouraged nineteenth-century surgeons in the belief that operations could be performed on the brain without the results necessarily being fatal. Almost immediately after the development of aseptic surgery Macewen and more extensively Bennett and Godlee acted on that belief. Second, the changes in Gage's behavior contributed substantially to the view that mental changes could serve as the localizing signs for frontal lobe lesions. Basing himself on a view like Ferrier's, Starr recommended so using the mental changes, and he and others acted on it. These developments offer no evidence of Gage's case contributing to surgical procedures for operating on the brains of psychiatric patients.

On the other hand, we should be alarmed at how the vagueness of the term "mental symptoms" allowed such disparate behaviors to be equated. Although this vagueness results partly from the limitations of the sensory-motor framework, another factor seems to be at work: the implicit assumption that behaviour *ought* to be rational. Were one in full control of one's behavior, one would always choose the mature alternative. Put simply, to be dull in thinking and generally weak, to be querulous, complaining and timid, or emotional and weeping at the sight of one's friends, or to be morose and indisposed to talk, or to understand everything but act purely automatically, or to be fitful, irreverent, obstinate, capricious and devise plans and abandon them almost as quickly, was to be irrational. Behaving irrationally meant a weakness of will, which meant, physiologically speaking, a weakness of the inhibitory process on which will depended. Behind the descriptions of the symptoms of these real patients can be discerned the dim figure of rational man.

Why place this will and the inhibitory process that sustained it in the frontal lobes? Ferrier's inhibitory-motor function was purely hypothetical, and he located it there because no other processes, especially sensory-motor processes, could be found in the frontal lobes. We shall see that this weakness in the reasoning of Ferrier and the nineteenth-century pioneers of brain surgery was to be repeated by the pioneers of psychosurgery and carried into the twentieth.

Notes

1. Details of these five cases are in Broca [1876] 1991; Macewen 1881, case 4, and 1888, case 1; Bennett and Godlee 1882–1885, 1884, 1885a, 1885b; Macewen 1881, case 3, and 1888, case 3; and McBurney and Starr 1893, respectively. I have been unable to solve the problem of priority over Broca's case of 1871 and Macewen's of 1876. Stone 1991 gives a full account of Broca's case, which was not published until 1876, the year of Macewen's operation. In the absence of contemporary records, I have listed them in what should be regarded as a claimed order of treatment. There is a more general treatment of Gage in relation to brain surgery in Macmillan 1996c.

2. Macewen's assessment of these factors is in Macewen 1888. By the time the first brain surgery was planned, the battle for the introduction of anesthesia into surgical practice was well over. I presume it was for this reason that Macewen did not include Morton's discovery of ether some thirty years earlier as a precondition.

3. In other of Macewen's early cases, which I have not cited, the symptoms were mainly motor. There is little doubt that in them also Macewen used both Jackson's and Ferrier's conclusions for localizing the lesions.

4. Macewen's (1888) overview contains his tribute to Ferrier. Ferrier (1873) for his preliminary results. Bartholow's experiments are in Bartholow 1874a. The controversy is partly covered in the *British Medical Journal* editorial (1874a), Bartholow's (1874b) contrite apology, and the *BMJ* editorial note (1874b). Bartholow's apology included an appeal to the Gage case: compared with the tamping iron, he had not expected the minimal stimulation he used with Mary Rafferty to cause deleterious effects. When Dupuy (1877a, pp. 85–86) revived the controversy, Bartholow (1877) replied again.

5. Horsley's first reported diagnostic use of electrical stimulation is Horsley 1884–1885; later reports are in Horsley 1886, 1887b, case 5. Horsley (1887a)

for the virtues of the method, and Keen (1888), Lloyd and Deaver (1888), and C. K. Mills (1889–1890, pp. 263, 270–272, 279–280, 283–284) for its adoption.

6. The first report of this pioneering operation and its sequel is in Bennett and Godlee 1884, 1885a. The full report is in Bennett and Godlee 1885b, and a condensed version in *Royal Medical and Chirurgical Society* 1885. The discussion to which Ferrier and Jackson contributed is in Bennett and Godlee 1882–1885, and Trotter's judgment of their achievement is in Trotter 1934. Power (1932), Trotter (1934), and Pearce (1982) all say that Jackson was present at the operation but in the contributions to the discussion, only Ferrier says he was there whereas Jackson's remarks read as if he were not. However, Jackson was supposedly close enough to the proceedings (psychologically at least) to have adapted Sydney Smith's jibe in something like the form of the joke that I have used as the epigraph to this chapter (Pearce 1982; cf. Jackson 1887).

7. Ferrier 1878a, 1878b for Gage. Macewen reports or discusses his case in three places (Macewen 1879, 1881, 1888). The stress on the "mental symptoms" occurs only in his 1888 overview of brain and spinal surgery. There is no mention of mental symptoms at all in the report of 1879, even though it is very much more detailed in all other respects, and they are not mentioned in the body of the 1881 report, especially in its concluding summary of "indications which led to a probable locus." For the moment, I accept Macewen's 1888 report as an accurate account of how he had weighed the diagnostic indicators nine years earlier.

8. Starr's series is Starr 1884a, 1884b. The other series, which are almost certainly not all that are in the literature of the period, are in Charcot 1876, [1876] 1878, [1876–1880] 1883; Pitres 1877; Bernhardt 1881, cited by Rylander 1939; Charcot and Pitres 1883; and Lewis 1883.

9. Macewen had already operated on his second case (here case 4) before Starr made his recommendation, of course.

10. McBurney and Starr's farmer patient is in McBurney and Starr 1893. Among the references they give for the number of frontal operations, Knapp's (1891) is described as containing "tables of all cases up to date of publication," and their other references are pre-1891. However, Knapp's table VIII and table IX list forty-six and twenty-six cases, respectively, making a total of seventy-two. Of these, eleven were cerebellar, and in thirteen the region where the tumor was located was not reported. McBurney and Starr mention another seven cases, some of which are post-1891, in their text, but even the addition of these (and their own case) does not result in a total of seventy-four cerebral cases. If the additional cases mentioned in their text are included, there may be eight frontal cases. Otherwise there are only six: the five from Knapp (three in table VIII and two in table IX) and their own.

11. Elder and Miles 1902.

12. In that his 1885 opinion was not much different from that of 1879, Gowers seems to have been skeptical from the beginning (cf. Gowers 1879, 1885, p. 146). C. K. Mills maintained the position he outlined in his address of 1889–1890, as a comparison with what he said in 1895 shows (C. K. Mills 1889–1890, 1895). I

do not know what Ferrier thought previously about the diagnostic value of changes like those Starr outlined and cannot determine whether what he said in his address marked a change of heart (Ferrier 1889–1890). Robertson's skepticism about localization, if not opposition to it, is in Robertson 1894 and 1896.

13. C. K. Mills 1889–1890 for the role played by the lack of relevant psychological categories.

14. Corporal G[eorge] W[ashington] S[tone] in Starr 1884a and U.S. Surgeon General's Office 1865, p. 15 and 1870, p. 205. My special thanks to Paul Sledzik, Curator of the Museum of the Armed Forces Institute of Pathology [AFIP], for beginning, and Grant Richards, 12th. Massachusetts Volunteers, for completing the identification of George Washington Stone and the particular action in which he was wounded. Corporal Stone's skull with the conoidal ball still embedded in it is AFIP specimen number 1108.

15. Starr 1884a for his interpretive summary of Burklin and the other cases. The original description of Burklin is in Prewitt 1873. Starr claimed that four of the cases of softening showed the characteristic change, but even though I have checked the original reports of all seven, I have been unable to identify the fourth. By exclusion it seems to be his case VIII, who is described in the original report, however, as suffering only "general debility" during the three weeks between his injury and death (U.S. Surgeon General's Office 1871, p. 123).

16. Ferrier 1878a and 1878b for inhibition and attention in relation to Gage and the other four cases.

17. Dandy 1933 for the "little peculiarities" and his opinion on the problems of tumor localization. His opinion was based on considerable experience in pioneering radical operations on the brain during the 1920s. Dandy there also spoke of "functions of the mind" being "stored" in the brain—a regression to a pre-Bain "cerebral closet" conceptualization that is worth noting.

11
Gage and Surgery for the Psyche

Such cases ... [open] ... the propriety of excising cortical areas as a method of treatment in insanity ...
—C. K. Mills's 1888 comment on an early brain operation for relieving hallucinations

There is a strong belief that Phineas Gage's case played an important role in the development of surgery for psychiatric conditions. However, we shall see that if his case played any role at all in the development of psychosurgery, it was because it corresponded to a number of observations that showed the frontal areas of the brain could be damaged or operated upon without marked effect on either the intellect or the vital processes. Nowhere does there seem to be evidence for any other contribution. Advocates of psychosurgery certainly did not argue that the kind of disinhibited behavioral change Gage had suffered accidentally was likely to benefit psychiatric patients were it induced deliberately.

I begin chapter 11 by considering the rationale for removing the areas of the brain thought to be responsible for the visual hallucinations and mood disorders of the first two patients on whom operations were performed for problems affecting the psyche. Both operations took place within three years of the Bennett and Godlee operation and used the same techniques. The Gage case played no role in their planning or execution. I then examine the bases of the operations Burckhardt and Lanphear conducted for treating more chronic and incapacitating psychiatric conditions and find that the Gage case was largely irrelevant to them also. The same is true of the radical resections like that used by Dandy on Joe A., and in showing that, I bring out the very gradual focusing of attention on the psychological consequences of those resections. An examination of the basis of the psychosurgical procedure known as leucotomy or lobotomy that Moniz invented and Freeman and Watts developed shows Gage to be irrelevant there, too. What the inventors wrote about their procedures, what some close observers have recalled about them, and what the more thoughtful histories of psycho-surgery spell out also attest this conclusion.

Surgery for Insanity

Shortly after beginning his 1888 address to the First Triennial Congress of American Physicians and Surgeons, C. K. Mills commented exten-sively on two then-recent operations as opening "a possible new field for surgical interference in insanity." The names of some of those involved are now familiar: the first was reported by Bennett and Gould in January 1887, and the second by Macewen in August 1888.

After a violent blow to the right side of the head, Bennett and Gould's patient had developed a scalp wound without apparent injury to the skull. Six weeks later he had the first of a series of unilateral left-sided convulsions with loss of consciousness that were to be repeated about once a week. After most of his attacks, he became so violent that eventually he was to spend three of the next six years in a mental hospital. Bennett reported that a nurse who witnessed one of his attacks observed that

on recovering, he was only partly conscious and very violent, rushed about the ward, shouted, called out to and threatened imaginary people, and, when held, struggled and hit out with his fists. In from half an hour to an hour he gradually calmed.... On interrogation he asserted he saw a bright red light in front of his eyes, soon after which he lost his senses. He had no recollection of any halluci-nations after the fits, but during them he certainly acted and spoke as if he saw people and other threatening objects.

Pressure on the scar which had formed at the site of the wound sometimes caused him to experience the light and to lose consciousness for a few seconds.

At the autopsy of an earlier case with similar hallucinations, Bennett had noted an injury to the "angular gyre." Bennett and Gould explored that area in this second patient but found nothing abnormal in the skull, the dura, or the cortex. During the next five months the patient earned his living in the same way as before the accident, some six years earlier, and had no further attacks. Neither Bennett nor Gould could explain why the symptoms had disappeared.

Macewen's operation was performed two years later. His patient had suffered a head injury, and he had eventually become melancholic and homicidal after a brief episode of psychic blindness. The operation exposed the angular gyrus and revealed a detached piece of bone exercising pressure "on the posterior portion of the supra-marginal convolution, while a corner of it penetrated and lay imbedded" in the brain. Macewen therefore replaced the bone in its proper position. The patient became "greatly relieved in his mental state though still excitable." He made "no further allusion to his homicidal tendencies."

C. K. Mills attributed the importance of these two cases to their opening up

the question of the propriety of excising cortical areas *in insanity* as well as of epilepsy, when certain subjective phenomena such as hallucinations of sight and hearing can be given a local habitation in the brain (emphasis added).

Mills could not know, of course, that a Swiss psychiatrist was already planning such operations, and that in a little over three months there would be an answer to his question.[1]

Burckhardt and Surgery for Psychiatric Patients

On 29 December 1888, Gottleib Burckhardt (1836–1907) commenced the first of a series of operations on six patients designed to modify symptoms that were the result of neither lesion nor trauma. In all six, Burckhardt undertook the procedures for purely psychiatric reasons, and he drew on an apparently extensive knowledge of localization for their rationale. Thus in operating on his first patient, Frau. Borel (his case 1), he decided to interrupt the pathways between the auditory and visual sensory areas and the motor areas. Borel was given to violent and impulsive motor behavior accompanied by verbal utterances initiated, Burckhardt thought, by visual hallucinations. Her movements were, he reasoned, due to a weakness of the natural barrier between the sensory and motor areas, and his operation would strengthen that barrier by removing a strip of cortical tissue between the two. However, the verbal utterances suggested the possible involvement of pathways to the verbal areas. Consequently the strip he removed was two centimeters wide and reached from the lateral part of the superior parietal convolution to the medial part of the supramarginal gyrus. Although Borel's behavior was less violent and impulsive after the operation, her verbalizations were still violent in tone and content and she still seemed to be hallucinating. In an endeavor to control these remaining symptoms, Burckhardt made four more excisions aimed at isolating the verbalizations, and after each one he judged there to have been improvement. She was, he finally reported, converted from a dangerous and excited demented person into a calm demented one.

Four of Burckhardt's other patients, his cases 3, 4, 5, and 6, had auditory hallucinations without accompanying motor behavior. Burckhardt therefore attempted to remove the supposed internal source of stimulation responsible for the hallucinations. In each he took this to be what he termed the auditory word field (Wernicke's area), but in one patient the auditory motor area (Broca's) was excised as well. Realizing that some form of aphasia might result, Burckhardt chose the risk of inflicting Wernicke's aphasia rather than Broca's because, he said, the person who could not say what he wanted was worse off than the person who didn't know that he didn't understand. Three patients had more than one operation and survived, but one died five days after the first operation. The survivors were somewhat improved, and aphasia was present only transiently or minimally after their operations.

Only in one of his operations, that on his case 2, did Burckhardt take frontal lobe function into consideration. The exception was the operation on Friedrich August N., a thirty-one-year-old lithographer. N. had been an intelligent student originally hospitalized many years earlier because of excitement and impulsive behavior, attributed at that time to masturbation, venery, and drink. After being discharged he had not settled and was admitted about a year before the operation, this time with "primary dementia." He was absorbed and without interest in his surroundings, had delusions of grandeur, was disobedient, and had episodes of excitement seemingly triggered by verbal-auditory hallucinations accompanied by the eyes and head turning to the right and the right leg being kicked out.

Burckhardt set out his diagnosis and operating strategy as follows:

> We are therefore dealing here with a completely developed chronic dementia in which stimulation turns the patient into an extremely troublesome and violent man. The task here, too, is to interrupt or obstruct the connections between the stimulating and executing areas of the cortex. I looked for the point of attack not between the central and sensory convolutions but between them and the forebrain because dementia paralytica brings with it a whole number of psychic symptoms that should, in my opinion be localised in the forebrain.

Burckhardt therefore decided to remove the lateral edge of the first and the foot of the second frontal convolutions, that is, excisions anterior to Broca's area. He carried out the operation on 17 April 1889, and although the patient seemed less excited and more interested in his surroundings, he developed epilepsy, and no more operations were performed.

Why Burckhardt decided that N.'s dementia was accompanied by more psychic symptoms than the disorders afflicting his other patients is no clearer than why he thought those symptoms involved the frontal lobes. He had an extensive knowledge of localization on which to draw a rationale for his operations. Burckhardt cited Welt and Jastrowitz on the frontal lobes but drew only on what they said about them to reinforce his very general argument that psychological functions were localized there. On the other hand, Burckhardt's operations were clearly influenced by his general argument about increasing the strength of the barrier between the sensory and motor areas and, as Fisher, O'Callaghan and Carroll, and Joanette have noted, by Goltz's observations of the placidity of dogs in whom the temporal cortex had been destroyed. Joanette adds that Mairet's argument that hypertrophy of temporal convolutions was responsible for auditory hallucinations may also have played a part. We note, however, that Burckhardt's operations on N.'s frontal lobes cannot be predicated on what Goltz or Mairet said about the temporal lobes.

We do know that Burckhardt did not mention Gage or cite anyone who wrote specifically on him, and did not draw directly on Ferrier's work on the frontal lobes. That is not to say Burckhardt did not know about Gage—it is most unlikely that Gage was not mentioned somewhere in the considerable literature Burckhardt cites—but we can be reasonably certain he gave no consideration to Gage's case in planning his surgery.[2]

Lanphear and Insanity Due to Softening of the Brain

By 1891 several reports had appeared on the surgical treatment of other forms of psychiatric disorder, and in 1895 Emory Lanphear described an operation of his own from about that time that was designed to cure insanity by removing brain tissue that had become soft because of a previous cerebral hemorrhage. Lanphear's patient had been left hemiplegic and partly aphasic, but the symptoms of which he complained were irritability, "a band-like sensation around the head," intense headaches, and uncontrollable impulses that had led him to make attempts on the life of his wife. Lanphear diagnosed softening in the region of the lower part of the Rolandic fissure, and possibly some part of the spheno-temporal lobe as well as some of the parietal convolutions. He explained to the patient that the operation he planned was "purely experimental" and had not even been proposed before. The patient agreed and the operation was performed on 27 June 1892.

On turning back the dura over the area to which he had been led, "there was disclosed a cloudy infiltrate in the pia and an apparent fluidity beneath" over the area of the third left frontal convolution. Piercing it caused a gush of about a pint of "broken-down brain and other *debris*" but no pus. The cavity was then washed and filled "as nearly full as possible" with "a sterilized salt solution," and the dura and scalp sewn up without drainage. The psychological symptoms disappeared almost immediately and had not recurred about three years later. The patient claimed better use of his leg, and, although his aphasia and arm paralysis had not altered, he was satisfied enough to send six other cases to Lanphear.

Lanphear's report also shows us that by 1891 surgical treatment of several other forms of psychiatric disorder had been attempted. Apart from Burckhardt's six operations and his own, Lanphear mentioned nine others: two for epileptic insanity (which he distinguished from epilepsy), two for syphilitic insanity, and five for general paresis (adding that for this condition "a large number of other operations have been recently published"). From the details he gave, the procedure involved trephining over the area the localizing signs suggested, breaking up adhesions and/or removing gummatous deposits in the dura and subarachnoidal space, and dusting the area with iodoform antiseptic powder. When this technique was applied early enough in general paresis, Lanphear believed it prevented "the spread of the trouble" from that part of the brain "which presides over the higher mental powers and ethical feelings" to motor and sensory areas. Lanphear, like Burckhardt, may have drawn on Gage for localizing these "higher" functions in the frontal lobes, but it is as clear that this was not a major consideration as it is that Lanphear was not operating on the frontal lobes themselves.

In concluding this section on the early surgical attempts to treat psychiatric disorders, the well-known but mysterious efforts of Ludvig Puusepp should be mentioned. In 1937 Puusepp reported that early in 1900 he had severed the connections between the frontal and parietal lobes in three manic-depressive patients. Because the success of the procedure was "rather poor," Puusepp abandoned it, and no one seems to have followed up on it. It is often implied that the influence that led

Puusepp to these operations was Burckhardt, but I have been unable to find out if the operations were so inspired or had some other rationale. Although Puusepp's work is often mentioned, Gage seems never to be associated with it in any specific way. If he was, it would be the last time before the beginning of the modern era of psychosurgery some thirty years later.[3]

Radical Resection as a Basis for Psychosurgery

A major contribution to psychosurgery came from the radical resections conducted by Dandy, who, by at least 1922, had concluded that 80 percent of brain tumors were nonencapsulated gliomata that invariably recurred. He therefore raised the question of whether radical resection of the lobes in which tumors were embedded should not be undertaken rather than merely removing the tumors *from* the tissue. By that time, he had successfully conducted ten such operations, removing all or substantial parts of the right and left frontal lobes, right temporal or right occipital lobes, and in two instances, both lobes. Even before Dandy's proposal, in August 1914, McCaw had already removed virtually the whole of a right tempero-sphenoidal lobe because of gangrene. Within the next ten years several more such radical operations were performed by O'Brien, Spurling, and Penfield and Evans, as well as a number by Dandy himself.

The Effects of Radical Resection

Two things are remarkable about these very radical early operations. The first was their seemingly slight physiological effects, the second was how little attention was paid to their psychological consequences. Although McCaw had devoted a paragraph to elaborating on the preoperative condition of his patient as a "worthless, irresponsible, irritable, and cruel fellow" who was "queer," "not mentally balanced," and "a moral and mental pervert," he used only about half that number of words to describe his improved postoperative "mental condition" and the fact that he had become a "reliable and fairly good citizen."

When making his 1922 plea, Dandy reported even more briefly and generally: "We have removed an entire right or left frontal lobe without any observable mental or other after-effect." Occipital removal had produced visual symptoms, but in the three cases in which Broca's area had

been removed, apparently completely, there was only a temporary aphasia. On Dandy's admittedly rather crude assessment, there was little or
no apparent change in mental state, and certainly nothing deleterious,
even when sensory and motor symptoms were present.

In the late 1920s and early 1930s more systematic and detailed studies
of the consequences of these radical procedures, including the psychological, began to be made and or reported. The beginning of the change
may be illustrated by the differences between Dandy's report on the three
cases of right hemisphere removal common to his 1928 and 1933
reports, and Joe A., on whom he operated in August 1930 but whose
case Brickner reported in 1934. Of Mr. R. F., on whom he operated
in April 1923, Dandy said in his preliminary report of 1928 only that
despite his being "repeatedly examined" before discharge, "there did not
seem to be any obvious mental impairment." In contrast, in 1933 Dandy
gave almost as much detail of the verbatim conversations, from which it
was possible to judge his conclusion about the mental effects, as he did of
the neurological sequelae. The same was true of Mrs. A. S., whom Dandy
operated on in October 1927, and, allowing for the fact that he died two
weeks later, the unidentified male patient Dandy operated on in March
1927. O'Brien's 1932 report of his patient, who was operated on in
August 1931, is at an intermediate stage. O'Brien provided an enormous
amount of postoperative neurological detail on his patient, although he
said little about her psychological state other than that she showed no
mental impairment or emotional instability.

One also notes that by his 1933 report, Dandy presented his cases in a
context of the value they had for knowledge of localization of function.
We saw in the last chapter that his conclusion about the results of tumor
analyses pointed to a paradox similar to that which Leny had noted.
Dandy similarly criticized the conclusions to be drawn from such degenerative processes as had led Broca to implicate the third left frontal convolution in aphasia, and from animal experiments, especially those Goltz
conducted. His conclusion? "The only accurate and safe data concerning
most cerebral functions can come from extirpations of parts of the
human brain."

But as Dandy said of his three patients:

The presentation of these three cases with extirpation of such vast areas of brain
tissue without the disclosure of any resulting defect is most disappointing. It is
still difficult to believe that some functions of the mind are not stored or at least
are not activated there.

Although none of the relatives of R. F. or A. S. had noticed anything deleterious, Dandy allowed, as we have seen, that those in frequent contact with the patients might have picked up such "little peculiarities of mental origin" as those shown by Phineas Gage.

Dandy also seemed to imply that more comprehensive and subtle mental examination might identify the effects of his operations. If so, his requirement was met over the next few years by the psychometric testing and mental state examination of some of the lobectomy patients seen between 1928 and 1931 by Penfield and Evans, in 1933 by Ackerly, and especially by the very detailed daily record of the behavior of Brickner's patient known as Joe A., whom Dandy operated on in August 1930. All but Ackerly's patient were reported on in 1932, at that year's Annual Meeting of the Association for Research on Nervous and Mental Disease.

By the early 1930s, then, attention was firmly directed to the psychological consequences of radical resection, especially of the frontal lobes. And of all the patients reported on up to that time, Brickner's patient Joe A. was the most important in Moniz's development of psychosurgical leucotomy.[4]

Brickner's Patient, Joe A.

Joe A. had been a successful stockbroker on the New York Stock Exchange until increasingly severe headaches began in the summer of 1929. Memory impairment and absentmindedness followed, and he went into a coma a year later. On his admission to the hospital, a frontal tumor was diagnosed. Dandy operated, and upon discovering that a meningioma had invaded the frontal lobes, removed almost the whole of the right and left frontal lobes. About a year later Joe A. came under Brickner's care at the New York Neurological Institute. He underwent comprehensive postoperation psychological testing, but the most valuable observations came from the extensive and almost daily observations made by Brickner himself or one of his associates in Joe A.'s own home.

Four aspects of Joe A.'s behavior were especially notable. First, on casual meeting he sometimes appeared mentally normal. On one occasion he toured the New York Neurological Institute in the company of two eminent visiting neurologists, who failed to recognize that there was anything wrong with him. Behavior of this kind was restricted to situations in which few demands were placed on him and in which he could get by with generalities. Second, almost everything he said and did was directed to showing his superiority over others. This "unremitting" self-aggrandizement was usually little more than crude boasting but also involved his ridiculing those with whom he was comparing himself. According to his friends, before the operation he never said anything bad about others and had been "anything but a braggart." Third, he frequently expressed hostility toward others, a tendency that sometimes led to "frankly infantile tantrums." Many of these were over self-care for, although he could care for himself, he required constant urging to ensure that he dressed and undressed himself, tied his shoe laces, bathed, and so forth. Fourth, Joe A.'s general conversation was "frequently interspersed with comments manifesting his sexual vigor," even though he made no sexual advances to women and had become almost incapable of normal sexual functioning. His sexual activity consisted of masturbation or ejaculating by rubbing his penis on his wife's abdomen.

In beginning his explanation of the changes, Brickner cited the inhibitory theses of Starr and Elder and Miles (which we have seen to have derived from Ferrier), Harlow's formulation about the balance between Gage's "intellectual faculties and animal propensities" having been destroyed, and several other interpretations that had it that frontal damage liberated instincts and impulses. He rejected all such explanations. Instead, he deliberately avoided what he called "the many sided term" of inhibition altogether, and just as deliberately he adopted the term "restraint." Brickner tried to derive Joe A.'s lack of restraint from a more fundamental loss, that of his synthesizing activity.

What Brickner termed a lack of synthesis was a fundamental inability to form complex associations from simple ones. Although Joe A. understood both old and new material, he could not "synthesize simple thought processes into more complex structures." Brickner started with the puerility that he claimed marked "practically every expression and act" of Joe A. Comparing the mental processes of children and adults, he claimed that Joe A. differed from a child in that he had knowledge but did not or could not use it. The child simply lacked knowledge. Joe A.'s more purely intellectual pursuits, including his puns, his jokes, and his associations, were also like the simple ones of a child. So also were his tantrums. Clearly, Joe A. had once possessed the knowledge that enabled him to behave in a socially acceptable way, and just as clearly still had it. In those situations where social relations were superficial, and vague generalities of speech and conduct adequate, he could still behave appropriately. More complex situations revealed his failure to use what knowledge he had. His difficulty was in relating the need for restraint to particular situations and behaviors where it would have been appropriate. His restraint was therefore not completely absent, merely weakened.

Although many of Joe A.'s symptoms had an emotional coloring, Brickner found "nothing to indicate an emotional disturbance in a primary sense." Nor was intellectual disturbance primary. The frontal lobes played no essential role in intellectual function; they merely added to intellectual intricacy, and were "not intellectual centers in any sense except, perhaps, a quantitative one." More generally, neither in those aspects of his mental life in which emotion was definitely present (e.g., the need to demonstrate his superiority), nor in those in which it was definitely absent (e.g., in arithmetical calculation) were any of the usual functions missing. In the former he merely lacked "usual adult restraint in concealing his apparently normal feelings"; in the latter he was simply easily distracted from pursuing an action or a line of thought to a conclusion. In this respect at least, Brickner echoed Harlow by concluding that because none of Joe A.'s functions was completely impaired, the changes "were fundamentally not qualitative but quantitative in nature."

Animal Experiments on Frontal Ablation

Beginning with Hitzig and Ferrier, the nineteenth century had seen a good deal of work on the effects of removing the frontal lobes on the general behavior of animals. Although different investigators used different methods, different descriptive terms, and different explanatory concepts, there was broad agreement about the effects of frontal ablation. With the exception of Bianchi's frontal studies, however, little work of this kind on complex animals like dogs and monkeys continued into the twentieth century—and Bianchi's work began in 1888, in the Ferrier era. Consequently, when interest in the psychological and behavioral effects of radical resection developed in the 1920s, Bianchi's highly regarded 1922 book on frontal function in the dog and monkey offered practically the only modern evidence to which the human observations could be related.[5]

Jacobsen and Fulton
Bianchi's work had been based on naturalistic observational methods and was incapable of identifying the effects of the operations in other

than a fairly gross way. Rather like Ferrier, Bianchi found it difficult to describe the resulting behavioral changes precisely. Partly as a consequence, in 1934, Jacobsen and his associates began experimenting with the effects of ablation on various kinds of learning and problem solving. They took advantage of a number of developments in comparative psychology and trained their subjects on tasks believed to be sensitive to frontal damage. After operating, they compared specific aspects of the animal's performance with what they had been like before.

Two of their chimpanzee subjects, the females known as Becky and Lucy, provided quite specific although unforeseen impetus to the development of psychosurgery. Both were trained on a number of tasks, one of which required delaying a response to a problem, and another assembling the elements of the solution to a problem while part of the solution had to be held in memory. In the delayed-responding experiments, the animals were first shown food being placed under one of two cups. A screen was then lowered preventing further sight of the cups. After a variable interval the screen was raised and the animals allowed to choose one cup. Normal chimpanzees could still make the right choice after delays of more than five minutes. The other problem required the chimpanzees to coordinate their movements between two platforms and use each of a number of sticks in a set order to reach some fruit. The learning began with a single platform and four sticks. Only the first short stick was within arm's reach but with it the next longest stick could be reached, and with it the third. With the third, the fourth stick and the fruit could be obtained. After mastering that problem the task was made more difficult by having two platforms with a single stick on one platform and the food on the other. The third level of difficulty had the sticks distributed differently between the two platforms such that the chimpanzees had to move alternatively from one to the other. The solution required the animal to solve the problem of which particular stick it needed to choose without the other sticks and the food necessarily being in sight.

After months of training, one frontal lobe was removed without performance on the tasks being much affected. After intensive observation and testing to make sure that that was the case, the other lobe was removed. Only at that point were there significant effects. They were very different in the two animals. Before the training began, Becky was described as volatile in temperament, loving, affectionate, and highly dependent upon reassurances from the humans around her. She coped reasonably well with the stick problem but had been unable to solve the delayed response problem at other than very short delays. Her failures gradually resulted in more and more severe "temper tantrums," and as time went on, she became more disturbed, finally refusing to enter the cage for testing. The first operation produced no change, but after the second she took part eagerly in the experiments and showed no upset at failure. She also became much less dependent on people. On the other hand, Lucy had been calm, unexcitable, and able to tolerate delay as well as occasional errors. However, after the second operation, she became prone to severe tantrums when she failed, as she inevitably did.

Jacobsen and Fulton took Becky's uncooperative behavior to be "as complete an 'experimental neurosis' as those obtained by Pavlov," that is, a generalized disturbance of behavior and conditional reflex activity induced by the difficulty of the task. It almost certainly was not such. However, that term and the changes induced by the ablation seem to have convinced some that frontal ablation either prevented a neurosis from developing or cured it. Moniz may have been one of many to make these mistakes. If he did so, in evaluating the significance of Becky's "cure," he and others who had similarly erred had to overlook how differently the same procedure had changed Lucy.[6]

Moniz and Frontal Surgery for Psychoses

The new operation for the treatment of psychoses called prefrontal *leucotomy* that Moniz announced in 1936 is now recognized as marking the beginning of psychosurgery. Soon to become better known as *lobotomy*, it severed, or at least disrupted, the connections between the prefrontal areas and the rest of the brain. On the three different occasions between 1936 and 1948 when Moniz discussed the basis for his procedure, he gave three slightly different sets of arguments, which he called "considerations," for it. His arguments are hard to evaluate because the kind of evidence he cited tended to vary and he failed to relate much of it specifically to his conclusion. Much of it was therefore of doubtful relevance. For example, he said different things at different times about the physiological "evidence" for the way in which the elements of the nervous system were connected: Cajal's concept of the synapse, Held's bundles, and the work of Pavlov. His citing clinical evidence about frontal lobe damage (e.g., Kleist's series of cases) showed a similar lack of relevance. The erratic nature of Moniz's arguments is quite well-known, but I do not believe that the logic that led him to the frontal areas has been adequately examined. When this is done, we shall see that Gage could have figured, at most, only incidentally in these considerations.

The basic considerations to be found in Moniz's three early publications can be fairly set out as follows:

1. Normal psychological functioning depends upon a proper and flexible functioning of the connections between nerve cells.

2. Mental disease is due to a derangement of connections. A "fixity" of the connections is the particular derangement that causes the persistence of the morbid ideas found in obsessional and depressive states.

3. Morbid ideas are "deeply submerged" in the complex of connections and continually stimulate the complex into "a continual state of live activity."

4. To alter the morbid ideas, the connections have to be altered.

5. Psychological activity depends on an increased number of highly varied neurons.

6. Psychological activity is especially associated with the frontal lobes, although it could not be said to be localized there.

7. Damage to the frontal lobes has only transitory effects, and there are never any deleterious psychological effects from it or from tumors that develop in them unless the corpus callosum is involved.

Moniz described in 1948 how he had then made a jump:

Guided by this reasoning, and having for over two years spent my every spare moment in reflection on the matter, at the same time weighing my responsibilities, I came to the decision that I would undertake to cut the fibers *joining the active neurons.* Inasmuch as I was convinced of *the importance* of the prefrontal lobes in mental activity, I *chose* this region for the experiments. (emphasis added)

Although the general lack of logic in Moniz's argument was remarked on at the time and has frequently been commented upon since, especially by Valenstein, I do not believe the leap to the frontal areas has been scrutinized to the same extent.

Analyzing Moniz's run-up, we see that the last two considerations—the association of psychological activity with the frontal lobes and the transitory effects of damage to them—really provide his takeoff. Up to the fifth consideration, Moniz was not traveling in any particular direction, and the Gage case does seem to have given him an explicit final direction. Moniz does not mention Gage directly, nor are there references to him in any of the literature he cites. Of course, considerations six and seven may imply some knowledge of Gage. If Moniz did so use Gage, that use was, like his supposed preference for Becky over Lucy, an extremely ambiguous one: Gage did recover from his accident, but the changes in him could hardly be overlooked. In any case, considerations six and seven stand apart from Moniz's basic premises about the physiological basis of thinking and his assertions about what cutting the connecting fibers would do.

The first procedure Moniz used to disconnect the active neurons was to inject 0.2 cc of alcohol into the white fibrous tissue in each of the frontal lobes and destroy the nerve fibers there by dehydration. Moniz soon abandoned alcohol for a method that severed the connections mechanically. For this purpose he used a leucotome, an adaptation of a traditional surgical instrument, the trocar, that allowed tissue at some site in the body to be cut from the tissue surrounding it without doing other than minimal damage on the way to the site. Lima, Moniz's surgeon, drilled holes in top of the skull above each frontal lobe and inserted the leucotome a predetermined depth through one of them. When the plunger on the handle was depressed, a small wire loop was extended at the tip of the leucotome, so that when the handle was now rotated, the loop created a "core" of tissue disconnected from the tissue surrounding it. The procedure, at that point called leucotomy, was repeated successively through each hole. In Moniz's first operation, there was one hole above each lobe, and hence two cores. Very soon the creation of multiple cores, sometimes as many as four in each lobe, became standard.

Moniz fairly sprinted to publicize his results. On 3 March 1936, within four months of the first operation on 12 November 1935, he described the outcome in the first twenty cases at a meeting in Paris. Seven patients were said to be "cured," seven "ameliorated," and six "unchanged." By June 1936 his monograph had appeared, and he published five more articles by the end of the year, all on the same twenty cases. During 1937 another eighteen operations were performed and Moniz reported on them in another six papers and a book that appeared that year. Most responses to Moniz's work were uncritically favorable, but some were not. Criticisms were made of the short follow-up periods, averaging, for example, eleven days after the last operation in four of the seven who were said to be "cured." The pre- and postoperation descriptions of the symptoms were brief, casual, and based on quite inadequate standards. It also turned out later that some of the diagnoses were altered after the operation. Some claims were totally unsupported; for example, Moniz offered no evidence for his assertion that memory and intelligence were unimpaired, and included patients who suffered severe negative changes in his "unchanged" category. Hence Cobb wrote "the reports are so meagre that one cannot judge the work.... Only 1 of the 20 cases is given in enough detail to allow the reader to judge for himself as to the diagnosis and the result." Valenstein describes how eleven years later, Diego Furtado, a neurologist who was coauthor with Moniz of a paper on the method presented in 1937, dismissed the therapeutic results in the series as "slight."

Not surprisingly, Moniz made no assessment of whether the operation changed the fixity of the connections. If Moniz's "considerations" can be taken as an index, he had no head for theory, and would not have known where to begin to test that proposition. What he had so loosely strung together around this most central of his propositions was far from constituting a theory. Many said his belief in fixity was naive. According to Valenstein, as early as 1937, at the first discussion of Moniz's results, Sobral Cid, the psychiatrist who had reluctantly allowed Moniz access to his first few patient subjects, went further to brand it as "pure cerebral mythology."[7]

Freeman and Psychosurgery

As far as I can determine, the one person who gave the Gage case any consideration in the development of psychosurgery was Walter Freeman, an American neuropathologist, and that was primarily at a press conference prior to announcing the results of his first operations on the frontal lobes. Gage neither figures in Freeman's publications prior to 1942, when *Psychosurgery*, which he coauthored with Watts, appeared, nor appears in Freeman's unpublished *Autobiography*, written in 1970.

Early in 1936, Freeman came across Moniz's first paper, obtained the monograph as soon as it became available, and discussed his work with James Winston Watts, a neurosurgeon colleague. Both were convinced of the value of Moniz's procedure, and decided to use it themselves. They ordered leucotomes and commenced operating as soon as they had mastered the technique. Because Freeman and Watts believed the operation destroyed cell bodies as well as nerve fibers, they decided *lobotomy* was a more appropriate name, and had no hesitation in developing operations that damaged more of the white matter than had Moniz. They also coined the term *psychosurgery*.

The press conference at which Freeman mentioned Gage was held on 21 November 1936, a few hours before he presented his paper on the results of the first prefrontal lobotomies. Freeman's account of what he said to the reporters reads as if Gage were an afterthought. The City Editor of the *News Post* (Baltimore) knew that Thomas Henry of the *Washington Evening Star* had prepared a story in conjunction with Freeman, and he had been pursuing Freeman for details for his own story. Freeman had not been prepared to speak to him, and gave the following account of the remarks he made:

on the morning of the meeting on which our presentation was to be given I stayed away from the lecture hall most of the time but Griffiths sought me out, took me to the press room, and told me to talk while he took notes. Three other reporters came in at the same time. I got all wound up and proceded to give a lengthy history of the functions of the frontal lobe; the results of the crowbar being driven through the skull in a man some sixty years ago; the symptoms resulting from disease of the frontal lobes; the war wounds and their effect on character; the experimental evidence produced by physiologists in their work on monkeys; and finally the work of Moniz. Then I pleaded that it was time for the paper to be given and I really had to be there. So with diversion and delaying tactics I escaped, and, at the same time, gave Mr. Henry his chance. He had come in during the time the interview was progressing and at first looked a little shocked but caught on as I went into detailed consideration of inconsequentialities.

Circumstances had virtually forced Freeman to make more of Gage for the press than he intended but we know that Gage remained inconsequential enough not to figure in the story by Henry or in those by anyone else from the press conference. Although Freeman probably also mentioned Gage to Waldemar Kaempffert, the science writer who later publicized the operation, Gage is not referred to in his or other accounts.

We cannot be sure what Freeman told the press about Gage. I think it likely he said only that his case showed that frontal damage could cause mental symptoms, and that trauma to the lobes was not life threatening. Certainly all he and Watts said in the first edition of *Psychosurgery* was that Gage was "the most famous" case of accidental injury to the frontal lobes that was followed by "mental symptoms." Although Freeman described the Gage case in some detail, drawing directly on Harlow's 1868 paper, he did not expand on the reference to those or other symptoms. Nor did he connect Gage's case to the new operation. Then as if to emphasize Gage's irrelevance, reference to him was dropped from the second edition.

Additionally, when Freeman and Watts published *Psychosurgery: Intelligence, Emotion and Social Behavior following Prefrontal Lobotomy for Mental Disorders* in 1942, they explicitly rejected Moniz's thesis that psychoses were due to fixed connections or abnormally stable synaptic patterns. Stereotyped thoughts were not basic to the psychoses, and they proposed an anatomically better-supported substitute. Histological studies showed the frontal areas were connected to the thalamus and hypothalamus, and physiological studies identified the two latter structures as central to emotional life. They thought lobotomy interrupted the connections between the cognitive and emotional "areas" of the personality, a disconnection noticeable in the blunted affect and lowered anxiety it often produced. Although the frontal lobes retained their importance in their theory, it was in a very different sense from Moniz. And Gage was important to neither.[8]

The Histories of Psychosurgery

In the general neuroscientific, psychiatric, and psychological literature it is widely believed that the Gage case gave rise fairly directly to lobotomy. Those literatures often simply juxtapose the topics of Gage and lobotomy, sometimes in an explicit context of brain "therapies." Connections are also established through citing Gage as an accidental lobotomy or by drawing attention to the similarity between the changes Harlow saw in Gage and the symptoms seen after psychosurgery. Others set out an explicit although single line of development from Gage to Moniz *via* Joe A. and the Jacobsen monkey experiments. There are less complete lines around which is woven the claim that lobotomy resulted in "thousands" or "tens of thousands" of Phineas Gages. In one paper a Gage-Brickner-Moniz line is separated from the Jacobsen-Moniz, and the former is judged to be a "possible" influence and the latter as "probably no less important."[9]

Actually, most accounts of psychosurgery that cover something of its history mention Gage not at all or only in passing. No one accords him a prominent place. This is as true of the shorter papers as it is of the major histories. My tracing the role of Gage in the following brief chronology of the significant steps in the development of psychosurgery draws on my own reading of most of the original works, filled out by some details from the major works, especially from that of Valenstein.[10]

Moniz claimed to have spent several years thinking about psychosurgery before arranging for the first leucotomy to be performed. There is, however, no evidence, published or otherwise, that this was so. He was well known as a neurologist, having invented the diagnostic technique of cerebral angiography (the injection into the carotid artery of substances opaque to X-rays that would reveal the defects in cerebral blood flow caused by tumors and the like). Although not a psychiatrist, Moniz saw many psychiatric patients whose problems he was inclined to explain and treat somatically. His more general belief was that progress in psychiatric treatment had to be somatically based.

In August 1935 Moniz attended the Second International Congress of Neurology in London, primarily to present a large exhibit on angiography. His exhibition was close to Freeman's on ventriculography and the two met for the first time. Both attended an all-day symposium on the frontal lobes. In it, Brickner and Penfield described the long-term effects on the personalities of the small number of patients on whom they had performed radical frontal lobe resections in order to remove tumors, and Jacobsen presented his work with Fulton on frontal ablation in chimpanzees. Brickner gave a full report on Joe A. and repeated his conclusion that Joe A.'s functions were impaired quantitatively rather than qualitatively. Moniz seems to have regarded this difference as unimportant and judged Joe A. to be better off than most psychiatric patients. He evaluated the effects on the other patients in a similarly sanguine way, apparently ignoring those aspects of the reports that elicited caution from others. I have the impression that it was because Brickner's "quantitative" description matched some slightly later remarks by Penfield about the relative lack of impairment of one of his patients that Moniz came to "consider" that frontal lobe damage was transitory and psychologically nondeleterious.

Jacobsen's presentation included the essentially incidental observations that bilateral removal had made Becky calmer and able to tolerate failure, but Lucy had changed the opposite way. According to Fulton, who was chairing the session, after Jacobsen had finished, Moniz rose to ask whether the surgical methods that had prevented the development of what he took to be Becky's experimental neurosis could be used to relieve anxiety states in humans. In Fulton's account, these frontal ablation experiments provided Moniz with the rationale for his operation. As against this, Pressman argues convincingly that the story of Becky and the Moniz operation is little more than a founding myth actually created by Fulton. It is certainly true that Moniz did not acknowledge the Fulton–Jacobsen experiments in his first paper on the new procedure, and for a time seems to have denied them any role at all. Parable status would also explain the oddity of Freeman's quoting Fulton's description of how Moniz reacted to the Becky story rather than describing it as something he himself had heard in the discussion. About the only thing of which we can be certain is that Moniz began planning his operations immediately on returning to Portugal after the symposium.

On the other hand, Moniz acknowledged the importance of Joe A. from the beginning. He accepted Brickner's identification of Joe A.'s primary symptom as his inability to build up or synthesise complex mental structures from simple ones and singled out his overall conclusion for special endorsement: "Brickner considère les fonctions psychiques de ce malade plus altérées en quantité qu'en qualité." If Moniz's consideration of Gage is somewhere submerged in that of Joe A., he must have aligned the two cases even more grossly than Ferrier and Starr did in their comparisons.

Many of those who conducted radical resections for the removal of tumors explicitly rejected the comparison with Gage. Thus when Bond asked Ackerly if he had compared the "mental results" in his 1933 case "with those in the Harvard crowbar case," Ackerly replied:

I think that there was so much irritation from scar tissue in that case that it makes it difficult to compare it with the cases we have had recently—those of Dr. Brickner, Dr. Spurling and others where there are clean-cut amputations of frontal lobe tissue rather than traumatic scar tissue.

He went on to point out that in his patient (whom he referred to as Spurling's case because Spurling had done the operation), there were three quite different sets of "mental signs" in each of the three stages of the operation.

Even with the cleaner operating techniques it was still difficult to compare any one of the 1930s patients with another. For example, Penfield believed the changes in his patients were "difficult to correlate" with those of German and Fox. Similarly, Brickner was very reluctant to compare Joe A.'s behavior with that of lobectomized animals. He was prepared to say merely that Joe A. resembled "in a very general way, some of the reported instances of animals with bilateral frontal lobe extirpation." It is reasonable to suppose that he and Penfield would have shared Ackerly's doubt about the use of Gage as a standard, a comparison even less warranted because Gage did not figure in their presentations at all. Fifteen years later, when all the 1932 pioneers were present (together with Freeman and Watts) at the 1947 "anniversary" meeting of the Association for Research in Nervous and Mental Disease to discuss the frontal lobes again, no one mentioned Gage.

The personal accounts of those with first-hand knowledge of some of the early cases of prefrontal lobotomy confirm the impression that the Gage case did not contribute to psychosurgery directly. Thus E. R. Hilgard, Emeritus Professor of Psychology at Stanford University, who carried out conditioning studies on one of the patients on whom German and Fox performed a unilateral lobectomy for the relief of epilepsy, told me that all he recalls knowing about Gage in the 1930s is that he survived the massive damage. Walle Nauta, Emeritus Professor of Neuroanatomy at the Massachusetts Institute of Technology, who worked for many years on the anatomical connections of the frontal lobes with other brain structures, and with Teuber and others on the Columbia-Greystone Associates project assessing the effects of psychosurgical lobotomy, confirmed this impression. The report of that project expresses the same opinion. On the other hand, Jasper's published historical perspective on lobotomy begins with Gage. Jasper learned about Gage as a graduate student of psychology in the late 1920s when Harlow's "charming account of the effect of lesions of the anterior frontal lobes" gave him, he said, his "first impression" of their importance. However, after describing his own work and that of his colleagues, Jasper concludes with his only other mention of Phineas: that it was with his case that the observations on frontal function began. Hence despite his title and opening remarks suggesting a connection between Gage and lobotomy, Jasper gives the very strong impression that Gage's case provided only a background to the development of the procedure.[11]

Conclusion

There is no evidence that the changes in Gage were among the considerations that gave rise to psychosurgery. Frontal symptoms were not relevant for the psychiatric surgery conducted by Bennett and Macewen, by Gould, or by Lanphear, and none of them implied that the Gage case came into their considerations. Neither does it seem to have played more than a minor role in Burckhardt's consideration of the one operation where he thought frontal pathology was present. It also seems unlikely that knowledge of it was a factor in the operation planned by Moniz, and it was more important to the publicity campaign Freeman conducted than to his version of Moniz's procedure. Consequently there is no evidence that Gage's case contributed directly to psychosurgery. That is, no one argued that psychiatric patients would benefit from having disinhibited behaviors like his deliberately induced in them. As with surgery for the brain generally, what his case did show came solely from his surviving his accident: major operations could be performed on the brain without the outcome necessarily being fatal.

It is also very evident from the way Burckhardt and Moniz weighed the evidence in planning their psychosurgery, and from the way symptoms were evaluated in diagnosing frontal tumors, that the very indeterminacy in defining sensory-motor functions allowed almost any argument to be mounted, however illogical, speculative, or distorted, to situate almost any psychological function in the frontal areas. What we see historically in the varied and somewhat inconsistent descriptions of frontal lobe functions are functions that could not be fitted into that framework. That there is still variation and inconsistency in assigning functions to the frontal lobes today is because, I think, there is still no adequate alternative to the sensory-motor framework.

The most that the Gage case indicated was that radical operations on the brain were possible. Why had his symptoms failed to provide a reliable guide for conventional frontal lobe surgery? Partly it was because there were many cases of tumor in which there were no symptoms at all, or only very subtle ones, and partly it was because there was no comprehensive and agreed-on theory for interpreting such changes as did occur. Evaluating the effects of radical resection was similarly difficult. Although sensory-motor physiology and psychology seem to have provided the most popular explanatory concepts, not everyone used them. For example, Brickner preferred "restraint" over "inhibition" because the latter was too vague and general ("many-sided"). Consequently is it surprising that the changes in Gage were given no consideration in the development of psychosurgery? Establishing anyone's parentage with certainty is always difficult and is made more so when descent cannot be traced through the maternal ancestral line. Becky and Lucy have to be ruled out as the mothers of leucotomy—they do not even seem to have shared the role of foster-mother. The father of Moniz's leucotomy seems easier to identify—it is probably Joe A. About Gage's relationship we can be quite certain: he was at most on a remote side-branch of the ancestors of surgery for the psyche.

Notes

1. The two cases on which C. K. Mills (1889–1890) comments are in Bennett and Gould 1887 and Macewen 1888.

2. The sequentially numbered cases are reported in Burckhardt 1891, and I have to thank Elfreide Ihsen for translating the relevant parts of Burckhardt's monograph-length paper for me. Burckhardt's rationale and operations are sometimes described differently, but I cannot see where my account, which is consistent with Lanphear's (1895) contemporaneous reference, is in error. Whitaker, Stemmer, and Joanette (1996) note the extent of Burckhardt's knowledge of the localization literature, and Fisher (1951), O'Callaghan and Carroll (1982), and Joanette (1990) all note the importance Burckhardt gave Goltz's findings.

3. Lanphear 1895 for his procedures. For Puusepp himself see Walker 1951 and Lichterman 1998. Typically brief mentions of his work are in Fisher 1951, Tow 1955, and O'Callaghan and Carroll 1982. Valenstein (1986 p. 44) gives slightly more detail, including the date of 1900 for the frontal-parietal severance and 1910 for a later treatment in which Puusepp applied chemicals under the dura to the brains of paretics with notable improvement.

4. Dandy's argument for radical resections is in Dandy 1922, and his later amendment to 60 percent barely changes its force (Dandy 1966, p. 485). McCaw 1919 for his radical procedure, with the other examples being Dandy 1928, 1933; Spurling 1929; O'Brien 1932; Penfield and Evans 1934, 1935; Brickner 1934, 1936; and Ackerly 1935. Association for Research on Nervous and Mental Disease 1934 for the 1932 annual meeting. By 1922 imaging techniques had reduced the reliance on localizing signs: X-rays (1901), ventriculography (1918), pneumoencephalography (1919), and positive contrast myelography (1921). Angiography came (from Moniz) in 1927. My datings for these techniques are from Walker 1951, Dandy 1966, and Bull 1982.

5. Brickner's shorter account of Joe A. is Brickner 1934. There is also a longer account in Brickner 1936. Bianchi 1922.

6. I have not been able to see what Jacobsen said about Becky and Lucy in his 1935 report to the London symposium, but a later version is in Crawford et al. 1948. That and other chimpanzee work is in Jacobsen, Wolfe, and Jackson 1935, and Jacobsen with Elder, and Haselrud 1936. Denny-Brown 1951 gives a good summary of the experiments without mentioning "experimental neurosis," and Willett's (1960) negative appreciation of the therapy of such neuroses by lobectomy is basically correct but for the odd reason that he does not believe in the concept of experimental neurosis. Among those who endorse the "experimental neurosis" interpretation are Browder (1941), Tow (1955), and Adey (1974). One of Fulton's blunders over the concept is in Fulton 1949b, and Valenstein (1986, p. 112) cites another.

7. See Valenstein 1986, chap. 4, 5, and 6, for much of the detail I give about Moniz's operation; the various "considerations" are in Moniz 1936a, 1936b, [1948] 1954, and others in Freeman n.d.; Moniz's "jump" is in the last of his publications listed here. Willett 1960; O'Callaghan and Carroll 1982, pp. 9–10, 216–218; Shutts 1982; and Valenstein 1986, pp. 80–100 for Moniz's arguments; none comment particularly on his forward leap. Valenstein (1986, pp. 118–121, 163–164) mentions the contemporary theoretical discussions, and the many reports of frontal operations, other than Moniz's, that suggest the frontal lobes had become "popular" by the early 1930s. Cobb's reservation is in Cobb 1940, see also 1943.

8. Valenstein (1986, chap. 7 and 8) is also the source of much of my detail about Freeman and Watts. Freeman's own account of his work in psychosurgery is in a carbon copy of an undated and untitled typescript held by the Paul Himmelfarb Health Sciences Library of the George Washington University Medical Center. Evidently there were at least seven chapters, but chapters II and III are now missing. Unfortunately they seem to be the very ones in which Freeman discussed the factors that led him to adopt and develop Moniz's operation. Further, because the carbon paper between the first and the copy page accidentally folded back as one of the pages of chapter IV was being typed, some crucial information is missing from Freeman's description of the press conference. The incomplete and defective copy of Freeman's typescript seems to be the only one in existence. I have to thank Franklin Freeman, Walter Freeman's son, for his efforts in trying to find the original or another copy, and for telling me that his father did not write about Gage in his unpublished *Autobiography* or his pre-1942 published work. Incidentally, Valenstein (1986) gives the title of Freeman's manuscript as the *History of Psychosurgery*, but the Himmelfarb Library catalogues it as *Adventures in Lobotomy*. The editions of *Psychosurgery* are in Freeman and Watts 1942, pp. 43–45, and 1950, chap. 2. Freeman gives the last name of the city editor of the *News Post* (Baltimore) both as Goodrich and Griffiths but, as the printed copy reveals, the *News Post* article was written by Alexander Gifford. The press conference reports are in the *News Post* (Baltimore), 20 November 1936, p. 30; the *Washington Evening Star*, 21 November 1936, pp. 1, A2; and the *New York Times*, 21 November 1936, p. 10, col. 1; and Kaempffert's are in the *Saturday Evening Post*, vol. 213, 24 May 1941, p. 18, and the *New York Times*, 7 June 1937, p. 1, cols. 4 and 5. The *Morning Sun* (Baltimore), 21 November 1936, pp. 1, 6, has a much longer report that, because it mentions the many criticisms made during the discussion, is more interesting than any of those in the other contemporary newspapers, but it does not mention Gage either. I am very much indebted to Jeff Korman of the Enoch Pratt Library, Baltimore, for finding this and the *News Post* item.

9. Simple juxtapositions are in Zimbardo and Ruch 1979; Singer and Hilgard 1978; McMahon and McMahon 1982; and Shutts 1982 has a therapy context. Gage as an accidental lobotomy is in Eckstein 1970; C. U. M. Smith 1970; Coon 1986; Morris 1996; Plotnick 1996; and the Gage-lobotomy similarity is in Rosenzweig and Leiman 1982. The Gage-Jacobsen-Moniz line is in Fulton 1949b

(but not 1949a or 1951); Wooldridge 1963; Adey 1974; Brown 1976; Mowbray, Rodger, and Mellor 1979; Dimond 1980; Shutts 1982; Restak 1984; and Carlson 1994, 1995; lesser lines are in Levitt 1981; Eckstein 1970; and Brown 1976; and the separation of the lines is in Damasio and van Hoesen 1983.

10. Incidental treatments of the history of psychosurgery are in Rylander 1939 and Columbia-Greystone Associates 1949; short histories are in Fisher 1951 and Meyer 1974; major works are by Greenblatt, Arnot, and Solomon (1950); Denny-Brown (1951); Robin and Macdonald (1975); Shutts (1982); Valenstein (1986); and O'Callaghan and Carroll (1982).

11. The Congress is discussed by Shutts (1982) and by Valenstein (1986)—who uses Fulton as his primary source. The Becky-Moniz parable is in Pressman 1998, ch. 2; and the quotation of Moniz from Fulton is in Freeman n. d. The resection patients are in Ackerly 1935; Brickner 1934, 1936; and Penfield and Evans 1935; and the chimpanzee experiments are in Jacobsen et al. 1936, and Crawford et al. 1948. Joe A. is cited in Moniz 1936b and 1954, but Jacobsen's work only in the latter. Penfield's doubt and Brickner's caution are in the discussion of German and Fox 1934, and Ackerly's reply to Bond in the discussion of Ackerly 1935. The 1947 "anniversary" meeting is Association for Research in Nervous and Mental Disease 1948. Hilgard reported on case 4 in German and Fox 1934; Nauta carried out a considerable amount of work of his own on the frontal lobes as well as with the Columbia-Greystone Associates (1949) project; and Jasper 1995 for his recollections.

12

Gage, Inhibition, and Thought

Bennett did not ... substitute the physiological statement of the psychical facts for the facts themselves.

—Bramwell, *Hypnotism: Its History, Practice, and Theory*, 1903

We have seen that one of the main problems in interpreting the changes like those in Phineas Gage was that there was no explanatory framework into which they could be placed. The orthodox sensory-motor framework was patently inadequate, and some of those who declared that Gage was without symptoms may have done so because they implicitly equated symptoms with sensory-motor functions. Those who tried to use the mechanism of inhibition had the problem that the behaviors were too diverse to be accounted for by that mechanism. Ironically the problem is seen most clearly in its first application to the four patients with whom Ferrier compared Gage. It reappears in the diverse behaviors in Starr's series, in the "mental symptoms" of the patient that he and McBurney operated on, and in the symptoms, different again, described by Elder and Miles. Was it loose thinking that led these workers to class such diverse symptoms together and to believe a single mechanism explained them? Answering this question requires us to consider the origins of the concept of inhibition itself and the context in which it was formulated. There we find why there was such a readiness to use the failure of an inhibitory process to explain such a wide range of behaviors.

Brunton's definition, formulated toward the end of the nineteenth century, conveys what was meant by "inhibition" in the early part of that period. Basically it is the same as that used today:

By inhibition we mean the arrest of the functions or organ by the actions upon it of another, while its power to execute those functions is still retained and can be manifested as soon as the restraining power is removed.

Inhibition in Brunton's sense seems to have become popular in physiology in the 1850s, although "arresting" or "restraining" functions had been recognized in physiology some years before. The same concept, if not the term, had been used even earlier in psychology and philosophy.

However termed, and whatever observations they seemed to encompass, inhibitory phenomena and inhibitory concepts posed two problems. One was the difficulty of understanding how stimulation—a positive action—could restrain, arrest, or even prevent some other action or function from occurring, rather than provoking further action. Physiologists mainly had this difficulty. The other came, as Roger Smith has argued so persuasively, from the complex individual and social processes in which inhibition seemed to be involved. Control of social behavior, especially through obedience to authority, the individual's control of impulsive behavior, especially sexually impulsive behavior and excessive drinking, and morality itself all seemed to call on inhibition. Those who wrote on these problems—philosophers, psychologists, moralists, and physiologists alike—tended to use a concept of inhibition that fused social, individual, and physiological processes.

I begin chapter 12 by considering physiologists' experimental observations and outline the main problems with their concepts. This is a consideration of inhibition in isolation, so to speak. Then I turn to the use of the concept in reflex theory and the psychological concepts with which it was aligned. At this point the admixture of physiology, psychology, morality, and social prescription becomes most marked.[1]

Inhibition in Physiology

Physiologists had observed processes that seemed to involve inhibition prior to the 1850s, but their reports of them tended to be ignored. A good instance is provided by Charles Bell's footnote to his explanation in 1823 of how stimulation of the fourth cervical nerve caused, "on certain occasions," the superior oblique muscle of the eyeball to relax. So much did this observation run counter to the usual view of the effects of stimulation that he felt impelled to expand:

The nerves have been considered so generally as instruments for stimulating the muscles, without thought of their acting in the opposite capacity, that some additional illustration may be necessary here. Through the nerves is established the connection between the muscles, not only that connection by which muscles combine to one effort, but also that relation between the classes of muscles by which the one relaxes while the other contracts.

He also observed that a flexor muscle contracted when the tendon of the opposite extensor was stretched. For such reciprocal connection to be possible, Bell hypothesized that "there must be particular and appropriate nerves to form this double bond to cause them to conspire in relaxation as well as to combine in contraction." Were there such a relationship between the muscles of the eyelids and the superior oblique, "the one will relax while the other contracts." The theoretical importance of Bell's observation was virtually ignored for three quarters of a century until, according to Meltzer, Sherrington rediscovered it.

The discovery of what seemed to be more direct forms of the inhibitory effect of stimulation is usually credited to Volkmann. In 1838 Volkmann caused the beat of a frog's heart to weaken, with some beats being missed altogether, when he electrically stimulated the vagus nerve leading to the heart. This negative effect was said to have so surprised Volkmann that he rejected his own observation. Fulton, for example, put it that Volkmann was "convinced that excitation of nerve always provoked increased activity of the tissue it innervates [and] dismissed this chance observation as due to some error of technique." Seven years after Volkmann's observation, the Webers stopped the action of the heart completely. Importantly, they reported that "the heart, whose beat is by this means interrupted, is not contracted as in a tetanic convulsion, but remains relaxed and has a flat appearance." Muscular relaxation like this was so contrary to expectation that their observation was given a "primarily skeptical or even hostile" reception. It was not so much the Webers' facts that were in dispute, as had been the case with Volkmann; what was difficult to assimilate was that an excitatory nervous impulse could arrest or inhibit some process at the place of its termination.

Neither Volkmann nor the Webers tried to find a locale for the inhibitory process: Sechenov took that step. He first confirmed the Webers' results, and then the observation made by them and others that separating the brain from the cord intensified spinal reflexes. Sechenov measured the time it took for a decerebrate frog to withdraw its leg from an acidic solution. He found the speed depended on the solution's acidity: the stronger the solution, the quicker the response. In an intact frog, one with the brain still connected to the cord, the speed was slower. Sechenov then used what he described as a "very simple" experimental procedure to find where in the brain the source of the slowing was located. Beginning at the upper levels of the brain, he worked downward, successively sectioning the brain and cord and measuring the speed of withdrawal at each section. He then applied various chemical and electrical stimuli to the exposed sections and measured the reflexes again. Whether the stimuli were applied at the level of the brain, the midbrain, or the cord, the speed of response was slowed in the same way as in the intact frog.

Sechenov attributed the inhibitory effect "to the excitation of some special mechanisms which are absolutely different from the sensory and motor apparatuses of the organism. In other words, the mechanisms inhibiting the reflexes are of a specific nature." The slowing was greatest at the level of the optic lobe, the very place at which separation had caused the greatest increase. Sechenov placed the inhibitory mechanism there. Although he made his discovery in Claude Bernard's laboratory in 1862, and demonstrated the phenomenon to equally eminent physiologists in Ludwig, Preyer, Brücke, and Du-Bois Reymond in that year—all of whom he says found it of great interest—it had almost no impact on physiological thinking.[2]

Even for what appeared to be relatively simple experimental results like these, nineteenth-century physiologists found it very difficult to agree on what kind of process could account for them. More complex phenomena provoked even more disagreement. From about 1860, major reviews appeared at about ten-year intervals devoted to the heroic task of arriving at some kind of resolution. The reviews resulted only in a reaffirmation of the complexity of the disparate facts and an agreement that the theories were vague, difficult to investigate, and impossible to reconcile.

The reviews are striking in their unwillingness to grant that stimulation could produce inhibition. Meltzer made by far the best statement of this aspect of the problem at the thirty-year mark. He began by saying that inhibition had had "to fight on general grounds at every step for the establishment of any new fact, and has still to fight for recognition as an independent vital force." When summing up he said:

Our knowledge of the laws of life had a one sided- development. The active manifestations of life aroused our curiosity; the phenomena of contraction, secretion, sensation presented problems and were studied. The absence of these phenomena was no problem. Rest of a muscle did not require an explanation. A muscle is at rest, it was implicitly assumed, when there is no cause for its contraction. Thus all the laws and conceptions which were formulated upon this one-sided basis are obstacles to the progress of the conception of inhibition. Had there been more such unbiased minds as that of Charles Bell, to whom vital arrangement for an active relaxation of the muscle was a self-understood requirement, inhibition would have been firmly established long ago.

Not until Loewi's work of 1921 was it granted that the inhibitory effect of vagal stimulation might be due to the liberation of what he termed *vagustoff*, now called acetylcholine, and it was another five years before that hypothesis was confirmed.

Contemporary discussions and reviews attest to the continuing problem of what it was that inhibition could explain. Partly that difficulty comes from the continuing tendency to equate physiological inhibition directly with psychological processes that were originally assigned to the brain. Will is among the most important of them.[3]

Inhibition, Will, and Reflexes

A place had been prepared in the brain for the will well in advance of the physiological concept of inhibition. Many physiologists believed nervous functions were subordinate one to another, with the cerebral hemispheres having the premier role. For example, it was easy for Flourens to place the functions of the hemispheres above those of locomotion that he placed in the cerebellum, of respiration in the medulla, and the more primitive functions of the spinal cord and nerves. Once inhibitory phenomena had been identified with willing, it was just as easy to locate an inhibitory mechanism in the brain.

Marshall Hall's theorizing shows these preliminary steps especially clearly. Hall concluded his first *Memoir* of 1833 by saying:

One part of this inquiry is altogether untouched,—the influence of the mind and emotions, and the corresponding parts of the nervous system, upon the organs which are the subject of reflex functions.

Hall did not mention inhibition here. Nor did he do so in his second *Memoir* of 1837. However, having observed that strychnine increased reflex activity in hemiplegic limbs but decreased it in nonaffected limbs, he raised the possibility that reflexes were controlled, not by a physiological process, but by the will:

Is it that, for the want of the stimulus of volition ... the irritability is greater in the paralytic than in the other limbs ... and that the muscles of the paralytic limbs are therefore more susceptible of the action of the [reflex] stimulus, and its augmentation under the influence of the strychnine?

The *Table of the Nervous System in Relation to Motion* Hall provided shows that by then he had explicitly fitted his system into Flourens's hierarchical schema. Two years later Hall answered his question about the will affirmatively and still without reference to inhibition. However mysteriously the will exercised its control, it did so very directly, as Müller showed when he integrated the main points of Hall's reflex doctrine into his general physiology.

Once reflexes had been assigned to the "lower" centers and their appearance made dependent on the strength of the influences above them and once inhibition was discovered, it was relatively easy to attribute a weakness of will to a failure of inhibition. Reflexes were responsible for involuntary, automatic, and nonconscious functions; behaviors that were irrational, automatic, unconscious, and overemotional could be attributed to them. Their appearance in the otherwise rational subject therefore indicated a loss of cerebral influence. Those of the early physiologists who had experimented on inhibitory phenomena and tried to explain psychological functions took that path almost immediately. Of them, Volkmann was the first.

At about the same time as his experiments on vagal inhibition Volkmann observed that some reflexes appeared only after decapitation. He immediately implicated the loss of inhibition as the cause of the reflex action and equated inhibition with attention and will:

With the concept of inhibition it becomes clear that the brain contains the cause for the hindrance in the activation of the nervous principle ... That deficient psychic influence supports [its] activation ... And conversely that the influence of the mind possibly hinders this activation. The psychic forces, on which everything seems to depend here, are attention and will.

Generally in the nineteenth century those physiologists who explained particular psychological processes also localized an inhibitory function or its equivalent in the brain, and vice versa.[4]

Inhibition in Psychology

The first extensive use of the concept of inhibition in psychology was made by the German philosopher-psychologist Johann Friedrich Herbart (1776–1841). Having rejected associationist psychologies, Herbart needed to explain how ideas, or *Vorstellungen* (presentations), became connected with one another. *Hemmung*, now translated as inhibition, forced dissimilar presentations out of consciousness but allowed similar ones to combine. Herbart treated each presentation or idea as if it were a force possessing an inhibitory energy because, as Dunkel put it:

If there were no such mutual resistance, all presentations would merge into one, and the content of consciousness would be a unity rather than that manifold of varied elements with which experience presents us.

Herbart especially needed to be able to say how aggregates of presentations were reflected upon, identified as familiar, recognized, explained, and related to new perceptions. That is, Herbart was concerned with how presentations were "apperceived."

Herbart's psychology was predominantly educational, and what took up most of his book was a practical program of steps by which he believed teachers could build up the apperceptions of their pupils. Inhibition as such played a minor role in Herbart's conceptualization of the control of psychological processes, and he did not place inhibition into the traditional hierarchical framework. In Herbart's theory, inhibition was not a separate mechanism, equivalent to the will itself, as it was in conceptualizations like those of Volkmann. For Herbart, inhibition contributed to morality via the will only insofar as it helped build up the apperceptions from which the will itself was fashioned. Although Herbart's conceptualization is consistent with Brunton's definition— ideas forced out of consciousness continued to exist but their conscious manifestation was arrested—his predominantly nonhierarchical, detailed, and purely psychological conceptualization contrasts strongly with the controlling and physiologically based later accounts.[5]

Inhibition as a physiological controlling or restraining mechanism meshed with and reinforced notions of moral and social control. Smith has argued that concerns over the control of personal behavior and social processes were of at least of the same importance as what could be determined about inhibition in the physiological laboratory. The many nineteenth-century references to inhibition

involved argument by analogy from physiological or physical processes to psychological ones, just as belief in the arresting power of the will over the body encouraged argument in the opposite direction.

Smith also points out that the context in which inhibition was introduced was one in which the intellect was supposed to rule the passions, rational control was the hallmark of the mind, and the will had always to win out over impulse. Known in Western thought since at least Plato's time, this context practically guaranteed that anything other than purely rational behavior could be attributed to the failure of inhibition, whether considered physiologically or psychologically. Particularly striking instances are provided by the way in which inhibition was used in one very influential German theory of insanity and in the physiologically based theories of hypnosis.[6]

Inhibition and the "Insanities"

One of the first to make major use of inhibition in interpreting the "insanities" was the German alienist William Griesinger (1817–1868). His approach is especially interesting because it was based on a combination of reflex doctrine and Herbart's psychological concept of inhibition. As early as 1843 Griesinger had written on the relevance of inhibition and reflex theory to "insanity." Those ideas and Herbart's concept were central to his *Mental Pathology and Therapeutics* of 1845. The brain was for Griesinger, as it was in Laycock's theory, "an immense reflex apparatus" in which sensory excitations were "transformed into impulses of movement." Psychical life therefore commenced "in the organs of sense" before passing out "into the organs of movement." Griesinger located "the intelligence" in the brain as a powerful, complex, and ruling "third element" between the sensory and motor components of the reflex.

Griesinger turned inhibition into a psychological ego mechanism:

All mental acts take place within the intelligence. This is the special seat of thought and all the various mental acts which were formerly designated separate faculties (imagination, will, emotions, &c) are only different relations of understanding with sensation and movement, or the result of the conflict of ideas with themselves.

So aligned, the will acted as part of "intelligence" to regulate what happened between sensation and movement.

Here Griesinger added Herbart's psychology of inhibition to the reflex doctrine. When sensory impressions from within the body, such as those from appetites and instincts, called up ideas appropriate to their ends, they led immediately to movement provided that those ideas were not opposed by other groups of ideas. In the healthy adult, the most important opposition came from the group of ideas constituting the "I," or ego. Griesinger conceived of all groupings of ideas, including the ego, as forming *via* the apperceptive inhibitory process Herbart had proposed. For Griesinger, the ego consisted of a uniform set of ideas about the self or "I" that attempted to inhibit all ideas not in accord with itself. He proposed that the "I" was "weakened or destroyed" by "almost all pathological states of the brain," that is, in almost all mental diseases.

Griesinger based three "essentially distinct groups" of mental diseases on the three components of the reflex: the "sensitive [i.e., sensory], motory, and mental (perceptive) anomalies." There were thus "three leading groups of elementary disturbances—intellectual insanity, emotional insanity, and insanity of movement." Griesinger further distinguished depression and mania as the two fundamental abnormal states. Depression involved "morbid production, governing, and persistence" of emotions and emotional states. The "fundamental affection" of "the morbid influence of a painful negative affection" generated states of mind that were not controlled by the ego but

constantly and in every way intrude ... they can no longer be removed by outward mental excitation ... and ... instead of being controlled by the group of perceptions of the I, they affect us tumultuously and excite a lasting state of painful internal disquietude.

Depressive states did not consist of "inaction and weakness, or in the suppression of the mental or cerebral phenomena which accompany them." Rather they were caused by "very violent states of irritation" that the weakened ego could not control.

The corresponding fundamental affection in mania was a derangement of the motor side such that psychical movement became "free, unrestrained, and considerably increased." If the increased mental activity manifested itself directly, this "free development of volition" took the physically restless form of simple mania. But it could be transformed into another form where "extravagant volition" dominated by "delirious conceptions" hid behind an outward calm. Some manic behavior and thinking was impulsive and not willed, but most, Griesinger believed, was truly volitional, involving the transformation of an idea into an unopposed action. On recovery, patients sometimes said they had not tried to behave or think differently.

Absent in both the manias and the depressions was "the third element" of intelligence, and with it the will. Consequently Griesinger's conception of inhibition as a weakened force located in the ego explained the apparently very different symptoms of depression and mania. Others may have used the concept of inhibition differently, but they were successful, perhaps not to the same degree as Griesinger, in bringing a wide range of symptoms under it. None would have been surprised that the childish dementia of patients like those of Baraduc, the incapacity of Selywn's to apply himself to any mental activity, the passivity of Lepine's, the automatic behavior of Davidson's, the depressive reactions of a Burklin, or the impulsiveness of a Gage were grouped together as different forms of irrational behavior. Once inhibition had been equated with rational control, all these behaviors were clearly manifestations of the same inhibitory weakness.[7]

Inhibition and Hypnosis
From some time in the middle of the nineteenth century, a view began to emerge that hypnotic behavior was automatic, independent of cerebral control, and the result of the hypnotized subject having surrendered his or her will to the hypnotist. With these notions came a theory or, rather, different versions of a theory that hypnosis was marked by the absence of physiological controlling mechanisms located in the cortex. The essence of this kind of theory seems to have been formulated in 1851 by Bennett, who proposed that the psychological phenomena of hypnosis were due to the failure of one set of ideas to inhibit others. He proposed that the monotony of the hypnotic induction procedure caused the paralysis of some of the nerve tubes of the white matter of the cerebral lobes and a resultant exaltation of others. Paralysis caused a loss of inhibition because it resulted in abnormal connections between the different "cerebral ganglia." Smith cites the 1881 theory of Heidenhain and Bubnov as an exemplar of this mixed psychological and physiological conceptualization.

Characterizing hypnotic thinking as automatic and conducted with other than full efficiency overlooked three things. First, Franz Anton Mesmer, with whom the modern study of hypnosis begins, does not seem to have observed these automatic or "lower" processes in hypnosis. In fact, he and many of his followers believed that hypnosis enhanced psychological functions. Second, some experiments seemed to show actual improvements in intellectual ability during hypnosis. For example, hypnotized subjects often performed complex calculations of elapsed time more accurately than normally. Third, it was especially difficult to retain a theory of automatism in which the manifestations of hypnosis included what seemed to be intelligent and completely conscious secondary personalities having full control over their voluntary functions. Phenomena such as these had been well known in the hypnosis literature for years, and it was exceedingly superficial to describe them as automatic. Psychological or physiological, inhibitory theories were contradicted by the facts. There was (and still is) no evidence that hypnosis is based on significant alterations in physiological functioning.[8]

Noninhibitory Theories of Loss of Control

If we ask what alternatives there were to inhibitory explanations of the control of behavior, we find one of the main ones in the work of Anstie as it was developed by Hughlings Jackson. As a solution it not only did not avoid the problem of the dual analogy that Smith has identified, it actually exacerbated it, perhaps even rested on it.

Anstie wanted to know what alcohol, ether, and chloroform did when they were used, as they were, in the stimulant regimen that was supplanting antiphlogistic therapy. His clinical and experimental observations led him to conclude that none of these substances caused excitement by direct stimulation. He interpreted their effects in the early stages of administration as the result of the removal of a higher-level controlling mechanism:

The simplest explanation may be found in the supposition that, in the absence of any extraordinary circumstances, the apparent exaltation of certain faculties should be ascribed rather to the removal of controlling influences, than to positive stimulation of the faculties themselves, or of the physical machinery by which they work.

Hughlings Jackson explicitly adopted Anstie's conclusion in his later theory of the ways in which the levels of the nervous system functioned in relation to one another. Jackson actually coined the phrase "Anstie's principle" for the "over-action of lower centres as a consequence of loss of control from inaction of higher centres." Higher centers controlled the lower just because they were more complex and had had evolved later. Neither Anstie nor Jackson needed to attribute apparent increases in lower-level functioning to a loss of inhibition or to locate any kind of inhibitory process in any particular part of the nervous system.[9]

In Mercier's 1888 attempt to resolve the problems of inhibition and in the discussion of it, we see how Jackson's shift to explaining control by successively evolving levels of the nervous system did not avoid analogies being drawn between psychological, social, and physiological processes. In his paper, Mercier made much of an analogy between the way defects of inhibitory regulation and control of nervous processes paralleled defects that could arise in an army were various of its controlling centers put out of operation. For example, the loss of the commander-in-chief might result in "a languor, a want of initiative, a failure to take advantage of opportunities" on the part of the army, an outcome paralleled "by the heaviness, the dulness [*sic*], the defect of intelligence on the part of the individual" suffering from a loss of the highest level of nervous regulation. There might also be "uproar from absence of the controlling authority" as an effect of "the removal of the highest functions in the one organisation or the other." And suppose the commander-in-chief should begin

to become highly excited and to issue orders in great excess. The result will be an excess of activity on the part of the army at large.... The analogous process in the individual is universal convulsion.

As if to show the independence of the physiological concept of inhibition from Mercier's analogy, Hughlings Jackson commented, "I have nothing to say on the nature of the inhibitory process," but repeated a significant analogy of his own.

Hughlings Jackson's analogy came from his 1884 *Croonian Lectures*, in which he had drawn a parallel between modes of governmental control and the hierarchical, evolution-dissolution control of the nervous system his theory required:

If the governing body of this country were destroyed suddenly, we should have two causes for lamentation; (1) the loss of services of eminent men; and (2) the anarchy of the now uncontrolled people. The loss of the governing body answers to the dissolution in our patient.... The anarchy answers to the no longer controlled activity of the next lower level of evolution.

The mixture of moral, social, and ideological factors these analogies reveal partly explains the ease with which Mercier, Jackson, and other investigators moved between physiological and psychological concepts of inhibition. But at the same time as widening the scope of inhibitory and quasi-inhibitory explanations, they practically guaranteed that the physiological nature of inhibition would be clouded and its understanding held back. The same was true of inhibition in the psychological sense.[10]

The Fate of Ferrier's Inhibitory Thesis

Ferrier's inhibitory motor function had a very short life. The second edition of *The Functions of the Brain*, published ten years after he had announced it, and eight after he had used it to explain the changes in Gage, made no suggestion that the brain had an inhibitory-motor function or that attention had a physiological basis. It simply omitted the "Diagrammatic Summary" of the first edition of *Functions*, which had contained the figure locating the inhibitory mechanism in the frontal lobes (my figure 9.2) and the explanatory text that accompanied it.

Ferrier went much further. He now denied positively that there were inhibitory processes of any kind in the nervous system. Thus although he discussed the effects of stimulation of the vagus nerve on the heart again, and in more detail, he now expressed doubt about the nature of the mechanism. He also completely dismissed Sechenov's postulated inhibitory centers in the brain:

It is not, however, necessary to assume, as Setschenow [sic] and others have done, that there is anything specific in this restraining or inhibitory action of encephalic centres, or that there are special inhibitory centres in the brain.... Setschenow's experiment and volitional inhibition appear to be only individual examples of the general law that reflex action is liable to be arrested, or interfered with, when the centres engaged in it are solicited at the same time from other quarters.... Setschenow's experiment is in all probability merely the influence of irritation of sensory centres and tracts, which are undoubtedly present in the optic thalami and optic lobes.

Ferrier also argued against Jackson's notion of an evolutionary-based hierarchical control:

This hypothesis receives no confirmation from the facts of experiment, nor does it appear to me to be at all necessary to explain the facts of either normal or abnormal "mentation." We have in the sensory and motor centres of the cortex the substrata of the respective forms of sensory perception and ideation.... It seems more reasonable to suppose that there may be higher and lower degrees of complexity or evolution in the same centres.

This modification was as much of Hughlings Jackson's thesis as Ferrier was prepared to accept.

We can narrow the time during which Ferrier abandoned his concept of an inhibitory-motor mechanism to some time after 1879 or 1880 but before 1886. The German translation of the 1876 or first edition of Ferrier's *The Functions of the Brain* came out in 1879. Heinrich Obersteiner, the translator, explained in his Preface that Ferrier had approved of his incorporating additional material in the translation. This material was, in essence, Harlow's illustrations and the description of Gage and other cases of frontal damage from his *Gulstonian Lectures*, originally written two years after *Functions*. As in the first English edition of *Functions*, chapter 11 contained the Bain-Ferrier theory of thinking, and chapter 12 the "Diagrammatic Summary." Hence up to at least 1879, Ferrier must have believed in his inhibitory-motor thesis. Otherwise he would not have allowed Obersteiner to illustrate it so strikingly. Because it is precisely the outline of the thesis, and the "Diagrammatic Summary" together with its explanatory text, that were omitted from the second English edition of *Functions* of 1886, Ferrier must have changed his mind about inhibition before then but after 1879.

Two reasons suggest themselves for Ferrier's *volte-face*. First, his inhibitory mechanism was not immediately relevant to any of the details about the localization debate in general or that relating specifically to aphasia. Second, and to me more important, at some point Ferrier had to come to terms with the obvious weaknesses of an inhibitory-motor system for which he had no direct evidence ("no motor manifestations," "negative" facts, "not actually motor"). Ferrier did retain one aspect of his initial thesis, that of unwanted actions being suppressed by attention. The new explanation was just as plausible as the old. As his comments on Sechenov indicated, the phenomena of inhibition were now individual instances of the fact that a center could not be stimulated simultaneously from more than one place. At the beginning of the twentieth century, Sherrington put forward a similar conception of inhibition. For him, inhibition was due to unlike pairs of reflexes (e.g., those extending and flexing the same muscle) having only sequential use of a final common path. The activity of any one member of the pair necessarily prevented the activity of the other.

Ferrier and Sherrington probably did not realize that their retreat from an independent inhibitory mechanism took them back, conceptually speaking, to the time of Gall. In Gall's system, where two or more faculties competed, whichever was the most powerful, that is, the biggest or most developed, decided the issue. The thief who returned to the woman he had robbed and untied the rope with which he had tried to strangle her had organs of Murder and Compassion smaller than that of Acquisitiveness. Only one faculty could be in operation at any given time.[11]

Frontal Functions and the Sensory-Motor Framework
Ferrier was the only nineteenth-century physiologist to suggest a definite sensory-motor function for the frontal lobes, but in doing so he stretched the sensory-motor framework to its limits. We can understand therefore how C. K. Mills could simultaneously propose that the frontal area be renamed "a higher psychically or inhibitory lobe" and also class it as "one of the so-called latent districts of the brain." From a narrower standpoint we can also appreciate Deaver's explanation in his anatomy text that "the two principal regions of the hemispheres are the motor and

the sensory areas" and the region in front of the coronal suture was known as "silent" because lesions there did not "give rise to any localising symptoms." Even today these terms, and the nonspecific functions to which they refer, are found. For example the illustration of the brain in the text by McNaught and Callander leaves the frontal areas blank, but the legend to them reads "Large unchartered areas of the cerebral hemispheres are probably concerned with mental processes such as intelligence, memory, judgement, imagination, creative and conscious thought." Guyton and Hall do maintain consistency between legend and text, with the former reading "Planning complex movements and elaboration of thoughts."

Silent the frontal areas may have been from the point of view of sensory-motor physiology but, as Martin explicitly brought out in the eighth edition of his textbook, they were higher only by default:

By a sort of process of exclusion, the rest of the cortex being allotted (though on unsatisfactory evidence) to motion and sensation the frontal regions have been supposed to have special connection with the higher intellectual faculties.

It is likely the frontal lobes were sometimes labeled "latent areas," as for example by Donaldson, for the same reason.

Some of the solutions to this paradox are not without their humorous side. W. Mills, for example, tried fiat rather than exclusion. He gave a comprehensive summary of nearly all the experimental and clinical work on localization without discussing the frontal lobes at all. Then he simply labeled them "Higher psychically" in his figures 366 and 387. Ballantyne tried the opposite tactic. He termed the areas "silent" in his text but left them unlabeled in his diagrams.

Conclusion

The sensory-motor blinkers were still much in evidence toward the middle of the twentieth century when frontal lobe changes were described in detail but only vague generalizations about them formulated. Thus Howell had it that the frontal lobes were necessary "for intelligent responses that depend on the utilisation of past experience or immediate memory" and Lucas that they were required "for completeness of mental expression." Attributing such vague and varied functions to the frontal lobes, or labeling them indifferently as "the silent areas" or "higher psychically" showed only that they had defeated attempts to incorporate their functions into the sensory-motor conceptualization as soundly as they had resisted the earlier efforts to stimulate them into producing movements.[12]

Many of the other nineteenth-century physiological explanations of psychological processes also localized an inhibitory function or its equivalent in the brain. Smith gives as examples Spencer (rationality), Lloyd Morgan (learning and intelligence), Brunton (control of impulses and emotions), Carpenter and Obersteiner (attention), and Barlow and Maudsley (will). Each specified the relation between inhibition and psychological processes vaguely, but all seemed confident that a failure of inhibition was responsible for irrationality, failures of learning or intelligent reasoning, impulse control, overemotionality, inattention, and lack of will. What Ferrier, Starr, and Elder and Miles did in grouping very different patients together was very little different.[13]

The story of the development of the concept of inhibition did not end at the end of the nineteenth century. Different kinds of inhibitory phenomena continued to be brought under the one rubric, and the methods for investigating them are still difficult to master. That there are inhibitory nerves, inhibitory neurons, and inhibitory transmitter substances is readily accepted today. Equally it is widely agreed that not all of them always have inhibitory effects. Whether stimulation causes inhibition on a particular occasion appears to depend on the activity of other nerves and neurons and on which other substances are also released.

A Digression on Bain, Ferrier, and Freud

Bain foreshadows so many of Freud's conceptualizations that considering them is a worthwhile digression. Eight aspects of Freud's conceptualization of thinking and of other more general psychological processes are very close to those of Bain, and necessarily to Ferrier's, of course. Freud shares the first three with them and with many of those interested in neurology during the last century:

1. Freud and Bain took a view of the relation between mind and brain that was similar, although not identical, to the psychophysical parallelism adopted by Hughlings Jackson and Ferrier. The difference was that for Freud and Bain mental processes were "*dependent* concomitant[s]" of the physiological, and not merely the concomitants they were for Jackson and Ferrier.

2. Freud's theorizing about the mind was solidly in the tradition of the reflex and sensory-motor physiology of Hall, Müller, and Laycock. His first model of the mental apparatus was, in fact, a simple variant of the mechanism originally proposed by Hall, and each of his subsequent models of the mind had à similar basis.

3. Possibly like Müller and Laycock, and to some extent like Jackson, Freud believed that the nervous system acted to discharge surplus excitation. At times Bain also alludes to a tendency of the nervous system to dispose of excess energy through movement, and, like Freud, notes that that discharge is pleasurable.

The last five aspects have a striking resemblance to specific concepts of Bain:

4. Like Freud, Bain gave the dominant role in development and learning to the avoidance of unpleasure, rather than the search for pleasure.

5. Freud's concept of a sexual drive was based on a periodic physiological process that made imperious demands for discharge and only gradually found its object. It is not very close to those of his contemporaries who wrote on sexuality, but it is almost identical to Bain's and Ferrier's.

6. Freud and Bain shared the view that criteria for the sense of reality are the difference between the effects of movement on a real perception and a recollection, as well as the attenuated level of nervous energy used during the latter.

7. Freud's view of conscience was very like Bain's. Conscience was due neither to God's will, nor an innate moral sense, nor self-interest, but reproduced "a facsimile of the system of government as practised around us," best studied during the child's learning. It was forged initially from a connection between "disobedience and apprehended pain, more or less magnified by fear."

8. Freud's puzzling references to the contribution that "secretory" neurons make to emotional experience and its revival find a parallel in Bain and Ferrier, perhaps even becoming comprehensible through what they say about secretions being parts of emotional reactions.

9. Bain had it that conflicts between motives occurred so often that "the inner life of every one is a sort of battle ground, or scene of incessant warfare."

The reflex suppositions underlying Freud's thinking in the *Project for a Scientific Psychology* and chapter 7 of *The Interpretation of Dreams* are quite explicit, and the same is present, although less obviously, in *The Ego and the Id* and the posthumously published *Outline of Psycho-Analysis*.[14]

In *The Interpretation of Dreams* Freud said his model of the mental apparatus fulfilled

a requirement with which we have long been familiar, namely that the psychical apparatus must be constructed like a reflex apparatus. Reflex processes remain the model of every psychical function.

The apparatus he then described has a sensory system at one end and a motor one at the other, with excitation usually traveling from the former to the latter. Originally, and as a theoretical fiction, this simple reflex apparatus could only discharge the excitation impinging on it. Having no internal energy of its own, and displaying no spontaneous activity, it acted only because it was driven by energy arriving in filtered form from the external environment or in muted form from the organic drives, especially the sexual. It was a nervous system governed by what Freud termed the "primary process," which, in this respect, was substantially different from the systems pictured by physiologists and philosophers like Müller, Laycock, Bain, Hughlings Jackson, and Ferrier.

Unless the perception of the objects that satisfied the organism's internal needs left traces of the experience behind it, there would be no possibility of experiences accumulating that would allow that object to be refound should the need arise again. Were there only a trace, the energy could only be expended in undirected motor activity (e.g., crying, restless movements) or in reviving the memory of the object as a hallucinatory percept. Traces alone could not guide or direct actions capable of refinding the object. Appropriate action would result only if discharge were delayed long enough for the memory of the right action to be found by searching through all or most of the memory traces. There also had to be some way of judging whether the image of the object found through the action was "real" or hallucinatory. The apparatus therefore had to move from the primary process mode of immediate discharge to a "secondary process" that enabled it to tolerate delay in disposing of the energy and to distinguish between the real and the hallucinated. This secondary process was a function of a system located just before the motor end of the apparatus, where its inhibitory powers enabled it to control access to movement. It also attended to processes going on within it by adding extra excitation to them and so making them conscious.

Within the reflex systems of the *Project* and *The Interpretation of Dreams*, Freud conceptualized consciousness, attention, voluntary activity, and willing in almost the same way as Bain and Ferrier. Thus motor images aroused action, the motor paralysis of sleep was equivalent to a paralysis of the will, attention was due to extra excitation being added to already existing excitation, and the "key" to voluntary movement was the critical agency controlling attention, consciousness, and voluntary conscious movements.[15]

Freud's notion of a secondary process that inhibited action while the memory traces were searched is clearly very close to those of Bain and Ferrier. He first publicly set out the relation between inhibition and realistic thinking in *The Interpretation of Dreams*, in which he presumed that

under the dominion of the second system the discharge of excitation is governed by quite different mechanical conditions from those in force under the dominion of the first system. When once the second system has concluded its exploratory thought activity it releases the inhibition and damming-up of the excitation and allows them to discharge themselves in movement.

The conceptualization appears even earlier, in the unpublished *Project for a Scientific Psychology*, and is prominent in all of his subsequent theorizing.[16]

A particularly clear formulation is in the posthumously published *Outline of Psycho-Analysis*, in which Freud said the constructive activity of the ego consisted of

interpolating between the demand made by an instinct and the action that satisfies it, the activity of thought which, after taking its bearings in the present and assessing earlier experiences, endeavours by means of experimental actions to calculate the consequences of the course of action proposed.

Even the mechanism by which Freud's apparatus was able to differentiate between the real and the imagined was eventually based on the same kind of mechanism as Bain had proposed. In the *Project*, the presence of a real object caused a special set of neurons to discharge and produce alterations in consciousness. Freud never developed this somewhat ad hoc mechanism much further, and he settled for one based mainly on the effects of movement. What was real was external and could be made to change and disappear through movement; what had arisen internally and was hallucinatory was not so affected.

Freud's mechanism of inhibition has a very different basis from Ferrier's. In his only detailed account, that in section 14 of part I of the

Project, Freud's diagram shows how a quantity of neural energy, Q_n, or neural excitation, which were it to traverse the path between neuron a, recording a memory of an unpleasant event, and neuron b, which he termed a "key" or "secretory" neuron, unpleasure would be produced. However Q_n was diverted to neurones α, β, γ, etc., because they were the permanently excited neurons constituting the ego. In Freud's theory of thinking, excitation coming from the ego to the "side" or "lateral" aspect of the main direction of neural transmission inhibits action. Although Freud's theory of thinking was based on the inhibition of action, the inhibition itself resulted from excitation. As with Ferrier's final position, there was no room for an independent process of inhibition.[17]

Phineas Gage and Sigmund Freud

Could Freud have known about Phineas Gage and the theories of Bain and Ferrier? Freud may have known about Gage, because his case was cited so frequently in the neurological literature. But it is certain that he had read about Gage directly. In his *On Aphasia*, Freud cited two cases from the chapter on aphasia in Walter Hammond's textbook on nervous diseases. Hammond described Gage in the introductory part of the chapter, and sixteen pages later set out the two cases Freud cited. Although we saw in chapter 9 that Hammond's appreciation of the centrality of the Gage case to aphasia was ambiguous, he did give references to Harlow's 1848 paper and the extensive report by Jackson in 1870 in the Warren Museum *Catalogue*. Then there is the copy of Theodule Ribot's 1891 *Les Maladies de la Volunté* (Hinterberger Collection, item number 633) in what purports to be part of Freud's library, the Hinterberger Collection in the Special Collections of the Health Sciences Library, Columbia University, New York. In it, Ribot mentioned the Bain-Ferrier theory of the will as inhibited movement and used the changes in Gage as the main illustration of it. Ribot had already given a very full account of Bain's conceptualization in his *English Psychology* of 1874, and attested to its uniqueness. There is no direct evidence of Freud's reading either of Ribot's works, but he could not have avoided reading about Gage in Hammond's.

One tantalizing piece of evidence makes it reasonably certain that Freud knew about Ferrier's work on localization directly, and through it also knew about Gage. The Hinterberger Collection contains translations of the 1876 or first edition of Ferrier's *The Functions of the Brain* (item

40), the book form of Ferrier's *Gulstonian Lectures* of 1878 (item 41), and the English edition of the 1890 *Croonian Lectures* (item 39). The first two of these works contain a surprising amount of information about Gage in relation to the Bain-Ferrier theory.

Of the three Ferrier books, only item 41, the *Gulstonian Lectures*, is annotated. On the title page there is the name "Dr. Freud," which appears quite clearly, and a word that is more difficult to read but appears to be *halbbund*. The book is indeed "halfbound" and, although Eissler does not include the *Lectures* among the list of books he believed Freud to have signed, the handwriting does appear to be Freud's. The annotation itself could be either an instruction from Freud to the printer to "half bind" the book for him, or the printer's record of the instructions from "Dr. Freud," or a later bookseller's description. Whether this is so or not, the book declares itself unambiguously to belong to Freud's library. The German translation seems to follow the English original very closely throughout and certainly does so in the sections on Gage's case, both in itself and in relation to the hypothesized inhibitory functions of the frontal lobes. These *Lectures* rescued Gage from the virtual obscurity of the *Proceedings of the Massachusetts Medical Society* and were the first forum in which the changes in Gage were discussed in terms of a frontal inhibitory function. We have only to assume that Freud read this particular book (and we know he did not always read those he acquired) for him to have known about both the Bain-Ferrier theory of thinking and about Phineas Gage.

But Gage also figures prominently in item 40, the German translation of the first edition of Ferrier's *The Functions of the Brain*. He is in fact much more prominent than in the English original, where his case was used only to illustrate the possibility of extensive frontal damage without "manifest symptoms." We saw earlier in this chapter that Obersteiner, the translator, had Ferrier's permission to add material about Gage from his *Gulstonian Lectures*, originally written two years after *Functions*. Chapter 7 of Obersteiner's translation begins, like the original, with section 48, which introduces the methods of investigation. However, the sections in it dealing with Gage have been altered completely. Harlow's figures from the Gulstonian lectures are included together with his detailed report of the changes; they are those with which Ferrier rebutted Dupuy's attack. Similarly, although section 78 of the translation also deals with the changes produced by ablation of the frontal lobes in the monkey, it now includes all the human cases previously mentioned only in the *Lectures* and, as in them, Gage is again placed first. Chapter 11 also sets out the Bain-Ferrier theory of thinking as outlined here and includes all the quotations I have used. Chapter 12 is the "Diagrammatic Summary" of the English original, complete with the diagram from section 106 and the text from section 111 describing the frontal local-ization of the inhibitory-motor centers. Consequently, once again, if Freud actually owned or read this version of Ferrier's *The Functions of the Brain*, he had to know of the Bain-Ferrier theory of thinking as action inhibited by an inhibitory-motor function localized in the frontal lobes and of Gage as the most compelling contemporary human evidence for it.

Not too much weight should be put on any claim, which I am not making of course, that Alexander Bain, David Ferrier, and especially Phineas Gage were *the* sources of Freud's theory of thinking. But that they may have influenced him seems to be at least a reasonable possibility.[18]

Notes

1. Brunton 1883 for the definition; Smith 1992 for the argument.

2. Bell 1823, Meltzer 1899. Volkmann's experiments are in Diamond, Balvin, and Diamond 1963, pp. 20–22, and their reception in Fulton 1966, p. 295, Meltzer 1899, Sherrington 1906, p. 288, Brazier 1959, p. 36, and Smith 1992, p. 77. The Webers' experiments are in Weber and Weber [1845] 1966 and their reception in Diamond, Balvin, and Diamond 1963, p. 22. Sechenov's experiments and their reception are in Sechenov [1862] 1968; [1866] [1965a?], p. 519; and [1904] 1965b, pp. 107–108; and Diamond, Balvin, and Diamond 1963, pp. 28–30.

3. Typical nineteenth-century reviews are by Althaus (1873), Brunton (1874, 1883), A. James (1881), Mercier (1888–1889), and Breese (1889). Reviews and discussion from the twentieth century are by Dodge (1926a, 1926b), Pilkington and McKellar (1960), Diamond, Balvin, and Diamond (1963), and Macmillan (1992a, 1996b). Some of the history is in Hutter 1961 and Wiersma 1961. Meltzer's appreciation is in Meltzer 1899; Loewi's discovery is from Bacq [1974] 1975, p. 15.

4. Flourens in Smith 1992, p. 39. Hall [1833] 1837a, sec. 139, pp. 39–40; 1837b, p. 105, sec. 213, p. 102; 1839. Müller [1833–1842] 1833–1840, p. 934. Volkmann's 1838 paper is cited by Smith (1992, p. 77).

5. Herbart [1834] 1891; Dunkel 1970, p. 135; cf. Herbart [1834] 1891, chap. 3, sec. 22.

6. Smith's 1992 two-way characterization of the arguments is on pp. 144–145.

7. The first edition of Griesinger was published in 1845, but the edition I quote is the second, published in 1861 and translated into English in 1867. The reflex theses, the role given opposing ideas, and the ego or "I" are in bk. 1, chap. 1, sec. 14–36, pp. 16–60, and chap. 4. Insanities generally are in bk. 1, chap. 4, sec. 36, p. 60, and bk. 3, Introduction, sec. 110, p. 207. The depressions are in bk. 1, chap. 4, sec. 37, pp. 60–61, and bk. 3, Introduction, sec. 110, pp. 207–210, and chap. 2, sec. 130, p. 273. The manias are in bk. 3, chap. 2, sec. 130, pp. 273–275, secs. 134–135, pp. 282–283, and sec. 141, pp. 305–307.

8. Bennett in Bramwell [1903] 1956, pp. 294–295, 303, and Heidenhain and Bubnov in Smith 1992, pp. 126–129. Bramwell also describes hypnotic phenomena very comprehensively.

9. Anstie 1864a for his experiments (his conclusion is on p. 78). The therapeutic context is in Anstie 1864b, 1865. Jackson 1874b for the formulation of "Anstie's principle," but also see Jackson 1875, 1884. Unlike Diamond, Balvin, and Diamond (1963, pp. 33, 36, 38), I do not believe Anstie's thesis rests on a concept of inhibition. Apart from Jackson, Anstie's argument seems to have gone unnoticed, possibly because of its therapeutic context. No points central to his thesis were made in the reviews I have found (e.g., "Review of *Stimulants and Narcotics*" 1864a, 1864b, 1864c).

10. Mercier 1888–1889 and J. H. Jackson 1888–1889; cf. 1884.

11. Ferrier on the vagus (Ferrier 1886, pp. 98–100; cf. 1876, pp. 29–32), on Sechenov (Ferrier 1886, pp. 70–71; cf. 1876, p. 18), and on Jackson (Ferrier 1886, p. 460). Sherrington 1906 for the common pathway, Macmillan 1992b for the substitution of attention, and Macmillan 1992a for the parallel with Gall. In lecture 6 of his *Croonian Lectures*, Ferrier (1890a, 1890b, 1890c) gives almost no consideration to the frontal lobes, saying their function "is still obscure." There he also rejects ideas generated by the muscular sense as a necessary precursor to movement. Naturally I cannot agree with the assertion of Diamond, Balvin, and Diamond (1963, p. 47) that the Gage case was one of the factors that led to Ferrier's abandoning his inhibitory hypothesis.

12. C. K. Mills (1889–1890; cf. 1895) first proposed the names in his address. Deaver 1901, vol. II, p. 499, for his variant; McNaught and Callander 1983 and Guyton and Hall 1996 for diagrams and legend; Martin 1898, p. 631; cf. 1890, for exclusion; Donaldson 1896, p. 702 for "latent." W. Mills 1889, pp. 521–535, and Ballantyne 1915, pp. 363–364, for other labels, and Howell 1937, p. 237, and Lucas 1940, p. 94, for vague functions. See also Mader 1990, Carola, Harley, and Noback 1992, and Creager 1992 for typical modern examples of the comprehensively vague legends or descriptions offered students.

13. The same can be said for the applications others made of Ferrier's or similar theses. Perhaps the most famous of these applications are those by Wundt and Freud. Both seem to have known of the Gage case through Ferrier, although Wundt's application seems to have owed as much to Herbart's conception as to Ferrier's (Hildebrandt 1991), and Freud's eschewed any notion of an independent inhibitory process (Macmillan 1992a, 1992b).

14. Mind and brain in Freud [1891] 1953a, pp. 54–56; Wallace 1992, pp. 244–250; Macmillan 1991, pp. 109–111, and 1997, pp. 104–105. Discharge of excitation in Jackson 1879–1880; Macmillan 1990, 1991, pp. 175–180, and 1997, pp. 171–176; Bain 1855, pp. 73–80, and 1859, pp. 355, 387, 442–444, 476–477. Unpleasure in Bain 1855, pp. 291–296. Sexual drive in Bain 1855, pp. 249–254, and 1859, pp. 54, 371–372, 494–495; Macmillan 1991, pp. 300–305, and 1997, pp. 302–308. Reality sense in Bain 1855, p. 373, and 1859, p. 410. Conscience in Bain 1859, pp. 287, 313–315. "Secretory" neurons in Bain 1859, pp. 9, 14, 17, 28, 164, 229; Freud [1895] 1966, part I, sec. 14; Macmillan 1991, pp. 462–464, and 1997, pp. 471–474. Conflict in mental life in Bain 1859, pp. 419, 439. As is well-known, Freud's conception of language is very like that of Jackson, and there might well be similarities between it and those of Ferrier and Bain.

15. Freud [1895] 1966, pp. 337, 384, and [1900] 1953b, pp. 538–541. Exactly the same notions are in *The Ego and the Id* and the unpublished *Outline of Psycho-Analysis*.

16. Freud [1900] 1953b, pp. 566–567, 598–599; [1923] 1961a, p. 55; [1925] 1961b, p. 228.

17. Inhibition and delay in Freud [1940] 1964, p. 199; inhibition by the ego in Freud [1895] 1966, part I, sec. 14.

18. Freud's *On Aphasia* (1953) and Hammond 1871, pp. 174–176. For Freud's "library" see Lewis and Landis 1957, Bakan 1975, and Eissler 1979. I have to thank Marvin J. Taylor, then Special Collections Librarian, Health Sciences Library, Columbia University, for examining Freud's copies of the works of David Ferrier, comparing the handwriting, and suggesting how the annotations can be interpreted. I have also to thank Richard Hollinger, the current Special Collections Librarian, for allowing me to examine the works later.

13

The Popular Stories

... too monstrous for belief ...
—J. B. S. Jackson, *Warren Museum Catalogue*, 1870

As a kind of preliminary to the examination in chapter 14 of the stories told about Phineas Gage in various scientific works, I here consider some rather different ones. These portrayals derive from the small place that Gage has in fiction, semifiction, and popular culture. I believe they are worth analyzing because of their resemblance to those told in the scientific literature. I begin with an unusual story: Gage's treatment as it has been passed down in the family lore of the descendants of Edward Higginson Williams of Proctorsville, the first physician to attend Gage.

Gage in the Lore of the Williams Family

Every nineteenth-century published account of or reference to Gage's treatment of which I am aware credits the treatment to Harlow. However, on 1 February 1923, in a letter to a Springfield, Vermont, newspaper, a contrary version appeared. It claimed that Harlow had not begun the treatment at all and had stolen the whole glory from the Proctorsville physician, Edward Higginson Williams, who had. The writer was Edward H. Williams, Jr., the eldest son of the Proctorsville Williams, who had indeed been the first physician to see Gage and whom Gage had greeted with his famous "Doctor, here is business enough for you." Five years later the president of Jefferson Medical College repeated the claim. Eventually it was incorporated into a biographical entry on Williams in a history of Philadelphia and lives on strongly to this day as part of the Williams family history. At the 1998 commemoration of the 150th anniversary in Cavendish of the accident to Phineas Gage, Williams's great-great-grandson, the Rev. Edward H. Williams, IV, told me how he had frequently heard the story as a child when he visited his grandfather. He also remembered how his aunt would "fairly bristle" at the name Harlow and always include "and he never came for two days" in defending her grandfather's claim to priority.

What do we make of the claim? My comments about it are in two parts. In the first I try to clarify just what was claimed; in the second I try to evaluate the claims. Edward H. Williams, Jr., began his letter with an account of his father's education. His first career was in engineering, and he first worked on the Michigan Central Railroad. During that time he contracted a severe fever and what was thought to be asthma and gave up engineering. He then trained as a physician at Woodstock Medical College in Vermont and at the Bellevue Hospital in New York before setting up in practice in Proctorsville. Without too much medicine to practice, and having studied the rudiments of surveying under Hosea Doton, who was by then the engineer in charge of construction for the Rutland and Burlington Railroad, "he employed his spare time by running transit or level on the new road." In that capacity he became acquainted with Phineas Gage.

On the 13 September 1848, "an extremely hot day," an Irish railroad hand stopped Williams as he was driving home. He told Williams that

Mr. Gage wanted to see him. On being asked what was the matter he said "he is hurted, doctor, he had a tamping bar blown through his head." To further questions he said, "he is waiting for you at the hotel beyant."
When Dr. Williams drove up he found Gage sitting on the lowest step with his feet in the road; with his elbows on his knees; holding his head between his hands and spitting blood. On being asked what was the matter, he did not speak but raised up his hat with one hand showing the hole in his skull.

The letter continued with an account of how Williams had had Gage carried up to the third story of the hotel, placed on a rough operating table made of a pile of mattresses, washed, and made comfortable. He was not expected to survive but when he showed unexpected vitality,

Dr. Williams trephined and cleansed the wound. Owing to the entrance hole through the roof of the mouth, there was good drainage. Then a fungus-growth appeared around the edges of the wound and these were cut away. Then Dr. Harlow appeared and, as he was the surgeon of the company, the case was placed in his hands.

And when it came to reporting Gage's recovery:

According to medical etiquette the physician in charge makes the report and according to the medical rules this was a case under Dr. Harlow. This was an anomalous case—a unique case—and it seems that Dr. Harlow wished to take the whole glory. He did not do this at once, as it was well known to the teachers and pupils of the medical school at Woodstock that Dr. Williams was the first to reach and treat Gage.

When these matters came out in a distorted form, Dr. Williams let them alone, as the facts were known.

Soon after Gage's accident, Williams regained his health and resumed his career as an engineer. Eventually he became a partner in the Baldwin Locomotive Works in Philadelphia, a company that made railway locomotives used throughout the United States and in many countries around the world.

Alba B. Johnson, president of the Board of Trustees of Jefferson Medical College, added to the story in his commencement address at the University of Vermont on 18 June 1928. Having commenced work in 1876 for the Baldwin company, Johnson knew Williams personally and said he had heard him speak of Gage as an old friend, but it was not until after Williams's death that he learned of his role in Gage's treatment. In Johnson's version of the incident, Williams is homeward bound in 1846 when he finds Gage sitting by the roadside in Cavendish itself. He has him carried to the hotel, cleans the wound, trepans the skull, and "from time to time as fungus growth gathered, the Doctor took it away and eventually Gage recovered." Johnson did not mention Harlow, either directly or by implication, but he included among the facts well known to the Woodstock faculty and Doton "that Dr. Williams had done all the surgical work."

In February 1930, in an account of Gage's case for which he seems to have been interviewed for a Philadelphia newspaper, Johnson added what amounts to a caricature of Williams's treatment. Johnson was commenting on a Ripley "Believe It or Not" cartoon portraying the accident that the paper had published. The long interview quoted extensively from the commencement address before adding that Norman Williams had once asked his brother how he had performed the operation. According to Johnson, Williams told his brother:

The parts of the brain that looked good for something, I put back. Those that were too badly injured and looked as if they would be no good, I threw away. I kept the wound clean, sewed it up, and Gage got well.

This account of the "treatment" is placed between two paragraphs from the address and, like them, is also placed in quotation marks so that it reads as if Johnson were being quoted verbatim.

No details of a treatment like this are given in the short biography of the one-time Proctorsville physician that Edward H. Williams, IV, compiled in 1981 from letters, newspaper clippings, and recollections of conversations with E. H. Williams, Jr., and E. H. Williams, III. What his account does add is that Gage's

> became a noted case—the first in American medical annals, of trephining, a procedure but recently described in a European medical journal. Dr. Williams cared for Mr. Gage for the first two days until the company doctor, Harlow, by name could be summoned from Rutland. This man later claimed the entire responsibility for the case, which Dr. Williams took no special pains to challenge, since Dr. Harlow was the doctor in charge, and there were many at the Woodstock medical college who knew the facts.

In July of 1998, the Butler family Website included the whole of Edward H. Williams IV's compilation.

The story of the case in the biographical note in the Philadelphia history concentrates on the attempt to deprive Williams of the kudos:

> The case was one of the most celebrated in medical annals, and for its successful achievement Dr. Williams was given full credit by all those who knew of his, the first and most important, connection with it at the time—although the regular railroad surgeon, to whom the case was turned over and who made the official report of it, sought eventually to take the whole glory of the successful outcome.

Putting to one side some of the obviously incorrect minor points, such as the date of 1846, which is probably a typographical error, and others, such as the uniqueness of trephining in the United States, which may be due to a misunderstanding on the part of a nonmedical member of the family, what do we make of this challenge?[1]

There are four points central to the claim. Dr. Williams

1. comes upon Gage not long after he has been injured as he is sitting either on the side of the road near the site of the accident, or on a step with his feet on the road outside the hotel.
2. has Gage taken upstairs where he cleans the wound, trephines the skull, dresses and/or drains the wound, and cuts away the fungus.
3. looks after Gage for some two days until Harlow comes.
4. defers to Harlow as the railroad surgeon.

Williams's own account, written in December 1849, describes the circumstances and place of his first seeing Gage differently:

Dr. Harlow being absent at the time of the accident, I was sent for, and was the first physician who saw Mr. G., some twenty-five or thirty minutes after he received the injury; he at that time was sitting in a chair upon the piazza of Mr. Adam's hotel, in Cavendish. When I drove up, he said, "Doctor, here is business enough for you."

In other words, Williams did not find Gage sitting on the road as he was driving home. Nor was he sitting on the lowest step of the tavern with his feet in the road when Williams arrived.

Williams's letter is also at variance on the second point:

Soon after Dr. Harlow arrived, Mr. Gage walked upstairs, with little or no assistance, and laid down upon a bed, when Dr. H. made a thorough examination of the wounds, passing the whole length of his forefinger into the superior opening without difficulty; and my impression is that he did the same with the inferior one, but of that I am not absolutely certain; after this we proceeded to dress the wounds in the manner described by Dr. H. in the Journal.

On Williams's own account he did not attempt to treat Gage in any way before Harlow arrived.

A reasonable estimate of the time Williams had Gage solely under his care is at variance with point three. About an hour elapsed between Williams's arrival, at about 5 P.M. ("some twenty-five or thirty minutes after he received the injury"), and Harlow's ("I did not arrive at the scene of the accident until near 6 o'clock, P.M."). This interval is shorter than any in the claim and also rules out Williams's treating the fungus—as a product of infection, it could not have developed so quickly. Trephining would not have been appropriate. Well-known for some hundreds of years, it was a technique in which pieces of bone were removed from the skull in order to relieve pressure on the brain—and we can be reasonably sure that Gage did not need more openings in his skull than he already had.

What Williams and Harlow wrote about who was first in attendance is identical: in his 1848 report, Harlow clearly acknowledged that Williams was there first, Williams also said this in the 1849 letter, and Harlow repeated it just as clearly in 1868. It may also be worth noting that in both his reports, Harlow refers to "my friend Dr. Williams." Similarly, although Williams's letter was addressed to Bigelow, it was Harlow who had requested a description of what he had seen, and Williams opened his reply by saying that "I hasten to do so with pleasure." I do not sense any antagonism or disagreement between the two in these remarks.

The picture of Harlow as having some prior claim on the case because he was a railroad surgeon warrants two comments. First, physicians were commonly retained by railroad companies, but I have been unable to establish whether this was true of Harlow (I also do not recall the point being made other than in this claim). Second, even if he was on a retainer, one would think the seriousness of Gage's injury would warrant over-riding any "medical etiquette." What those proprieties might just account for, however, is Williams's seeming passivity during that first hour. But was he really passive? Would Williams really have had time to do much more than he said he had, that is, examine and assess the extent of the fracture, obtain Gage's story, and examine the slit in the cheek? Working together, it seems to have taken Harlow and Williams about an hour and a half to complete the examination and initial treatment. An hour for Williams by himself to establish the facts may not be unreasonable. Gage's story of how he came to be injured was, after all, a most unusual one, and may well have found the unbelieving Williams as unprepared as Harlow.[2]

Before I met the Rev. Edward Higginson Williams, IV, his niece, Mrs. Susan Czaja, asked her uncle if the family possessed any original material on the dispute over Harlow's priority. Through her, the Rev. Williams told me he had "never seen any first-hand account" and drew on "just what his father and grandfather told him." In Cavendish I had some long conversations with Rev. Williams and he confirmed what Mrs. Czaja had passed on to me. None of Dr. Edward Higginson Williams's medical manuscripts seem to have survived. Had there been such, and had they come into the possession of his son, E. H. Williams, Jr., they were prob-ably lost in the fire that completely destroyed his Woodstock home in the winter of 1921. The only written material bearing on the claim seems to be that which I have drawn on here.

Semifiction

Stories of the Gage case have been presented in a number of TV series. Sometimes the presentation is part of a straightforward discussion of brain function, sometimes it is a dramatic reconstruction, and sometimes it is narrative and drama. In this section I discuss examples of each type of story.

1984: Gage and Emotional Control

One part of the 1984 eight-part Canadian TV documentary science series, *The Brain*, is devoted to a dramatized version of Gage's accident and its consequences. The film was made to accompany Bloom, Lazerson, and Hofstadter's 1985 book, *Brain, Mind, and Behavior*. As with the book's treatment of Gage, the episode's main focus is on the limbic system's role in emotion. Within that framework the changes in Gage's behavior after the accident are reenacted and explained.

After an explanatory introduction, Gage is shown at work with his gang outside Cavendish. Some members of the gang are arguing about whom a young lady of the village really favors. Their quarrelling leads Gage to intervene and calm them down. In a voice-over commentary, the presenter describes Gage as an intelligent, well-balanced man who is modest, reliable, and in charge because he makes careful, well-balanced decisions. An animation shows the frontal intellectual part of the brain controlling the emotional limbic system.

The explosion takes place as Gage is distracted by the quarrel breaking out again. After he falls to the ground, the gang carries him to the village, where Dr. Williams attends him. At various points in the action the presenter's commentary tells the viewer that the connections between his frontal lobes and the limbic system have been damaged, that the limbic system is now free to fire emotional messages, and that the release of endorphins has probably diminished Gage's pain. Gage resists being taken inside the hotel and does not recognize Williams.

Harlow appears (out of nowhere) to assist Gage into the hotel, but Williams removes the bone fragments and joins his fingers together in his exploration of the damage between the two holes in Gage's skull. As the commentator repeats that the brain has been freed to fire its emotional messages, the hotel maid is shown walking downstairs at the same time as Gage is convulsing and apparently hallucinating. When Gage asks Harlow to let him have his dog, Biff, with him, one of his gang tells Harlow that Biff died (implying that Biff's death was some time before the accident). As Gage walks across the town center, the presenter tells the viewer that Gage survived physically but never regained his "emotional and intellectual self-control, balance, and judgment." He goes on to say that Gage's ability to communicate with others decreased, that he developed a special affinity for animals, that his gang believed he was now "a man out of control," and that what was destroyed was "the balance between his emotions and his intellectual faculties."

Gage is then shown outside the hotel, where he learns from the member of his gang who has been promoted to his job that he is no longer foreman. The gang members leave him, saying as they walk away that

Gage is not the man who was Gage, that he is like an animal, and that he has the emotions of an animal in a man's body. Gage is next seen asking for his job back in a railroad official's office, where he is told that although he had been the surest, the most efficient, and the most capable foreman, the company will not give it to him. Thereupon he fights with the official. The presenter ends the episode with an announcement of the whereabouts of the skull and tamping iron and states that physical changes in the brain affect behavior. By way of foreshadowing the next episode, Bloom is introduced to make a brief comment on the role of chemicals in mediating emotions.

The episode pictures no long-term postaccident changes. The lack of emotional control, immediately and in the short term, are placed centrally. It is, of course, an aspect of Gage's behavior about which Harlow says almost nothing. Consistent with this particular emphasis, Harlow's reference to the balance between Gage's intellectual faculties and animal propensities being destroyed is represented as referring to the balance between his emotions and his intellect. There is also, of course, nothing in Harlow about Gage having convulsions and hallucinations, or on his becoming aggressive enough to start fights.[3]

1991: Gage and the Physical Treatment of Psychiatric Disorder
Jonathan Miller discusses Phineas in about the middle of Episode 3 of his TV series *Madness*. The episode is devoted to the evolution of physical treatments of psychiatric disorder and begins with Miller watching a videotape of a delusional patient being interviewed. After the titles, it goes on with an extensively illustrated discussion with a psychiatrist about the form of electroconvulsive therapy he uses. Miller then turns to the early confinement of the insane, using the Vienna Fool's Tower as an illustration, and brings out how the view that asylums should have curative functions emerged only gradually. Lavater's studies of physiognomy, and various pictorial representations of the "insane," are next dealt with in the context of what the study of faces seemed to reveal about patients. Miller then contrasts brain explanations with "humoral," before turning to early methods of treatment, including restraint, Benjamin Rush's chair, swings, showers, and the like. He explains their rationale, making the point that all were directed to treating the brain as a whole, and suggests that all those methods subjected the brain to some sort of trauma that "presumably" jolted it into restoring its functions.

The invention and introduction of shock treatments (insulin and electroconvulsive therapy) is then discussed, and many illustrations of the administration of both are given.

Miller then turns to the apparent paradox that the functional architecture of the brain was known earlier than these holistic treatments. After outlining Gall's doctrine, he turns to the relation between disease and language functions identified by Broca and Wernicke. It is immediately after this that Phineas Gage is introduced. Miller remarks that "Once you began to entertain the idea that the brain is a system of physiological offices interacting with one another, and that certain morbid interactions might cause clinical symptoms, and possibly insanity, the stage is set for surgical intervention." Over a picture of an explosion taking place in a railway cutting, accompanied by the sounds, he continues, "It would be hard to regard the accident that befell Phineas Gage as a surgical manoeuvre." After relating the basic facts of the accident accurately, Miller says of Gage, "It's only by hindsight that he's acquired an almost mythical role in the history of psychosurgery."

Dr. Ken Tyler then joins Miller in discussing the case in the Warren Anatomical Museum, mostly in front of the cabinet displaying Gage's skull and the tamping iron, or over closeups of the skull itself. Except for having Gage survive for thirteen years, Tyler gives an accurate account of the case, noting that the "mental manifestations" were noted as early as 1848 when Harlow then promised a report on them. Tyler then illustrates the "minimal site" of the damage to the brain had the tamping iron followed the path he believed it had taken, explaining "And I think you can see it's really devastated almost all of the frontal lobe on one side."

A discussion then follows about the difference between what happened to Phineas and a typical stroke patient. When Miller asks "So this is a disorder of person, rather than of a person's bodily parts, really?" Tyler answers:

Yes. I think the key feature here was that Gage wasn't Gage; that the things that make someone a unique personality had been either subtly, or in many cases not so subtly, altered. It was as if he was a different person. Then, all of a sudden, this man who is almost a model citizen, suddenly can't hold a job, isn't to be trusted in the presence of women, because he might offend their delicate sensibilities with his profanity or his inappropriate remarks. He couldn't follow any sort of a plan; it was as if he darted from job to job, or thing to thing. And I think that at this point, this suddenly fit in so well with what was coming to be understood about what the frontal lobes of the brain might do.

Miller's voice continues immediately over a close up of Gage's life mask:

The therapeutic implications of this bizarre accident took a hundred years to emerge. In 1949 the Nobel prize for medicine was awarded to the Portuguese neurologist Egas Moniz, by which time literally thousands of patients had been subjected to the operation of lobotomy, which Moniz had inaugurated more than ten years earlier.

Miller goes on to discuss and illustrate the introduction and spread of lobotomy, especially in the form proposed by Freeman and Watts, but without further mention of Gage.

One notes that although Miller introduces Gage in the immediate context of the brain having independent offices, the overall context is one of physical treatments of psychiatric disorder, especially lobotomy. It is also notable that it is Miller who introduces the topic of lobotomy, that nothing Tyler says is related to it, and that what Miller offers is nothing more than an assertion of a connection between Moniz's operation and the changes to Gage's personality.[4]

1998: Gage as Narrative

The TV film made by Anne Georget with Hanna and Antonio Damasio is an illustrated narrative rather than a dramatized reconstruction. Essentially the film brings together two different kinds of material: Gage's story and an account of the attempted reconstruction of the damage by Hanna Damasio and her colleagues.

Gage's story is told mainly through the "voice" of John Martyn Harlow, in voice-over mode, reading or summarizing his own case notes and Bigelow's summary. Oddly, the film does not mention the discrepancy between Bigelow's and Harlow's reports. Because it adheres so closely to Harlow's account, the facts about the accident and the storminess of his recovery are presented in a way that is generally accurate and simultaneously interesting and extraordinarily imaginative. The film contains some minor errors: the population of Cavendish is slightly overstated, the wrong date is given for Harlow's beginning practice there, modern explosives and "modern" patent medicines are pictured, the time of the explosion is given as 4 P.M., what appears to be the September countryside is covered in snow, part of Harlow's quoting from Bigelow is illustrated with Harlow's woodcut, the newspaper coverage is represented as greater than it was, and Gage's date of death is given as 1861 (despite the producers' knowing that 1860 was the correct date).

The major inaccuracy is the emphasis given Gage's "wanderings," which are depicted as beginning almost from the moment of his physical recovery in April 1849. This part of the film is introduced with the sentence "M. Gage semble incapable de se fixer, il erre visitant Boston et la Nouvelle Angleterre." (M. Gage seemed incapable of settling down, he wandered visiting Boston and New England.) As this is being said, a trace of Gage's supposed journey appears on a map of New England of the period. He is then described as working in Hanover for a year before leaving for Chile, where he remains, looking after horses and driving a coach, until his health begins to fail. In 1860 he rejoins his family in San Francisco. This segment of the film ends with Harlow learning that he was then (apparently in 1860) employed on farms, was always dissatisfied, and frequently changed his employer. His convulsions apparently begin in 1861 and lead more or less immediately to his death.

Only in the direct comments by Hanna and Antonio Damasio is there anything different from what Harlow said about the psychological changes. Antonio Damasio claims Gage to be like a particular patient in whom he had first seen that "the problem in reasoning and decision making was somehow connected to a disturbance of the ability to have emotion and feeling." Other patients of his had a "very similar" pairing of "the flattening of the ability to react emotionally" with a "tremendous disturbance of the ability to reason and decide." Hanna Damasio describes the reconstruction against a background of the computer images she and her colleagues generated. Neither she nor Antonio Damasio localize the damage in any very specific part of the brain.

Harlow's account actually contains nothing about Gage's emotionality, and certainly nothing about his inability to "have emotion and feeling," or the flattening of his ability to react emotionally. Consequently, the parallel between Gage and the characteristics of the patient Antonio Damasio describes does not seem to be based on anything Harlow said. Although Hanna Damasio shows the trajectory for the tamping iron she and her colleagues chose, she does not give detailed reasons for its choice. Nor does she say how it differs from the other reconstructions, including Harlow's. She also implies that it was "bien plus acceptable à l'époque" [very acceptable in that era] to localize language in the brain, but placing morality there was "une autre histoire" (another story).

The film's strength is its amalgamation of Harlow's narrative with a strong and highly imaginative visual sensibility. Its weakness is its dubious comparisons with the behavior of Antonio Damasio's patient.

Such a parallel has the same dubious relevance to understanding Gage as that drawn in the WNET/13 film between Gage and patients with limbic system damage. In so "explaining" behavior that Gage did not exhibit, both films succeed in illustrating one of the striking features of stories about Phineas Gage: the fitting of almost any theory to the small number of facts we have about Gage.[5]

Fiction

Gage's place in fiction proper begins only twelve months after Harlow's last report. In 1869 a short story clearly based on the Gage case appeared. By 1998, exactly 150 years after the accident, at least one playwright had a play about Gage that had progressed to the rehearsal stage, and another four writers were serious enough in their plans for film scripts to have written to me for factual information. In between, I know of four other fictional accounts: two short story–like accounts, a "yarn," and the musings of the main character of a novel on the significance of the frontal lobes. Although there may be more such works, I do not imagine that what they say is very different from those I do know. And the parallels between what they do say and what the scientific literature says is surprisingly close.

1869: Gage the Apparition
The earliest fictional treatment of Gage known to me is that by Noah Brooks entitled "The Man with a Hole in His Head," which appeared in a San Francisco literary magazine within twelve months of Harlow's 1868 report. The main characters are Obed Murch (Phineas Gage), Dr. Peletiah Otis (John Martyn Harlow), Priscilla Dolkins (first wife of Gage-Murch), Mrs. Dolkins (Priscilla's mother), and Phoebe Morey Murch (second wife of Gage-Murch).

The story is introduced with Gage-Murch, born in Penebscot, Maine, searching for gold just outside of Mooney Flat in the Sierra Nevadas, when an accidental explosion blows his tamping iron through his skull. "Twenty-two inches long and one-half of an inch in diameter," it creates "a clean hole ... from under his chin to the top of his head ... [going] through bone, muscle, brain, skull, and scalp." Gage-Murch is taken home to his cabin, where Priscilla urges that Dr. Harlow-Otis be sent for. While they wait for him, Gage-Murch lies "motionless but not quite breathless." After Harlow-Otis has completed his examination, he tells those waiting that he believes Gage-Murch will survive because "the iron was small and smooth; it parted the formations of the brain, cut no large blood vessels, did not injure the cerebral organs, and left him only sense-less." Regaining consciousness later that night, Gage-Murch recovers rapidly over the next month, during which time he is pained only by the hole in his mouth. The hole in his head is covered by a silver plate, over which the scalp regrows.

The story really starts with the bargain struck between Gage-Murch and Harlow-Otis over payment for his services. Times being hard, Harlow-Otis asks for Gage-Murch 's skull in lieu of his fee, and Gage-Murch and Priscilla agree. Harlow-Otis gives Gage-Murch a receipt that does not mention the bargain, because a formal document would be no better than his word attested by Priscilla. The "curious facts in [Gage-]Murch's case got into the newspapers, and two medical journals recorded the singular fact of a man's brain being perforated by an iron rod without any fatal result." Gage-Murch resumes work, actually pros-pering, and living comfortably and contentedly in a larger town, until Priscilla is "taken down" with a fever. Medical help is sent for and, sur-prise, Dr. Harlow-Otis reappears as the town's physician. Gage-Murch feels uneasy but Harlow-Otis reassures him that his own time has not yet come. Not so with Priscilla, who dies but not before reminding Gage-Murch of his bargain.

Priscilla's death unsettles Gage-Murch, who returns to sawmilling in Maine and marries Phoebe Morey. She, being "light, trifling, and super-ficial," urges him to return to California, taking her with him. He resists until Dr. Harlow-Otis sets up practice in the little village, not knowing Gage-Murch is also a resident. Gage-Murch then offers to pay the bill but Harlow-Otis refuses. If he slips "off the hooks" before Gage-Murch, he will lose, but "that is my risk, not yours." His frequent visits unsettle Gage-Murch: "He would look almost savagely at him, muttering to himself: 'He's waiting for my head. Don't he wish he may get it.' " Finally Gage-Murch and Phoebe leave for California.

During the next few years, Phoebe's "fickle disposition" leads her to become discontented wherever they go. Gage-Murch moves "about rest-lessly from place to place, never staying very long anywhere." Phoebe drags him around from mine to lumber camp, to ranch, and to inn, but wherever they go, Dr. Harlow-Otis follows, as "he was so attached to the man whose life he had saved." Gage-Murch is always aware of the doctor's presence, even when he lives in the next town. If Gage-Murch meets him as he goes about his medical work, he grumbles "in his set teeth 'There goes the man that's waiting for my head. Let him wait.' " After a bad attack of colic, during which he is unexpectedly attended by Dr. Harlow-Otis, Gage-Murch goes mining in Idaho, leaving Phoebe in the care of Mrs. Dolkins, Priscilla's mother, now resident in San Francisco. Dr. Harlow-Otis establishes a good practice in the city before Gage-Murch eventually returns to share his abode with his former mother-in-law. Gage-Murch meets him in the street and asks if he is still waiting. "It was [Gage-]Murch who had followed [Harlow-]Otis this time. And there was an omen in it."

Finally, Gage-Murch's time to die does come. He is "brought home on a stretcher, dumb with apoplexy and gasping for breath." Dr. Harlow-Otis attends and he and Phoebe both hear Gage-Murch's last words, "Don't you call 'time' on me yet, Doc. You may have my head tomorrow." The bargain is news to Phoebe, and Harlow-Otis foresees trouble. She is "a flighty weakminded woman, without the least consideration for the requirements of science and totally ignorant of anatomy. Besides, the foolish woman appears to have loved her husband." She objects so strenuously to the bargain that Gage-Murch goes "to Lone Mountain ... taking his head with him." Phoebe and Mrs. Dolkins disagree so much on the bargain and many other matters that Phoebe moves out of the house. Years go slowly by, with Gage-Murch's body "mouldering in the grave," until Dr. Harlow-Otis marries Mrs. Dolkins. She brings "small dowry beyond a little furniture and a small bit of iron which had once been blown perpendicularly through a man's head.... It was [Gage-Murch]'s tamping-iron." Three years after Gage-Murch's death, she gives permission for his body to be exhumed and the skull removed. She does so on the rather mixed grounds that she is his mother-in-law, the mother of the wife who was party to the compact, the guardian of her daughter's good name, and custodian of the body. Phoebe's wrath is "dreadful to behold." Knowing that Dr. Harlow-Otis has promised "an eminent professor of anatomy in an Eastern college that he should have the skull for the college lectures and the college museum," she commences legal proceedings to prevent this from happening but is unsuccessful. In a "stout box, under an enormous pile of freight, [Gage-Murch]'s skull was travelling to New York, ghastfully grinning to itself all the way."

The last part of the story is set at night, in the library of Corinthian College. The night watchman has been asleep and wakes to find the door to the adjacent anatomy museum open when it should be closed. Making his way to the museum he sees "a strange, dark figure gliding stealthily along.... The Shape stopped by one of the cabinets; and then he saw it was the headless figure of a man." The Shape removes a skull that is impaled on an iron rod:

It slipped the gibbering, bony skull up and down on the rod that pierced it from chin to crown, as if it were amused at the curious sight; then the awe-struck watcher heard from the fleshless lips of the skull: "Yes, you bet that's me!"

Brooks concludes, "Unless the watchman dreamed a horrid dream, he had seen the Spectre of the Man with a Hole in his Head."

The first notable feature about Brooks's account is its use of the framework provided by some of the facts about Gage. Murch's skull and tamping iron do end up in a university anatomy museum, two articles about him do appear in medical journals, both of which emphasize the singularity of the accident not being fatal, and eventually Murch does die in San Francisco. Brooks may also be making reference to a real event in using a title that mimics the museum advertisement incorporated in Blackington's story. The second feature is the emphasis on Murch's being unaffected and unchanged. He virtually recovers by himself, the accident itself produces no change whatever in his personality and behavior, and the problems that beset him are the result of his wife's fickleness and the pressure of the "bargain" struck with Dr. Otis. In following Bigelow's 1850 interpretation rather than Harlow's account of 1868, Brooks matches perfectly those many contemporaneous medical comments on Harlow's 1868 paper in which the changes were overlooked. We will see that that view continues to be represented in the scientific literature. The Otis-Murch bargain also has a modern parallel there: one modern author has Gage selling his skeleton to more than one medical school.[6]

1956: Gage and the Gypsy
Having already drawn on the apparently factual parts of Blackington's "The Man with the Hole in His Head" in chapter 5, I focus here on the more clearly fictional aspects of his Yankee yarn. Blackington opens with Phineas emerging from a fortune teller chilled with the prophecy:

You are in immediate danger! Before the sun sets tomorrow, *the icy fingers of death will touch you*. But you will survive. You will go on the stage, and a hundred years from now, people will still be talking about you.

The next day, a Saturday, Phineas has his accident.

With the exception of some invented dialogue, the adoption of the wrong day for the accident, and Phineas's recollecting the prophecy on the way to the tavern, Blackington's yarn follows Harlow's account reasonably closely up to the time he tries to resume work. Blackington has it that the contractors do not give Phineas his job back because it has been given to another. Gage then goes to Boston, lives in a tent on the Common, and exhibits the nature of his injury by passing the tamping iron through a skull that has had two holes made in it. After Gage has spent periods with the museums of Austin and Stone and of Barnum, Bigelow examines him. "Day after day" Phineas gains publicity in the press and in the medical community, and does well financially from it. Nevertheless he becomes restless, "roaming from circus to side show and back again," until he settles to work as a "horse handler for Jonathan Currier." While there, Phineas joins a man who is "buying horses for a stage-line in Chile," traveling with him "to look after the animals, and after a year among the mountains back of Valparaiso, he graduate[s] to stage driver, skilfully handling six or more spirited steeds as they hauled a lurching coach up and down the tortuous mountain roads." His health fails, he sails "on a clipper ship" to live with his mother, but is in such "broken health" that he can do only light work. He dies "suddenly," but no cause of death is given.

When the news of Phineas's death reaches Boston, "the medical men" there forward a request to the family asking that the skull be preserved. They agree, and the skull and tamping iron are placed in the museum. Blackington begins his conclusion with a return to the prophecy:

While the gipsy fortune teller did prophesy that Phineas would "go on the stage and travel to far places," after his brush with death, she omitted to say that because of the accident he would gradually change from a simple country man to a loud mouthed boisterous and very profane individual—so profane that the police drove him from Boston Common and even strong men of those rugged times quaked when they heard him.

Blackington's story also minimizes the effect of the accident by making Gage merely loudmouthed, boisterous, and profane. The importance of Harlow's treatment is implicit, but it is not Harlow who asks the family for the skull and tamping iron or who writes up the case. In one sense, Blackington almost writes Harlow out of his story. In this respect, his story parallels the review in the *Boston Medical and Surgical Journal* of Harlow's 1869 booklet form of his address to the Massachusetts

Medical Society. In it, the main focus is on Bigelow, and Harlow is hardly mentioned.[7]

1965: Gage the Puritan Turned Drunkard

From the beginning, Bernard Lamere's title, "Phineas Gage Had a Headache," minimizes the seriousness of the accident's effects. Lamere begins his seemingly factual account by stressing Gage's upright character:

Phineas was a bit of an oddity in the brawling lusty days of railroad building. Of puritan upbringing, he never used strong language, attended prayer meetings regularly, and didn't care for the demon alcohol. At a time when foreman were being killed or assaulted, he was liked and respected by his men, who respected his fair treatment and knew that he would perform the most dangerous tasks himself.

The thirty drillers at work "on the morning of Sept. 13" accompany their hammer blows with the chant "Drill, ye tarriers drill." The accident occurs among holes "drilled the week before," just after Gage has placed "fulminate caps and fuses" in the hole and filled it with mud. The gang members are all Irish, some being named, but it is one referred to only as Patrick who helps Lem Goodrich support Gage on a three-mile trek to the steps of the Cavendish Tavern. Pat finds medical help "after a couple of hours." The doctor, who is not named, pronounces, "No man can live with a hole in his head; have him measured for a casket," apparently leaves, and is not mentioned further. Gage is carried upstairs, put to bed, and fed, although no one expects him to live. An account of the accident that appears in the Harvard Medical Journal draws "many scoffing letters."

Three weeks later Gage announces " 'My head isn't aching so much now, so I guess I will go back to work.' And he did." His personality was completely changed: "He took to holding forth in saloons, cursing and telling outrageous yarns which he maintained were factual." He is lured to Chile to work on railroad construction, where he dies in 1869. His will contains a request "that his head be detached from the body and shipped, with the bar, to a Dr. Harlow in the USA." This is done and Harlow gives the skull and tamping iron to the Massachusetts Medical Museum.

Lamere's account emphasizes self-cure. Gage seems to recover without treatment, and the absence of any medical details is consistent with Lamere's picture of the accident's having relatively minor effects. Gage is able to benefit financially from his accident, his capacity for work is unimpaired but, apart from his beginning to swear—as per Harlow—and spending time in saloons (apparently drinking) and telling outrageous yarns, Lamere leaves him virtually unchanged. His benefiting financially, his yarn telling, and his frequenting saloons—none of which are mentioned by Harlow or documented elsewhere—are also found in the scientific literature.[8]

1969: Gage and the Philosopher's Stone

The first part of Colin Wilson's novel *The Philosopher's Stone* centers on a search by Howard (Harry) Lester and Henry Littleway for the neurological basis of what Lester calls "the value experience, the childhood moments of universal 'newness' and happiness" to which poets cling. Lester seems to be searching for the basis of artistic creativity, Littleway for what it is that prevents aging. Their interests come together in the importance they attribute to the "input" state of the brain, the state in which, as Lester puts it, the brain "is passive, wide open, receiving impressions as an open flower receives sunlight."

By accident, Lester and Littleway hear that a serious head and brain injury has caused Richard O'Sullivan, a farm laborer, to stay in "a perpetual state of ecstasy." Closer investigation convinces them that he has acquired second sight. He has also changed from being athletic, vital, and given to practical jokes, to being dreamy, lethargic, and positively radiating benevolence and affection. They readily induce "value experiences" in him, and these have the effect of curing him of diseases with which they infect him. However, the experiments weaken him, possibly contributing to the brain tumor from which he eventually dies. Pondering what happens, Lester concludes that the value experiences "are merely moments in which man becomes conscious of what he already possesses." He seeks their basis in neurological processes that cause the brain to break its habitual mode of responding. He concludes that the possessor of a brain capable of snapping out of its habits at a moment's notice would live forever.

Without giving further reasons, Lester says he felt, from the beginning, that the answer to the basis of the value experience lay in the frontal lobes. He then sets out a kind of argument to justify that view. The frontal lobes have contradictory properties. On the one hand they are concerned with such higher faculties as "sympathy, tact, self-discipline and reflection," and although functioning as "some kind of extra storage," they are not affected by damage. He instances Gage and Joe A.—Brickner's patient—although he mentions neither by name. Gage is said to have lived for twelve years "in a perfectly normal manner, except that his behaviour was in many respects coarsened," and Joe A. is said to have become "boastful, and tactless, and ceased to care for his family." On the other hand, damage to the frontal lobes in children produces "a general loss of intelligence" and, since children experience more poetic states than adults, it can be seen why "the mechanism of the value experience should be concentrated in the frontal lobes."

Lester knows of the delayed response experiments on monkeys from which he draws the conclusion that although prefrontal damage does not impair monkey intelligence, "memory is to some extent affected." Consequently, he becomes convinced that "the centre for poetry and intelligence" is located frontally. He then begins an experimental program of direct electrical stimulation of the frontal lobes using a special type of electrode that amplifies the current for a very short time just before delivering it. During one experiment, a small piece of electrode breaks off and is left in the subject's brain. But "there was no real cause for alarm" because, "if a man can survive . . . after a crowbar has amputated most of his prefrontal lobes" the damage from such a small piece of the electrode would be "very small indeed." He and Littleway carry out experiments to assess the effects of frontal lobe stimulation on value experiences, aging, psychic powers, and the like. Lester himself undergoes the operation, experiences the effect of the "kick" the special electrode delivers, and, quickly learning to produce the effect by willpower, soon discards the electrodes.

This is all the use that Wilson makes of Gage. Unfair though it may be to Wilson, the rest of the novel is irrelevant for my purposes, concerned as it is with the psychic powers Lester and Littleway develop and the use to which they put them. Although Lester mentions prefrontal leucotomy as an "obsolete operation," the reasoning that leads him to the frontal lobes has the same gaps as Moniz's. Lester draws on the animal experiments on delayed response and those on Joe A., and he minimizes the alterations to behavior in both. He judges frontal damage to have little substantial effect and jumps to the frontal lobes as the place where he will find "the answer" as effortlessly as did Moniz. The only real difference is that Lester mentions Gage and Moniz does not. Lester's mention is, however, Moniz-like: Gage's behavior has not been seriously changed, merely "coarsened."[9]

Popular History, Folklore, and Popular Culture

Phineas Gage is mentioned in many popular histories of New England in both book and article form. While the broad outlines of his story are usually accurate, much of the important detail is not. Thus in his historical sketches, Hayes has the wrong date for the accident, has the minimum diameter of the tamping iron as half an inch, has Phineas being able to work for nineteen years after it, and Phineas's expressed wish for his skull and tamping iron to be preserved as the basis for the placement of both in the museum. Similar errors occur in Wheeler's history of Cavendish. She has Phineas causing the explosion by tapping a stick of dynamite with a crowbar. He walks three miles to a farm house, recovers despite the village doctor's pessimism, and works for years after. He wills his head to Dr. Harlow but she uses Bigelow's skull instead of Gage's to illustrate her account. Huban manages to have Gage dying in Chile twenty-one years after the accident.[10]

No American folksongs or ballads about Phineas Gage seem to exist. Nothing seems to have been passed down orally, either in general or railroad folklore. I found nothing in my own amateurish searches of broadsheet and ballad collections in New England, a result duplicated by inquiring of those having specialist knowledge (Richard Baumann, Roger deV Renwick, Edward D. Ives, and W. Edson Richmond). Tom Sabo of Cavendish, Vermont, who specializes in collecting and performing railroad ballads, knows of no songs or ballads about Gage.[11]

Two rock bands based on Gage's name do exist but I have been unable to determine why they were so named. "Phineas Gage" is the closest in name, but "Finneus Gauge" clearly has a similar origin. A relatively new group called "Slackdaddy" recorded a song in 1998 entitled "What's the Matter with Phineas Gage?" Although no one I know who has listened to the lyrics has been able to understand more than a few words, the group neither seems to sing anything of significance about Gage nor to answer the question posed in the title of the song.

Newspaper Stories

From time to time newspaper stories appear about Gage, sometimes in response to a report of a case of brain injury, sometimes apparently to mark the anniversary of his accident, and at other times without obvious reason. Most simply summarize the history but some are more complex.

Here I summarize one example of each of those types and one that continues, nearly 150 years later, the "miraculous" theme of the 1849 reports.

1930: Another Case
The first, from 1930, is an unsigned article from the *New York Sun*. It is a simple account of Gage written as a kind of comment on a case in which "a young boy was shot in the head and lived after a slug of lead was extracted from a wound that penetrated his skull and into his brain." It recalled, said the reporter, "another accident of some eighty years ago that undoubtedly will stand as the most remarkable case of its kind ever known to medical history." The account, clearly based on Harlow's 1868 report, is a very accurate summary that names Harlow. No real parallel is drawn between Gage and the case of the penetrating gunshot wound. It was sufficient that the brain was injured in both cases. Perhaps the most important point is the one implied by the subheading "Became a Freak" that introduces the last two paragraphs. The text says simply that "Gage took to travelling and for a time was with Barnum's Museum, where he displayed the wound in his head and the tamping iron that had made it." Merely being with Barnum was enough to make Gage a freak.[12]

1975: An Anniversary
Barney Crosier's 1975 article is of the "anniversary" kind. It opens with "Fall foliage and the whistles of steam trains always have a tendency to take Cavendish people way back into history—back far enough so they recall what was probably Vermont's most celebrated medical case of all time and a wonder of the world." The article is unusual for pointing to a number of the controversies surrounding the case. Although the account itself contains some unremarked and minor inaccuracies (e.g., the use of dynamite), Crosier often points out how the stories differ (e.g., whether Gage walked to the hotel or rode in the oxcart).

More interestingly, in referring to Gage's being attended at first "by a railroad surveyor, Edward Williams, who had had some medical training," he implies there may be an account other than Harlow's: that Williams had training in surveying is not mentioned other than in the story told by the Williams family. Of even more interest is Crosier's statement, one that I have not seen elsewhere, that in 1975 there was still some argument among Cavendish residents as to whether Gage swore before the accident. However, all agreed that he acquired an inflammable temper and the habit of swearing after it. Crosier says that from the change "doctors learned that that the front lobe of the brain ... was responsible for personality development," and this was "one of the clues that led ... to the 'lobotomy' that has been used in the past to cure mental problems." He judges the case to have "started physicians doing more research on the various parts of the brain."

Crosier's story matches some of those in the scientific literature by overestimating the Gage's importance to the development of psychosurgery and to studies of localization more generally. Further, given that Harlow seems to have spoken about Gage only once in public, Crosier rather astonishingly has Harlow as "a world-famous person who became rich with his lecturing" about the case. Perhaps this is another disguised reference to the challenge from the Williams family.[13]

1984: Gage as Information

Bill Lacey's 1984 article was not provoked by another case or by an impending anniversary. What is most remarkable about it is its accuracy. Lacey has told me that he based his article on transcripts of the papers by Harlow and Bigelow and on a conversation with Robert Leavitt, City Historian of Lebanon, New Hampshire. Clearly he absorbed the source material extremely thoroughly. In only two places does he go beyond what is in the papers, and here he may be incorporating information from Leavitt. He has Gage's family being so "appalled" by his condition on arrival in San Francisco that they write to Harlow "for whatever help he might be able to give." That is not quite as Harlow has it: he learns of Gage's return only after his death. Second, he refers to Phebe Jane as Phineas's "younger sister" when that, which is actually the case, is not in any of the papers.

However, the large and dramatic illustration that dominates Lacey's article contains one considerable inaccuracy. The skull shown with a tamping iron located in it is Bigelow's reconstruction and not Gage's. Lacey no longer has the illustration but clearly recalls its being on a heavy card stock about three inches by five inches, and that it was somewhat enlarged when printed. Its source? The "bizarre error," as Lacey described it in our correspondence, had been committed by someone at the Warren Museum who had sent the picture together with the transcripts. Unlike the authors of those scientific papers in which the

Bigelow skull is represented as Gage's, Lacey did not make this mistake because of his own carelessness.[14]

1998: Gage as Sensation Again

In 1998 the *Fortean Times* reported Gage in the context of an article on injuries to the brain that began with a case "that sent a shiver down the world's back." The *Times* is an odd journal founded by the equally odd Charles Fort to publicize odd phenomena that he believed science could not explain. It continues today, somewhat tongue-in-cheek, with the subtitle *The Journal of Strange Phenomena*. Its 1998 reference was in a report of an Allison Kennedy who had been stabbed in the head with a thirteen-centimeter (five-inch) hunting knife. After noting that she had recovered "more-or-less unscathed," the *Times* summarized another case of stabbing in the head, this time with a benign change in the victim's personality: he had been "a foulmouthed drunk" but was now "a quiet tee-totaller." Gage was then introduced showing a certain symmetry with these two cases, being described as "the first lobotomy." As the references show, the account of Gage's case and its interpretation clearly derives from the study by Hanna Damasio and her colleagues. Although that discussion is not particularly "miraculous," the other five cases are mentioned with such descriptors as "spectacular," "dramatic," or "grievous," leading to the introduction of Gage's case with the phrase "However, this is as nothing to the ordeal survived by . . ."[15]

Science, Newspapers, and the Warren

A 1972 paper by the late Dr. Harold Constantian of Worcester, Massachusetts, and the subsequent correspondence it generated illustrates well the interrelation between scientific and newspaper accounts. One day while wandering "aimlessly" through Woodstock, Vermont, Dr. Constantian came upon and visited the library founded by Norman Williams, where he discovered the story of Dr. Edward Higginson Williams's treating Gage. It encouraged him to investigate further and eventually to write the article that appeared in the *Worcester Medical News*.

The only source that Constantian specifically mentions is Bigelow's 1850 paper. From his own paper it can be inferred that his sources also included the 1923 *Springfield Reporter* letter from E. H. Williams, Jr., Alba Johnson's 1928 commencement address, Johnson's 1930 later caricature of the treatment in his comment on the Ripley cartoon, and a good deal of biographical material about Williams. Constantian reproduced Ripley's cartoon with its accompanying picture of Dr. Edward Higginson Williams from the interview with Alba Johnson reported in the *Evening Bulletin* (Philadelphia) of 15 February 1930. The article made no mention of either of Harlow's papers, although it should be remembered that Bigelow's account includes Harlow's 1848 account in its entirety. What Constantian says of Gage's postaccident history probably comes from the Warren *Catalogue*, as the reference to Gage's driving a stage coach indicates, but he does have detail not in it or other accounts. Thus he has Gage driving a coach "for a while" and traveling about "a great deal lecturing and exhibiting the bar, but usually driving or working with horses" before going to Chile. Perhaps this drew on some local knowledge of Gage, because Constantian also has him sitting "on a stool outside the door of the Boston Museum" for three months after his recovery. Although these descriptions are novel, I think that Constantian worked basically from the collection of material on E. H. Williams now at the Norman Williams Public Library.

Slightly less than half of Dr. Constantian's article is devoted to Williams's early education and career as an engineer, the remainder being a straightforward account of the accident to Gage and his injury, treatment, and eventual recovery. What is remarkable about it is that it does not mention either the claim of Williams's priority or that Harlow is supposed to have stolen the glory. Not only did the source material cover all these issues, but the Ripley cartoon that appeared with Johnson's expanded comments had had a picture of Williams placed over its bottom left-hand corner. Johnson made both claims in the article itself, and the short paragraph under the picture of Williams repeated the priority claim as follows: "Seeing this 'Believe it or Not' drawing ... several days ago, Alba B. Johnson ... recalled that the physician who treated the victim was Dr. Edward Higginson Williams." None of this sentence appears in Constantian's paper, although the first six words of it are on the copy of the photograph Constantian supplied to his printer. Was Constantian not convinced that either claim had substance?

The first two points to emerge from the article and subsequent correspondence are somewhat incidental. When Dr. Constantian was working on his paper, presumably in 1972, he saw "at the right of the cabinet" in which Gage's skull was displayed at the Warren "the skull prepared by Dr. Bigelow for demonstration purposes and pictured in the publication in 1850." Since then, the Bigelow skull seems to have disappeared. The second is the errors in Constantian's transcription of the inscription on the tamping iron: he gives Harlow instead of Gage as the depositor of the relic, and 1866 as the year of deposition.

The third point is in a letter to the editor in the February 1973 issue of the *Worcester Medical News* from David Gunner, then the Curatorial Associate at the Warren. Gunner first congratulated Constantian on his "scholarly article" and went on to blame Ripley for creating misunderstandings about the case. The cartoon itself "perpetuated the notion that that Gage lived for nearly thirteen years with a tamping bar securely positioned through his head," and the text had "formalized" the misnomer of the "Crowbar skull." Although he did not say that Ripley's drawing was closer to Bigelow's reconstruction than to the real skull, Gunner enclosed photographs of Gage's life mask and the skull itself. These accompanied Gunner's letter when it was published.

Fourth, some eight years later, in 1980, Burnham G. Gage of Natick, Massachusetts, wrote to Samuel Bachrach, then editor of the *News*, for information about his relative "who was listed" in Ripley and about whom he had been told the *News* had published an article. Bachrach replied, sending a copy of Constantian's article, and in the next issue reproduced Gunner's 1972 letter together with the Ripley cartoon (with its picture of Williams) and a photograph of the tamping iron. This time, the inscription was reproduced correctly (although in its usual truncated form).

The fifth point is rather more important. On 13 July 1973 David Gunner wrote directly to Dr. Constantian requesting a copy of the Ripley cartoon. After explaining that the cartoon "was of interest," he added, "more importantly, I am eager to have a 'portrait' of Dr. E. H. Williams." The Warren was reinterpreting the case and "Dr. Williams has never been adequately represented. . . ." If that reinterpretation was made, it did not lead to Williams's claim being included as a permanent part of the exhibit. The implied rejection of the claim is identical with that of Constantian, who, despite working primarily from Williams's sources, left the claim of his priority out of his article.[16]

Conclusion

If I have emphasized the errors in these accounts of the Gage case, it is because they also show up in the scientific literature to be considered in the next chapter. Both literatures contain the same minor errors about the work Gage was doing, report nothing about the accident's immediate impact and the stormy nature of his recovery (or play them down), misrepresent the changes to his behavior, and fabulate a subsequent history that, rather than having him working in a reasonably normal way, turn him into something like a drunken liar who drifts around as a circus freak. Whether Ripley is responsible or not, at least one "scientific" source actually has Gage surviving for twelve years with the tamping iron embedded in his skull. And although not identical, there is also a strong resemblance between Gage's fictional bargain over the disposal of his skull and the purportedly scientific report of Gage's making an advance sale of his skeleton to two different medical schools. All the errors have the same bases: ignorance of what Harlow reported in 1868 or flagrant disregard of what he did say in favor of fitting Gage into an existing theoretical framework (or both, of course).

Reinterpretation within an existing framework is the hallmark of the WNET/13 film, in which damage to the limbic system is used to "explain" behavior that Gage did not exhibit. It is also present in the comparisons Antonio Damasio makes with the behavior of his patient. Where Gage's history is presented accurately, as it is in both Bill Lacey's article and Anne Georget's French TV film, it is because the facts are presented as Harlow presented them. The same is true of the works to which I now turn.

Notes

1. E. H. Williams, Jr., letter to the editor in *Springfield Reporter* (Vermont), 1 February 1923; E. H. Williams, IV 1997; A. B. Johnson 1928, p. 4, and interview with him in *Evening Bulletin* (Philadelphia), 15 February 1930; Butler Website ⟨http://www.toto.com/butler/fam_tree⟩; Philadelphia biography (Collins 1941, pp. 160–161).

2. Williams's letter is in Bigelow 1850b, 1850c, and Harlow 1848, 1849, 1868, and 1869 contain his account.

3. WNET/13 1984. I have to thank Executive Producer Jack Sameth for providing me with a copy of the script of the episode.

4. Miller 1991.

5. Georget 1998.

6. Brooks 1869.

7. Blackington 1956 and "Bibliographical notices," 1869.

8. Lamere 1964–1965.

9. Wilson 1969.

10. Hayes 1907, pp. 331–332. cf. Hayes 1929, p. 340; Wheeler 1952, pp. 26–27; and Hugan 1956.

11. Folklore collections are Botkin 1944 and Botkin and Harlow 1953. Authorities consulted are listed under "Folklore" in appendix H.

12. "Hard to believe but absolutely true" (1930).

13. Crosier 1975.

14. Lacey 1984. I do not know if the basis of Wheeler's identical error in her history of Cavendish is the same (Wheeler 1952, p. 26).

15. McNally 1998; I have to thank Dr. Sheldon Benjamin for the copy of McNally's article and Paul Sieveking, Editor of *The Fortean Times*, for providing the publication details. H. Damasio et al. 1994. For Charles Fort, see Gardner 1981.

16. Constantian 1972. My belief about Dr. Constantian's sources is confirmed by my obtaining essentially the same collection from the Norman Williams Library (to which I wrote at his suggestion) as the collection of material he gave me in 1989. Dr. Constantian also gave me the photograph of the Ripley cartoon–Williams portrait in the form in which it seems to have been prepared for the printer, and the later articles and correspondence. The order of appearance of the articles and letters in the *Worcester Medical News* is September–October 1972, vol. [36?], no. 7, pp. 12–15; January–February 1973, vol. [38?], no. 3, p. 20; January 1980, vol. [45?], no. 3, p. 7. The copies of the *News* I have seen appear to have the wrong volume numbers printed on them. I do not know if Dr. Constantian had positive evidence for saying Gage "spent the years succeeding the accident displaying himself as a freak."

14

The Scientific Stories

A moral man, Phineas Gage,
Tamping powder down holes for his wage,
Blew the last of his probes
Through his two frontal lobes;
Now he drinks, swears, and flies in a rage.
—Author unknown

The scientific stories about Phineas Gage examined in this chapter provide some interesting parallels to the fictional accounts of chapter 13. Almost everyone agrees that science is different from art. We expect that an artist will convey the essentials of a serious subject with power and conviction, and, terming it artistic license, we forgive or allow that truth may be sacrificed for artistic effect. Very different rules govern scientific reports and interpretations; they represent things as they really are. One expects the scientist to investigate phenomena without prejudice, to collect data comprehensively, and to weigh conclusions judiciously. Phrases that would correspond to an essential feature of the endpoint of artistic endeavor, such as "scientific license" or "scientific effect," not only do not exist, it is hard to see what meaning they could have if they did. Yet we will see in this chapter that we are forced to draw on some such notions if we are to understand the pictures of Phineas Gage we find in much of the psychological, psychiatric, medical, physiological, linguistic, and general neuroscientific literature.

Gage in the Physiological Literature

Phineas Gage was mentioned in five of twenty-one physiological textbooks, mainly written for medical students, that I examined. Because his accident took place in 1848, it is perhaps not surprising that there is little mention of his case in textbooks of physiology published in the ten-year period that followed. For example, Todd and Bowman do not mention his case even though they discussed localization in a way that was reasonable for the time and Harlow's first paper and Bigelow's confirmation had appeared by then. But some authors seem not to have wanted the brain to have functions and reported nothing at all relating to localization, even when, like Dalton, they included chapters or sections on "The Brain."[1]

Up to the end of the nineteenth century and into the beginning of the twentieth, most textbooks of physiology discussed localization, but few mentioned Gage, even when the treatment of localization was reasonable or good for its time. The sixth and eighth editions of Martin's text are especially revealing. In both, but especially in the eighth, Martin gave very comprehensive and up-to-date coverage of the experimental studies of localization, but illustrated his point that the effects of disease were more important than experiment only with cases of aphasia. Gage also seems to have been omitted from works published outside the United States of America as frequently as from those in it.[2]

Similarly, most of the physiological texts that appeared in the first half of the twentieth century also failed to mention Gage, even when they included the clinical observations of Dandy and Brickner or the experimental work of Fulton and Jacobsen. Minimizing the role of the frontal lobes during this period was also common. For example, the early editions of Bayliss emphasized that frontal stimulation and extirpation had no effect, but the earliest, dating from 1915, could not have dealt with the work of Dandy. When Howell repeated without qualification Brickner's global summary that bilateral frontal lobectomy produced a quantitative rather than qualitative impairment, he also minimized the role of the frontal lobes. On the other hand, the 1923 edition of Huxley's text dropped the mention of Gage that been in every edition since the first in 1868.[3]

Five Nineteenth-Century Appreciations
What was said in the five texts that did discuss Gage is of interest. We saw in chapter 7 that in what might be the first discussion of Gage in the localization literature, Dalton (1859) situated his remarks on Gage between the insensibility of the brain and his account of Flourens. That he then drew only on Bigelow's 1850 account, with its benign outcome,

is understandable, if not completely excusable; but the way he continued to do so nearly thirty years later, in a considerably revised edition, is inexcusable. By then Harlow's account was already eleven years old, and even if Dalton did not cite it, he did draw on J. B. S. Jackson's entry in the Warren Museum *Catalogue*. But he did not use Jackson's summary of the changes in Gage. All he said was that Gage was "able to do the ordinary work of an ostler, coachman, and farm-laborer." When doing so, Dalton dropped the phrase he had originally taken from Bigelow that Gage was mentally "entirely unimpaired." By so dropping Bigelow's opinion and including Jackson's summary of the work Gage could do, Dalton suppressed what he did know about the changes. Dalton's continuing opposition to localization can be sensed in his remarks that the hemispheres functioned as a whole as the seat of "conscious intelligence" (as opposed to reflexes, simple sensations, and instinctive movements). Again, although he allowed some place for Broca's language function, his more general remarks about disease or injury of the brain were that they affected only the pre-Gall, cell-like psychological functions of intelligence, memory, and judgment.

Even when the changes to Gage were fairly fully reported, and in a developed context, it was possible to minimize their importance. Thus Stewart turned to the "famous" American crowbar case only after first discussing localization from Flourens to Munk and Horsley, then referring his student readers to the accompanying exercises on ablation and stimulation, and finally summarizing what had been concluded about motor, sensory, and language functions. He cited Gage as an example of damage "without any marked mental symptoms, except some restriction of mental power or loss of mental restraint." Although Gage had previously been decent, diligent, and capable, he had become fitful and vacillating, profane in his language, and inefficient in his work.[4]

Raymond had similar things to say. According to him, except for the loss of vision, Gage recovered completely, living for more than twenty years after the accident and able to work as a coachman and farm laborer. Further, despite knowing something of Harlow's second paper and identifying Phineas only as "Dr. Harlow's case," he used Bigelow's reconstruction as an illustration. Writing from Germany, Landois could perhaps be excused for the vagueness of his hints. In the Bigelow case, "the man's disposition and character was observed to have undergone a serious change," some of which "might be referrable to injury in the frontal region."[5]

Kirkes versus Hollander and Gage

There can be little doubt that much of the discussion of the significance granted Phineas was, like Dalton's, influenced by antilocalization sentiment. Nowhere is this more evident than in the treatment in successive editions of Kirkes's famous *Handbook of Physiology*, a text as famous in its day as Gray's *Anatomy* in ours. Kirkes brought out the first edition in 1848, and various editors took responsibility from the sixth edition of 1867 to the thirty-eighth of 1944. Either by himself or with Harris, Baker brought out editions six to thirteen, Halliburton editions fourteen to thirty-eight, and McDowall joined him from about edition thirty-nine. By then the work was actually Halliburton's *Handbook of Physiology* but was still referred to on the title page as the appropriately numbered edition of Kirkes's.

Kirkes's own edition of 1860 was probably the first that could have mentioned Gage, but it did not. The tenth London edition of 1880 covered studies like those of Ferrier and clinical inferences like those of Broca, but still made no mention of Gage. In fact, apart from aphasia and the sensory-motor functions, Baker said flatly, "Of the physiology of the other parts of the brain, little or nothing can be said." Not until Halliburton's 1896 London edition did Gage appear, in the overall context of a summary of the experimental and clinical findings concerning the sensory-motor areas. Gage was introduced as follows:

On referring once more to the maps of the brain, it will be seen that there is a large blank in the anterior part of the frontal region. This is left blank because its function is absolutely unknown. Extirpation or stimulation of this part of the brain produces no appreciable result. It has also been removed accidentally in man, as in the celebrated American crowbar accident; owing to the premature explosion of a charge of dynamite in one of the American mines, a crowbar was sent through the frontal region of the foreman's head, removing the anterior part of his brain. He, however, recovered, and no noteworthy symptoms were observed in him during the rest of his life. He, indeed, returned to his work as overseer of the mine.

Halliburton further concluded that the view that intellectual functions were localized in the frontal areas could not be correct, because, being dependent on sensations, they had to be "behind or within the Rolandic area."[6]

Halliburton's representation of Gage's case was vigorously disputed by Bernard Hollander, a British physician who, as a leading member of the British Phrenological Society, had maintained and defended the central truth of Gall's doctrine of localization from the nineteenth century into the twentieth. Hollander apparently wrote to Halliburton requesting a correction without success until Halliburton acceded in the 1909 edition. But he did so with what I think may fairly be said to be a lack of grace. The context was essentially the same, even to the point of the importance of sensations to the intellectual functions. Halliburton now went on to say:

This does not necessarily mean that the frontal convolutions have nothing to do with intellectual functions. The celebrated American crowbar accident is generally quoted as proof to the contrary; owing to the premature explosion of a charge of dynamite in one of the American mines, a crowbar was sent through the frontal region of the foreman's head, removing the anterior part of his brain. He is usually stated to have subsequently returned to his work, without any noteworthy symptoms. Recent examination of the records of the case has shown that this is not correct; when he returned to work he was practically useless having lost just those higher functions which are so important in the superintendence of other people.

There had, of course, been no "recent examination of the records." Further, whatever importance Halliburton was now prepared to give to the frontal areas he reduced in the next sentence by saying that observations on lunatics showed the parietal association area to be more important than the frontal. The thirty-fifth edition of 1937 retained this interpretation with a minuscule extension of Gage's psychological changes to include a loss of mental acuity, whatever may have been meant by that term.[7]

What is true of the textbooks tends also to be true of the many lengthy survey articles in the medical journals. Leonardo does not mention Gage in the neurological sections of his history of surgery, nor do any of the contributors to Walker's history of neurological surgery, and none of the three original papers about him is reprinted in collections like those in *Neurological Classics*. Hughes's early paper is an exception in that he mentions Gage and gives him the highest place. His is a somewhat idiosyncratic account of the damage, which he says is bilateral, and in saying that Gage was intellectually brighter after his injury than before. He is also one of only two writers to mention Gage's drinking: he was told that intemperance played a part in Gage's irregular life. Neither Browder's survey nor Walker's short history of neurosurgery mentions Gage, and his case was more often absent than present in standard U.S. histories of medicine. There were no papers about him in *Annals of Medical History* between 1917 and 1942, and only one in the *Bulletin of the History of Medicine* between 1939 and 1981.[8]

Gage in Early Textbooks of Psychology

What is revealed about Gage in the physiological literature is also found in the psychological. For example, chapter 2 of one of the most influential textbooks of psychology to be published in the United States in the 1800s, William James's *Principles of Psychology*, contained a very comprehensive review of the literature on localization. James was trained in medicine and psychology, and having assisted Putnam with some work on localization, had an extremely good grasp of the issues. Entitled "The Functions of the Brain," his chapter covered a wide range of experimental findings, including those of Fritsch and Hitzig, Ferrier, Goltz, and Munk, and he discussed the effects of brain injury in humans. An anonymous reviewer commented that it was "as well proportioned a sketch of the history of cerebral localisation as is to be anywhere found."

James concluded by saying:

I have now given, as far as the nature of this book will allow, a complete account of the present state of the localisation question. In its main outlines it stands firm, though much has yet to be discovered. The anterior frontal lobes, so far as is yet known, have no definite functions.

Neither Gage nor any other specific case was mentioned. Similarly, in the first ten years of the *American Journal of Psychology*, in that part of the review section on "Psychological Literature" devoted to the nervous system and localization, there was no reference to Gage.

Neither does Gage seem to have been discussed in many of the influential U.S., U.K., or non-English-language psychological textbooks that appeared between then and the 1920s. Thus Ladd, Wundt, Stout, Calkins, Kulpe, Angell, Pillsbury, Yerkes, Dunlap, McDougall, Warren, Kantor, and Lund do not discuss him. Not all of these authorities were opposed to localization. True, among them, Kantor, although not then much infected by the virus of behaviorism, made no mention at all of the brain or nervous system, and Yerkes, also then still immune, provided very little on either the brain or its functions, seemingly because he thought psychologists had no need for a knowledge of "neurology." But in 1901, Kulpe, who discussed the topic sympathetically, thought the results of the attempts to localize the brain's functions were "too uncertain to be useful to psychologists," and McDougall, who like James was medically trained, judged the doctrine of localization to be "rocking insecurely." Next to James's, probably the most detailed and sympathetic discussion of localization is that by Lund, and he does not mention Gage.[9]

Judd did mention Gage in what he termed a "speculative discussion" of localization in the frontal areas:

In certain cases large portions of this area have been destroyed without apparent interference with the individual's normal functions. There is a famous case known as the American Crowbar case, in which a common laborer, through an accident in blasting, had a very large portion of this frontal lobe removed by a crowbar passing through the roof of his mouth and out through the top of his skull. The individual in question continued to live with no serious interruption of his regular nervous or physical functions.

After Ribot's citation of Gage in his very influential discussion of the will as the most important of the cases revealing the physiological basis of volition, one might have expected Judd to refer to Gage in the same connection. But he does not.[10]

Half a century later, this neglect of Gage was still fairly common in the psychological literature. Thus, in the "Clinical Methods" section of the historical introductory chapter in his *Physiological Psychology*, C. T. Morgan mentioned only Broca. Similarly, Gage just squeezes in through a footnote, although an important one, in the section devoted to localization in Hilgard's masterly history of psychology in America.[11]

Gage in the Contemporary Literature

Two years after Harlow had presented Gage's skull to the Warren Anatomical Museum, J. B. S. Jackson estimated that it was "the most valuable specimen that has ever been added to the Museum, and probably ever will be," but complained that the skull had been given only a small amount of attention. The anonymous review of the *Catalogue* in the *New York Medical Journal* in 1870 implicitly endorsed his judgment of its importance. Nearly thirty years later Gould and Pyle ranked Gage's as "possibly the most noted" case of head injuries with loss of cerebral substance. At about the same time, Hughes described it as "the most remarkable contribution to the subject of brain tolerance of violence and the possibility of brain repair on record." Later opinions concur. About sixty years later, just past the middle of the twentieth century, Paul Yakovlev, then the Curator of the Warren, said that of its hundreds of exhibits "there are few which have attracted more attention and spread further the fame of the Museum in this country and even abroad than the skull and 'tamping iron' ... of Phineas Gage." Near the end of the twentieth century, on the eve of the 150th anniversary of Gage's accident, a spokesperson for the Harvard Medical School estimated that the museum still received one request per month to see the skull.[12]

Quantitative estimates of the importance of Gage's case have been made in the psychological literature. In 1974 LeUnes analyzed the references cited in then-recent abnormal psychology textbooks and found Harlow's 1868 report to be the earliest of only three nineteenth-century papers cited more than twice. With three citations, it was marginally ahead of the other two.

My own counts of presentations and discussions of Gage show that he appears in nearly 60 percent of the introductory textbooks of psychology published in the fifteen years before 1998. In arriving at this estimate I examined the most recent editions of some sixty introductory texts that had been published since 1983 and catalogued in the numerical range 130 to 150 of the Dewey system and that happened to be on the shelves of three Melbourne university libraries. The sample has no pretense to being random or complete, and the prevalence estimate it yields is certainly not accurate. First, in the Dewey system, the cataloguing and therefore the shelving of books is subject to the vagaries of the word order in the title. Thus a work titled *Introduction to Abnormal Psychology* tends to be somewhere within the 130–150 range, but *Abnormal Psychology: An Introduction* may be there or at various places among the medical or psychiatric textbooks, and the catalogue numbers given titles like *Cases in Abnormal Psychology* seem to be assigned at random. Second, Gage appeared reasonably frequently in the texts without benefit of a name or subject index entry for himself, or for "Harlow," "Bigelow," "brain," "brain damage," or "frontal lobes," and without Harlow's or Bigelow's papers being listed in the references. Short of a detailed reading of each work, one cannot be sure if he was mentioned or not.[13]

A Very Curious Feature

When we analyze what is actually said about Gage in the literature more generally, we find a very curious feature about the inaccuracies commonly found there. In a given account, the amount of error varies within its different parts; not all is equally in error.

Both Gainotti and Stuss recently described Gage as the classic example of the personality changes that are the hallmark of frontal lobe pathology, and Stuss drew attention to the fact that the changes to Gage are described in a contradictory way. My analysis of a sample of some ninety books, consisting of the post-1983 textbooks mentioned above together with a similar but smaller sampling of pre-1984 works, including textbooks, specialized monographs, and general works on brain and behavior, readily confirms this view. A finer analysis revealed the curiosity. If we divide the story into seven elements—the tamping iron, the nature of Gage's work, the circumstances of the accident, the damage done to Gage's skull and brain, his treatment and recovery, the changes to his personality and behaviour, and his subsequent history and fate—rarely did a single account contain major errors in more than three of these elements. Partly because of this variability, partly because not all the accounts include all seven elements, and partly because the amount of detail in each element also varies, it is impossible to arrive at meaningful quantitative estimates of overall accuracy or of accuracy of the components. Remembering that the general level of accuracy is low, the elements that seem to be more accurately reported are the dimensions of the tamping iron, the fact of the explosion, the length and difficulties of the treatment (if this was reported at all), and the fact that Gage's behavior changed after the accident. The most inaccurate components are those about his work before the accident, the details of the changes in his behavior, and his subsequent history.[14]

The basis of this variable accuracy is the authors' ignorance of Harlow's 1868 paper. They seem to have been content to summarize or paraphrase accounts that are already seriously in error. Contrariwise, where accuracy is achieved, it is by quoting or paraphrasing Harlow extensively (sometimes Bigelow). Usually the particular sources of the many grosser inaccuracies can only be guessed at. To take some of the more extreme instances, where does Brown find a Gage who simply goes to his room to lay down for a while after being only "a bit stunned" and seemingly recovers without treatment? Or Aitchison the Gage who survives for twenty years with the tamping iron embedded in his head? Why does Treisman tell us that Gage walks to "the surgeon's office" where he has the tamping iron removed? Smith pictures another Gage who recovers with enough residual wit to sell his skeleton, cash in advance, to several different medical schools some time before his death. Among the changes in Gage after the accident, Rosenzweig and Leiman include a curious lack of concern for matters he had formerly cared about, McMahon and McMahon that he had fits of temper when he did not get his own way, and Vincent a decline in sexual activity. As to working, Altrocchi gives Gage little inclination to any kind of work, Kalat implies he sought work but was unable to hold a job, and Hart has him "actively carrying on his own affairs" at the same time as being "an aimless drifter." Both Treisman and Smith have him becoming a drunkard or being frequently drunk, and, perhaps not surprisingly, Damasio and Van Hoesen then allow him to die "in careless dissipation." When he does, some, like Eckstein, manage to find evidence for an autopsy and its finding that the damage matches that of a lobotomy, or, like Altrocchi, that the damage had spread from the left frontal lobe to the right.[15]

Gage's Work

After sampling these rather spectacular inaccuracies it may seem churlish to mention the minor ones. I do so because they so neatly complement the major ones and, in most instances, equally neatly betray the writers' lack of knowledge of how Harlow and Bigelow described Gage's tasks. They also betray their lack of understanding of Gage's abilities and the circumstances in which he lived and worked. Thus although Gage is sometimes described as a miner or working in a mine, he is more usually described as building a road, rather than a railroad, by clearing rocks away, blasting a rock, some rock or large rocks blocking the tracks, or leveling the terrain generally. He does this by packing gunpowder into a crack in the rock, or by using dynamite and/or detonators, and makes a careless mistake over the sand during the tamping.[16]

The Tamping Iron and the Damage It Caused

Most of the errors about the passage of the tamping iron result from carelessness. These include having the tamping iron pass through the left eye, the attribution to Bigelow of the description of Gage as "totally changed," the representation of Bigelow's 1850 reconstruction as Gage's own skull, and a diagram in which the tamping iron emerges well behind the coronal suture, somewhere in the vicinity of the right parietal bone (although the text says "upper forehead"). But the most careless must surely be the reversed printing of Harlow's illustration so that the tamping iron appears to pass through the right side of Gage's head at the same time as the accompanying text describes a left-sided passage.[17]

With these aberrations about the tamping iron is linked a profound disagreement about just what damage was done Gage's brain. A goodly number of writers describe Gage as suffering only a head injury, a laceration of the brain, or an injury that resulted in diffuse damage. Others are vague or say nothing about the site of injury (e.g., "the brain" or in "the frontal region"). Some do specify a single lobe, either an unspecified frontal lobe or the left frontal lobe. But plurality is also indicated in having both frontal lobes damaged. Quantifiers are sometimes added to the claims of damage to both lobes. They range from being extensively or massively damaged, through being nearly obliterated, to being removed or extirpated.[18]

The Immediate Effects

The accounts of the more or less immediate effects of the passage of the tamping iron also show considerable variation. About half are quite accurate, consisting for the most part of direct quotations or paraphrases of Harlow, either from him directly or via Bigelow. Gage is correctly described as being knocked over, possibly not losing consciousness, walking with assistance to the oxcart, sitting in it as he was driven to the tavern, and waiting for medical assistance. If Harlow's treatment is mentioned at all, its length is usually stated correctly and its stormy nature summarized accurately. Minor errors, like Suinn's expanding Harlow's account of Gage giving a few convulsive movements to he "convulsed a bit," or Restak's "his body began to shake in a convulsive seizure," are relatively infrequent.[19]

Many other accounts show puzzling if not bizarre variations from Harlow and Bigelow. Thus although Hart has him not even fainting, Altrocchi has him stunned for an hour before he walked with assistance to the surgeon; Brown has him "a bit stunned" but recovering after lying down in his room "for awhile," apparently without treatment, and Treisman has the surgeon remove the tamping iron in his office after Gage walked there. Kalat implies some immediate but minor dysfunction in having Gage being without speech for part of the day; Kolb and Whishaw pass over the immediate effects, saying only that he walked to medical assistance after being stunned for a few seconds; C. U. M. Smith has him walking to a hospital, but like Rosenhan and Seligman, who mention only a loss of consciousness, says nothing about the infections or the treatment.[20]

The "Before" Picture

There is really only one source of information about what Gage was like before the accident, and that is Harlow. We have seen that his "before" descriptors are limited to Gage's being temperate in habit, having a well-balanced mind, being a shrewd, smart business man, executing his plans with energy and persistence, and being an efficient and capable foreman and a great favorite with his men. Again, the accurate descriptions given by others are based solely on Harlow, usually by way of quotation or paraphrase. Minor variations are seen in the omission of some of these characteristics, usually not more than one or two, and the addition of others that are not too discrepant from those Harlow gives.

Apart from those who merely include Harlow's characterization of Gage as a "shrewd smart business man" within a quote or paraphrase, only Levitt specifically singles it out. I assume this rarity of reference is because so little can be made of the phrase outside of the context of Gage's work in the railroad construction industry. Even Levitt modifies the phrase to a "shrewd efficient businessman," when, as we have seen, "smart" in the New England English of the time meant "clever" rather than "efficient." No matter. After making it Gage's *only* preaccident quality, he never refers to it again. To him as to most other writers, the context of Gage's work is a very dark continent indeed.

Others modify Harlow's preaccident picture considerably. From Gage being a great favorite with his men, he is painted as one who is "friendly" or "affable" in general. Other descriptors are then added, with the result that Suinn reveals a Gage who enjoys the respect and favor of his men; Plotnik one who is popular and friendly; Crider, Goethals, Kavanagh, and Solomon a considerate and friendly person, all round, that is, A. Smith's "genial fellow." More traits are added. Gage is also dependable and industrious (Bloom and Lazerson) and competent, and responsible (Hockenbury and Hockenbury). Other descriptions can be thought of as beginning with Gage's efficiency, and adding, as do Groves and Schlesinger, and Tavris and Wade, qualities that make him friendly and mild-mannered, or, with Altrocchi, considerate and well-balanced. Unsurprisingly, with transformations like these, Mowbray, Rodger, and Mellor make him reliable and industrious, Kalat steady and conscientious, and Carlson serious, industrious, and energetic.[21]

When Sdorow describes this Gage as hardworking, both Stevens and Myers as soft-spoken, and Lahey as polite and reasonable as well as hardworking, we see a Gage who is what the authors always knew or wanted him to be, namely, the brave, hardworking, responsible, conscientious, and excellent foreman pictured by Atrens and Curthoys, Ruch, and Vincent—even if Harlow did not use many (or any) of the above terms to describe him. But when Dimond sees a peaceful, happy, and tranquil Gage, I sense a very different tint to his glasses.[22]

The "After" Picture

Harlow restricts the characteristics he ascribes to Gage after physical recovery to the destruction of the balance between his intellectual faculties and his animal propensities: to his becoming fitful, irreverent, grossly profane, showing little deference for his fellows, impatient of restraint or advice that conflicted with his desires, obstinate yet capricious and vacillating, devising many plans and abandoning them, and a child in his intellectual capacity with the animal passions of a strong man.

Balance. Apart from its inclusion in the direct quotations of Harlow's summary, I found only four uses of Harlow's famous phrases about Gage's equilibrium or balance being destroyed, or his being intellectually a child possessed of adult animal passions. Levitt mentions Harlow's phrase but does not expand on it in any way. Luria, presumably the victim of a back translation into English from the Russian, has the disturbance as one of the balance between his "intellectual and animal traits," and he also mentions the release of Gage's "primitive animal instincts." With less excuse, Bootzin and Acocella and Bootzin, Acocella, and Alloy incorporate a similar notion into the way they describe the balance between what they term Gage's intellectual faculties and his instincts. Peculiarly, none of these authors goes on to make use of the concept that his balance was disturbed. Eckstein explicitly equates and restricts to sex the animal "passion" that is released by the lack of balance, and sex is the only animal propensity or passion that anyone else mentions. We actually know absolutely nothing about Gage's sexual life, and I have deferred discussion on what is said until later in this chapter.[23]

As distinct from his remarks on balance, a number of texts quote the other parts of Harlow's summary more or less fully. Peculiarly, there are also five lists of Gage's characteristics that are reasonably close to Harlow's, although they are not quoted from him. Thus Mowbray, Rodger, and Mellor quote an unnamed source to depict a Gage who is "a 'fitful, irreverent, profane, impatient, obstinate and vacillating,' fellow." Bootzin and Acocella and Bootzin, Acocella, and Alloy are reasonably accurate, with their Gage being inconsiderate, impatient, obstinate, and yet at the same time capricious and vacillating in decision making. They also have him beginning to engage in the grossest profanity and showing so great a change in temperament that his employers had to replace him. Altrocchi has Gage as grossly profane, showing little consideration for others, and no longer trusted to supervise others, as well as having some of the characteristics Harlow does give him. Lefrancois keeps most of the qualities but modifies or adds to them so that his Gage is moody, selfish, impulsive, and stubborn, and highly profane, even in front of ladies. Kalat has a Gage who is restless, unreliable, changing his plans suddenly, persisting to the point of obstinacy, and resisting advice or restraint opposed to his impulses, but is apparently neither profane, nor irreverent, nor lacking in deference. In most other instances there is a similar use of some part of what Harlow actually said with the addition of qualities that are different.[24]

Profanity. Profanity is almost always included in the characteristics ascribed to Gage. Nowadays this is more often placed with cognate terms like inconsiderate or phrases referring to a lost sense of decorum, rather than Harlow's irreverence and lack of deference. Elaborations of Gage's profanity are frequent, from the simple one of Myers, who has Gage irritable and profane, to the more complex of being unbearably or grossly profane as well as irritable (Shutts and Crider, Goethals, Kavanagh, and Solomon, with the latter adding "inconsiderate" for good measure). Others, like H. Damasio, Grabowski, Frank, Galaburda, and A. R. Damasio, simply refer to Gage's now-abundant profanity, or, like Fulton, have him indulging in profanity that would have embarrassed an eighteenth-century British sea captain. But the more considerable elaborations of his profanity begin with Stevens's bombastic and purposeless Gage who is continually cursing, move to the restless, profane, loud, and impulsive Gage of Bloom and Lazerson, continue with Plotnik's impatient Gage who curses his workers and refuses to make good on his promises, and finish with one who is a depraved child, capricious, lacking in respect, and proffering obscenities.[25]

Fitfulness. Similarly "fitful" is almost always included, although the terms now used are more likely to be restless, unreliable, or irresponsible. Often these qualities are only implied by reference to Gage's being "reliable" beforehand. Sometimes the Gage who results is, like Aitchison's, unpredictable, presumably in some general sense, as well as unreliable, or as Kalat has it, unreliable in his work and personal habits, following each whim of the moment, and unable to follow "any" long term plans. Other

Gages are represented as developments of the "personal habits" deficit and become so different from Harlow's description that we have difficulty in recognizing him: slovenly, unreliable, and feckless (C. U. M. Smith), exhibiting dramatic changes in his personal habits (Rosenzweig and Leiman), and slovenly, careless, and easily distracted (Atrens and Curthoys). In short, Dimond's peaceful, happy, and tranquil person of former days is now aggressive and violently quarrelsome, or has become Ruch's argumentative and untrustworthy one. A. Smith's once genial fellow turns into a capricious, obstinate, ne'er-do-well drunkard, and the mild mannered, friendly, efficient worker of Tavris and Wade changes into a foul mouthed, ill-tempered, undependable lout. He who had been Sdorow's friendly, popular, and hardworking foreman was now an ornery, disliked, irresponsible bully. Most of all, according to H. Damasio et al. and also to A. R. Damasio, he who had been the favorite of his peers and elders, who had made progress and shown promise, was now irreverent, capricious, and without respect for the social conventions by which he had previously abided. He often drank and brawled "in questionable places," and when he returned to San Francisco, he was under the custody of his family. As A. R. Damasio has it, Gage became a psychopathic personality who lied and could not be trusted to honor his commitments.[26]

Irritability. Whether Harlow implies "irritable" is doubtful in my view. But if cranky and inconsiderate are acceptable synonyms, as Fromkin and Rodman, and Fromkin, Rodman, Collins, and Blair seem to think, not much of Lahey's impossible to reason with, and unable to think rationally and plan, is. Neither, it seems to me, is Hockenbury and Hockenbury's substitution of bad-tempered for irritable, nor their addition of unreasonableness as well as stubbornness. McMahon and McMahon develop this theme rather more than anyone else. Their Gage not only makes elaborate plans that he then cancels and swears profusely "at any time or place," but loses control of much of what is called decorum, becomes like a child, and has fits of temper when he doesn't get his own way.[27]

Obstinate, impatient of restraint or advice that conflicts with his desires. Again, apart from being included in quotations from Harlow, neither Gage's obstinacy nor his being impatient of restraint or advice that conflicted with his desires is often commented on. When either is, it is in ways quite different from Harlow. It should be recalled that Harlow implies, and J. B. S. Jackson says explicitly, that Phineas was as obstinate after the accident as he had been before it. Perhaps obstinacy was not a consequence of the damage to his brain at all. Nevertheless, even without this qualification, the link Groves and Schlesinger seem to make between his obstinacy and his incapacity for planned activity seems arbitrary. Similarly, according to Levitt, his paying little heed to advice from others when it interfered with his own wants and desires had one special peculiarity: Gage experienced great difficulty in planning an action and carrying it through.[28]

Gage's Subsequent History

The part of Gage's story that is told with the greatest inaccuracy is what happened to him after the accident. Real events are exaggerated and events that are not documented anywhere are included together with others that almost certainly did not happen, while others that are important and that did happen are not mentioned. The core of what is said is based on his visiting the larger towns in New England and the period he spent with Barnum's Museum. Familiar elaborations, if not fabulations, are also found here. Gage drifts around in a more or less purposeless way, in geographically vague or unspecified locales, hardly ever just in New England. When he does not exhibit himself on his own, he does so as a circus or fairground attraction. Gage is motivated to do these things because he loses his job, cannot settle into another, and is unable or unwilling to work. The unreal events include the time and route of his travels, how he earned a living, and the circumstances of his death.

Hardly ever taken into account by the authors of these fables is the time available for Gage to have done these things. At the very most, the period could not have been longer than two years; it could have been as little as about nine months, but it was probably more like one year. The very earliest Gage could have commenced visiting the larger New England towns is January 1849, and we can deduce that he must have gone to work for Currier near the beginning of 1851, because he stayed there for nearly eighteen months, until August 1852. He worked as an ostler and possibly as a coach driver for Currier before going to Chile and worked at both occupations in Chile for seven years. However, we have seen that Gage was not physically fit enough for full work on the farm in May or June of 1849, and although well enough to search for employment in Montpelier in August, he did not go to Boston and see

Bigelow until November. In April of the following year the letter to the AMA Standing Committee on Surgery commented on his loss of bodily power. Had the visits commenced early in 1850, Gage could have been traveling, therefore, for only about a year—nine months if they started in the April.

Despite what Harlow tells us about his employment, and despite these time constraints, the once steady Gage never works again. He becomes a vagrant (Tow), a circus exhibit (Groves and Schlesinger, Tavris and Wade), or solo traveling attraction (Kalat). Our storytellers are uncertain if this is because he does not want to work (Altrocchi, Morris), or wants to work but cannot hold a regular job (Kalat, A. Smith, Lahey, and Hockenbury and Hockenbury), or simply because he cannot be trusted to supervise the work of others (Restak). Whatever the reason, he does not work. Although Kalat has him making a living on his own as he tours the country charging admission to see the holes in his head, H. Damasio, Grabowski, Frank, Galaburda, and A. R. Damasio have it that he "never returned to a fully independent existence." After having begged for a time, Restak says, Gage became "a pathetic sight" as he exhibited himself. According to Tavris and Wade, he was reduced to exhibiting himself as a circus attraction because he could neither hold a steady job nor stick to a plan. On the other hand, Groves and Schlesinger allow him to hold many jobs while traveling and seem to make his "even" participating in a circus a minor matter.[29]

The accounts of Ruch, Myers, and Bloom and Lazerson are so geographically challenged that not only do they not say where Gage went, but they leave out the travels altogether and mention only the freak or fairground part of the story. Those who are a little more specific about where Gage went are still vague. After he lost his job, Blakemore and Crider, Goethals, Kavanagh, and Solomon say he drifted around the United States and South America, exhibiting himself and the metal rod as a fairground attraction. Brown has him "drift" from Chile to San Francisco and spend some time as a Barnum Circus exhibit. A different voyage, geographical as well as psychological, is described by A. R. Damasio and Van Hoesen, who have Gage traveling "from New England to California" where he dies "in careless dissipation." Although Fromkin, Rodman, Collins, and Blair say Gage gained monetarily when he toured all over the country charging admission to his one-man circus, they have him dying penniless in an institution twelve years after the accident. Whenever and wherever Gage finally comes to rest, H. Damasio, Grabowski, Frank, Galaburda, and A. R. Damasio as well as Hockenbury and Hockenbury have him buried with his tamping iron.[30]

Functions for Interpreting Gage

That the variation in reports of the changes in Gage might turn out to be a function of the kinds of general functions attributed to the frontal lobes at the time his case was being considered would not be surprising. It is a hypothesis suggested by what I have read, rather than one that I have the time to test here. For example, establishing whether the cognitive orientation really dominated between about 1900 and 1930 would require an extraordinarily detailed analysis of the literature from that period. And it may not be necessary. What was patent behind the kinds of "mental symptoms" derived from Gage and applied in early brain surgery on the frontal lobes was the rational man of the Enlightenment. Consonant with that orientation, we find Gage interpreted within a framework specifying the importance of functions like making plans and executing them, that is, functions of a mental or cognitive kind.

Luria provides an important instance. He cites Harlow's as one of the first accounts of damage to the frontal lobes with marked personality changes and notes the disturbance of balance and what he calls the release of animal instincts. Later he includes Gage's case as a typical example of the disturbance of initiative and the critical appraisal of internally programmed action. Treisman combines cognitive deficits in long-term planning and initiative within a context of the frontal lobes being responsible for organizing social relations and social behavior. A different cognitive interpretation is that of Atrens and Curthoys, who conclude that patients with frontal lobe damage, among whom they seem to include Gage, exhibit distractibility, stereotyped behavior, and concrete thinking. A motivational component they add includes a combination of extroverted behavior and a lack of purpose and initiative.[31]

After the affective changes following lobotomy practically forced themselves to the forefront of brain and psychosurgery, it is fairly clear that the changes in Gage were interpreted anew. The actual emotional interpretation differed according to whether emotional control or the experiencing of emotion was being emphasized. When control was referred to, it was control of impulses and emotional reactions; when experience was under consideration it was usually to the depth of emotional experience or to anxiety reduction.

In the mid 1980s, Stuss and Benson judged Harlow's report to have provided a "brilliant beginning" to understanding the participation of the frontal lobes in emotion. Nevertheless, not until sometime in the mid 1960s and early 1970s were emotional functions given a substantial place. Thus sixteen years after originally mentioning only that Gage was more uninhibited and unrestrained emotionally, Mowbray and Rodger had the frontal lobes controlling emotional expression and experience. Their earlier opinion seems to have been linked with the notion that the frontal lobes controlled emotional expression by controlling impulsivity. Similarly Wooldridge summarized the literature to 1963 as suggesting that damage to the frontal lobes disconnected the intellect from the emotions, decreasing the amount of control that could be exerted over impulses, although decreasing motivation as well. By the 1980s, Changeux proposed that as well as their other functions, the frontal lobes had a role in regulating emotional expression, and Altrocchi interpreted Wooldridge to mean that the frontal lobes actually did so. Singer and Hilgard argued that because of their connections with the limbic system, the frontal lobes exercised control over the emotions and the instincts. They granted that, as association areas, it was not known how the lobes contributed to self-control and restraint, but Gage showed the lobes were concerned with conscious cortical control over behaviors influencing social interaction. Walsh's conceptualization seems to have been typical for the time. He described the changes as impulsivity, a lack of inhibition, and a lack of concern, and attributed them to the effects of severe bilateral damage. Beaumont similarly emphasized impulsiveness, but linked it more specifically to bilateral orbital damage.[32]

At the time that Stuss and Benson praised Harlow's work as a beginning, they also noted that correlating frontal lobe damage with specific emotional disorder had proved difficult. Bloom and Lazerson pointed to one reason: the mechanism of the connection could only be inferred. Rosenhan and Seligman conveyed strikingly the uncertainty over the connection in pointing out that the emotional response and personality functions typically revealed by frontal damage differed from the cognitive functions Luria had given the lobes. However, they also felt no explanation could be given of the relation between the damage to Gage's brain and the changes in his personality, suggesting only that the case highlighted "a possible role for hardware." Sdorow was even vaguer; for him the damage threw light on personality and emotionality.[33]

Weisfeld recently observed that by the end of twentieth century emotional interpretations had come to predominate over the earlier cognitive ones but many mixed interpretations remained. Sometimes these are both cognitive and emotional, as when Plotnik, following A. R. Damasio, attributed the changes in Gage to deficits in processing emotion and in decision making. Others, like Carlson, take a slightly different tack. Carlson uses "social" as a synonym for interpersonal behavior, and then relates orbito-frontal function to social-emotional behavior. Others again seem to integrate emotion with moral behavior. Thus Tavris and Wade list a number of cognitive functions, like making social judgments, setting goals, and making plans and carrying them through as making up what "is commonly called will." Also, following A. R. Damasio they argue that reasoning and decision making are dependent on normal emotions. They imply that the defects in Gage's will were due to "the flattening out of emotion and feeling." Probably without realizing the connection with Müller and Bain, Myers proposed that the removal of inhibitions caused by frontal damage was equivalent to a loss of moral compass. The weakness in all these lines of reasoning is, of course, that we know nothing about Gage's emotional life. And "flattening" does not sit well with those who emphasize his temper and emotionality.[34]

The Bases of the Errors

One has only to recall the limited circulation of Harlow's address, in both its periodical and pamphlet form, to appreciate that ignorance could be one source of the fabulations that overlay his original portrait of Gage. Little or nothing of what got into the secondary literature concerned the exact nature of Gage's work, the supposed damage to his brain, the details of the changes in his behavior, and what happened to him after recovery. And it is about those aspects that the ignorance is most profound. What is reported most accurately (and frequently) are the dimensions of the tamping iron, its general trajectory through his skull, and the mere fact that his behavior was radically changed. Miller's introduction to a partial reprint of Harlow's 1868 report contains an opinion consistent with mine when he says that Harlow's publications are not easy to obtain and are more frequently cited than read.

Ignorance of the Sources

Ignorance of those sections of Harlow's 1868 paper in which he described the damage, the treatment, and the subsequent history leads directly, in my view, to such things as the variation in the reports of the nature and locale of the damage and to such vague portrayals as that of Gage drifting about in a kind of geographical wasteland after he recovered. Interestingly, as compared with the papers of Beekman and Steegmann, in which the clear aim was also to reproduce or summarize most of Harlow's 1868 paper, only Miller covers the postaccident history in any detail. With the exception of Restak, many of the other works that quote the changes in detail from Harlow's 1868 report, or make comprehensive paraphrases of what he says, do so in isolation, without saying anything, or only a little else, about his postaccident history.

The most striking instance of this separation of the changes from any sort of context is Fulton's quoting Harlow's report of the changes in full but saying nothing about Gage's work or subsequent history until a few pages later, and then only briefly. The same kind of separation is responsible for the odd contrast found in Walsh's two texts. In both he gives reasonably accurate accounts of the changes, but in one is vague about the locale of the damage (frontal region) and shifts it in the other (frontal lobes). Walsh's source is Kimble's programmed introductory text, which contains much of Harlow's description of the changes (attributed only to a "medical journal of that time") but gives only the "frontal region" as the site of the damage.[35]

Gage as Other Patients

Some of Gage's alleged behavior clearly comes from attributing the characteristics of other cases to him. As we know, there are absolutely no data on Gage's sexual life, but when, for example, Vincent pictures him as suffering from decreased sexual activity while at the same time being disinhibited in his "moral attitudes" to sex, we sense he is virtually repeating what Brickner strongly implied about Joe A., what Russell actually said about one of his patients and Freeman and Watts said about some of theirs.[36]

Other characterizations of Gage's sexuality come from a more complex slippage in reasoning. Thus Dimond draws a parallel between Gage and an aggressive and violently quarrelsome patient of Welt's. A few paragraphs later Dimond places Harlow's 1868 paper in a set of papers apparently providing evidence for the facts that (1) frontal damage often causes the puerile sense of humor to which Jastrowitz had drawn attention, and named *Witzelsucht* by Oppenheim, and (2) leucotomized patients often become irresponsible over business decisions, exhibit abusiveness and uncontrolled profanity, and are promiscuous and overbearing in sexual behavior. Somewhat similarly, in the earlier edition of his text, Myers introduced Gage in the context of his being a classic case of frontal damage that left people more uninhibited, profane, or even promiscuous (the 1998 edition drops the reference to promiscuity). Crider, Goethals, Kavanagh, and Solomon make the same kind of connection, Beaumont comes very close to it, and I suspect a similar source for the unspecified alterations in sexual behavior that Fromkin, Rodman, Collins, and Blair include among the "major changes" to Gage.[37]

Many of Gage's other characteristics come from the brain surgery and psychosurgery literature of the 1930s. Gage's slovenly personal habits seem to come from Mettler's summary in the Columbia-Greystone Associates research of the changes lobotomy produced. After mentioning Gage, Mettler immediately describes a patient of Welt's who changed from a gay, polite, and cleanly person to a violently quarrelsome sloven. If one reads it quickly, it is easy to attribute Mettler's description of the changes in personal habits of this other patient to Gage. Similarly, when Zimbardo and Ruch say it was Gage's family and friends and not his doctor who noticed the changes, they are undoubtedly referring to what was sometimes said about the effects of some of the early operations in which whole lobes were removed to control epilepsy or the spread of tumors. For example, Penfield almost said this about the changes in his sister, and Rylander certainly did so in retelling the story. Gage's supposed general lack of concern (Walsh), his curious lack of concern for matters he had formerly cared about (Rosenzweig and Leiman), and his showing little emotion, losing his former values, and becoming unreliable in his personal habits (Kalat) almost certainly seep in from those sources.

Gage's childishness seems also to have its source in this other literature. In describing Joe A., Brickner drew a parallel between "the puerile quality of practically every act and expression" of his patient and the associations and behavior of children. He attributed puerility to Joe A.'s lack of restraint (Brickner's term for loss of inhibition) making it impossible for him to utilize the "adult" knowledge he had once had. Some years later, Brickner made the parallel even more explicit. However, where Brickner, and perhaps others, seem to have been referring to the functional similarity between the child lacking knowledge and the frontal patient having it but not being able to use it, later writers have made the comparison a global one. For them, Gage was simply childish. Thus Henderson and Gillesipie outlined childishness, the loss of the finer feelings, and intellectual and emotional decay as the main changes brought about by frontal lesions, and illustrated their point with Gage. Freeman and Watts may also be read as implying that there was a parallel between the kinds of changes seen in Gage and the "surgically induced childhood" sometimes seen for a short time after frontal leucotomy.[38]

The Gage who is a "child in his intellectual capacity" has become like a child or childish. Could this be the child who has the fits of temper? We have also seen how the not understood "animal passions" of yesteryear were replaced with the sex of today and the sexual life of others attributed to Gage. Could it be this combination of childlike intellect and sexual passion that turns Gage into a depraved child?

From the contexts in which the remarks occur, I also suspect that the observations of patients undergoing radical surgery or lobotomy are the source for what is variously referred to as Gage's inability to plan (Lahey), to make or follow any consistent life or long-term plan (Bloom and Lazerson, Kalat), or to make and carry out any plans (Carlson, Tavris and Wade). All of these descriptions seem to me to be slightly different from, if not actually more extreme than, Harlow's "devising many plans of future operation, which are no sooner arranged than they are abandoned in turn for others appearing more feasible."[39]

Gage as Metaphorical Alcoholic

There are two mentions of Gage's drinking in the nineteenth-century literature, and the picture of Gage as drinking heavily almost certainly has a more modern source. The earliest of the modern references that I came upon is that by Treisman, who gives Fulton as the source of his description of Gage as being "frequently drunk." However, neither in that work, nor another of the same year with which it may have been confused, does Fulton say anything at all about Gage's drinking. This second work of Fulton's makes a reference to the effects of alcohol. Endeavoring to convey what the behavior of chimpanzees was like once the frontal areas were removed, Fulton drew a parallel, rather as Elder and Miles had done with their patient, between "the fatuous equanimity of spirit" the chimpanzees showed and that of "the good natured drunkard." The parallel might just be the basis of Treisman's error.

Turning to the two nineteenth-century references to Gage's drinking, we find they do not provide strong evidence for any such thing. The earliest, from 1879, is that of Wilson and was found by Dr. Fred Barker. It occurs in the course of an attack on phrenology in which Wilson asserted that Gage's intelligence had not been affected, then claimed that few would attribute "the drinking habits which finally beset him" to his damaged brain. The other reference is one I found and is some twenty years later than Barker's. In 1897 Hughes, giving no source, wrote that Gage had led "an irregular life, in which intemperance played a part." We are entitled to be suspicious of Hughes's statement because he also says that whichever of Bowditch or Warren showed him Gage's skull at the Boston General Hospital in 1868 told him that Gage "was actually intellectually a brighter man after than before the accident."

No one who has written on Gage seems to have cited either of these references, including those who class him as an excessive drinker. I know that Dr. Barker regards the context of Wilson's remark, as well as the remark itself, as being very weak evidence that Gage was a heavy drinker. Nor is Hughes's saying that intemperance "played a part" in Gage's alleged irregular life quite the same thing as saying he was a drunkard. Together the references are far from compelling. Consequently, and in the absence of direct evidence, it seems to me that the twentieth-century attribution of excessive drinking to Gage is probably based on a misinterpretation of Fulton's parallel. No evidence exists for Gage's drinking and brawling in questionable places, being frequently drunk, becoming a drunkard, or dying in careless dissipation.[40]

Barnum's Museum as Circus

Rather in the manner that a Bartlett might have predicted, there are elaborations of Gage's postaccident history based on interpretations of those parts of the story, usually the vaguer parts, that can be fitted into an author's existing cognitive framework. Thus if the circus in which Gage appears is specified, it is Barnum's Circus—because Barnum is now remembered for his circus and not his museum. Beekman, Restak, and Steegmann provide excellent examples of this point. With the exception of giving "Barnum's Circus in New York" as one of the places to which Gage wandered, Steegmann quotes extensively from and accurately summarizes Harlow's 1868 paper. Similarly, at the same points of their otherwise detailed accounts, Restak says Gage "hooked up with P. T. Barnum and performed in fairgrounds and circus tents around the country," and Beekman lapses into the vagueness of having Gage exhibit himself "about the country." More generally, if Gage is an exhibit or a freak at an unspecified fairground, it is probably because it is in that kind of place that one sees (or once saw) exhibitions of freaks.[41]

One of the most interesting elaborations to fit Gage into an existing theoretical framework gives a pseudobiological explanation of the changes. Weisfeld argues that orbito-frontal damage generally causes an impairment in pride and shame, the loss of concern for conscientious job performance, and the loss of the most basic social courtesies. He then draws an analogy between Gage's behavior and that of monkeys with posterior orbito-frontal lesions. Lesioned monkeys lose their positions in their dominance hierarchies and show less aggressiveness and more inappropriate reactions to the ranks of their cagemates. Weisfeld supposes that these changes parallel Gage's reduced sensitivity to the reactions that others had to his reactions toward them and to explain the lack of deference he showed his fellows. Although Weisfeld does not refer to their work, other authors also mention a similar impairment in Gage's social and emotional functioning as a direct consequence of the brain damage. However others propose, equally plausibly, that these characteristics are secondary psychological reactions to the primary injury. Although all this is plausible, most of Gage's behavior here is supposition: recall that we actually know nothing about Gage's aggressiveness, and most of the other artists paint Gage as more aggressive, not less.[42]

Harlow as Frontal Lobe Theoretician

There is yet another attribution in the Gage case of knowledge obtained elsewhere, only this time the attribution is to Harlow rather than to Gage. Hanna and Antonio Damasio and their colleagues attribute to Harlow "the perceptive insight" that there were "structures in the brain dedicated to the planning and execution of personally and socially suitable behavior, to the aspect of reasoning known as rationality." They assert that Harlow's suggestions were not accepted at the time because (1) unlike the data through which the lesions in Broca's and Wernicke's aphasia were located, there were no autopsy data on the precise position of Gage's lesion, and (2) reasoning and social behavior, not being extricable from ethics and religion, were "not amenable to biological explanation." Expanding on this suggestion, Hockenbury and Hockenbury have Harlow suggesting or explicitly proposing that the frontal lobes were involved in emotional behavior, in reasoning, in the capacity to plan and think, and in decision making. They add a third reason for Harlow's theoretical ideas not being accepted: they were too close to the phrenological insistence that the brain did have functions.

Pleasantly plausible as this story may seem, absolutely nothing in Harlow's published or unpublished work is even slightly consistent with his formulating a theory of frontal lobe functioning, let alone an emotional/reasoning one. In his 1868 paper (reproduced in Appendix A), Harlow neither made an explicit case for "moral qualities" being localized in the brain nor put forward a theory that would explain how that could be. This was not because thinking along those lines was not acceptable at the time. Leaving the theories of Gall and the phrenologists aside, we have seen that a host of physiologists and psychologists from Marshall Hall onward proposed that conscience and the will were functions of the cerebral hemispheres. True, many of these were philosophical dualists opposed to localization, but many were not—think of Laycock and Hughlings Jackson, for example. Even if the keyboard on which Johannes Müller's pianist played was in the brain, recall that it was the role Müller gave spontaneous fetal movement that was eventually developed into a physiological theory of the will.

If Bain's merit was in his developing Müller's suggestion that the basis of the will was spontaneous movement, Ferrier's was in his founding its mechanism on inhibition. That Bain's and Ferrier's ideas were not accepted had nothing to do with resistance based on ethics or religion. Bain's notion of conscience as a reflection in the mind of the world around the child and its acquisition through fear was not objected to on these grounds, and it went some way to explain the acquisition of moral qualities. The most influential writers of the day, for example, Ribot in France and Wundt in Germany, accepted explicitly and wholeheartedly a physiological basis for the will itself.

The theories lacked a physiological mechanism that would explain how the brain performed such "higher" psychological functions. The vagueness of mechanisms like stoppage and inhibition practically guaranteed their explanatory failure. It is hard to see how ethical or religious objections could be relevant. Similarly with Ferrier's alternative: the attentional mechanism that he located frontally. Was it any more acceptable or unacceptable on religious or ethical grounds? Evidence is lacking that there were *any* attacks on either theory of will, let alone that attacks were grounded in ethical or religious considerations.

Nor is it really possible to argue that the localization of supposedly simpler functions like movement and language was more readily accepted at that time. Even in 1868, one could not be certain what was meant by their localization, and what the experimental and clinical evidence showed about movement and language continued to be as debatable as Damasio et al. claim the localization of moral qualities to have been. In fact, as Dupuy's criticism of work on the motor centers indicates, and as both the papers of Marie critical of Broca as well as the more than 1,200 studies Moutier considered in his massive evaluation of the aphasia literature show, whether movement or language was localized in any way was still being debated very vigorously at the beginning of the twentieth century.[43]

Conclusion

What we see in the pictures of Gage considered in chapters 13 and 14 is a very different person from the man Harlow portrayed in 160 words in his 1868 paper as "No longer Gage." Details of Gage's pre- and post-accident history are also very different from those in Harlow's approximately 150- to 200-word portrayal of the same events. Diverse as the many caricatures seen in the literature may be from one another, they have one thing in common: none is accompanied by supporting evidence. Carelessness aside, these supposedly scientific representations either are the result of ignorance of the true nature of their subject or are distortions generated by a theoretically driven vision of what Gage should have been like. Remembering that Harlow is virtually our only source of information about Phineas, their representations hardly attain the status of even partial truths.

Notes

1. Todd and Bowman 1856, Draper 1856. Todd had shown there was no anatomical basis to Hall's system of excito-motory nerves, and this may be why he did not mention him by name in the textbook he wrote with Bowman.

2. Non-U.S. texts or texts with non-U.S. authors include Vulpian 1866, Marshall 1868, Carpenter 1874, W. Mills 1889, Thornton 1896, Foster 1897, Starling 1897, Donaldson 1897, Rettger 1898, and Flint 1901. Martin's texts are Martin 1890, pp. 584–595, 1898, pp. 609–630.

3. Twentieth-century texts include Bayliss 1915, Howell 1937, Best and Taylor 1937, and Lucas 1940. Huxley 1923.

4. Dalton 1875, p. 423; Stewart 1899, p. 711.

5. Raymond 1905, p. 507; Landois 1887, p. 704.

6. Kirkes 1848; Baker 1880, p. 544; Halliburton 1896, pp. 267–268. The view that intellectual functions were localized posteriorly was quite widespread in the last century. Hollander cites five authorities for—including Bastian, W. B. Carpenter, Hughlings Jackson, and Schafer—and ten against. The editions of Kirkes I have considered are those published in London. The American editions, prepared variously by Dana, Rockwell, Coleman, Busch, and Greene, often had different pagination and content.

7. Hollander 1901, pp. 12–13, 1931, pp. 236–237; Halliburton 1909, p. 732; Halliburton and McDowall 1937, p. 720. In 1931 Hollander said that "in answer to my protest, in later editions, the case was left out altogether" by Halliburton. Phineas was grudgingly reevaluated in 1937, but I have been unable to examine editions of Kirkes between 1909 and then to see if the deletions actually occurred.

8. Neurological surveys are Leonardo 1943, Walker 1951, and Hughes 1897. Neurosurgical history in Browder 1941 and Walker 1959. Standard histories of medicine are Packard 1901, Garrison 1913, Viets 1930, and Mettler and Mettler 1947.

9. James's reviewer is "Review of Wm. James" 1890–1891, and James himself is James 1890, vol. 1, p. 62; Putnam 1875 for James as experimenter. The influential texts are Ladd 1894, 1898; Wundt 1897; Stout 1899; Calkins 1901; Kulpe [1901] 1909; Angell 1904; Pillsbury 1911; Yerkes 1911; Dunlap 1912; McDougall 1920; Warren 1920; Kantor 1924; and Lund 1927.

10. Judd 1907, p. 59; Ribot 1894.

11. C. T. Morgan 1943; Hilgard 1987.

12. J. B. S. Jackson 1870, pp. v, 149; "Bibliographic and Literary Notes" 1870 for the review; Gould and Pyle 1896, p. 551; Hughes 1897; Yakovlev 1958; and spokesperson Bill Schaller in *Burlington Free Press* (Vermont), 19 July 1998, p. 6B, col. 3.

13. LeUnes 1974. The oddity of the indexing and referencing of the Gage case may be partly responsible for McCollom's (1973) not finding Harlow 1868 among the pre-1932 papers in the general introductory textbooks he examined.

14. Gainotti 1996; Stuss 1996.

15. Brown 1976; Aitchison 1989; Treisman 1968; A. Smith 1984, p. 248, 1985, p. 337; Rosenzweig and Leiman 1982; McMahon and McMahon 1982; Vincent 1996; Altrocchi 1980; Kalat 1981; Hart 1975; Damasio and Van Hoesen 1983; and Eckstein 1970.

16. The representation of Gage as a miner may have its origins in the French literature. Although the French translator of the first edition of Ferrier's *Functions* avoided using "mine," one of the common French words for explosive devices, others did (e.g., Dupuy 1873, p. 32; Soury 1892, pp. 130–131). Soury

also used "une mineur"—one who sets off explosive charges—to describe Gage. This misunderstanding of Gage's work may also be partly based on a confusion of Gage with Joel Lenn, who was a miner. The other errors are in Tow 1955; C. U. M. Smith 1970; Robin and Macdonald 1975; Altrocchi 1980 (quoting Wooldridge 1963); Treisman 1968; McMahon and McMahon 1982; Crider et al. 1983; Fromkin and Rodman 1983; Dworetzky 1988; Fromkin et al. 1990; Sdorow 1990; R. E. Smith 1993; H. Damasio et al. 1994; Carlson 1994, 1995; and Hockenbury and Hockenbury 1997.

17. Carelessness: left eye (Adey 1974); Bigelow's description, but with Gage "totally changed" (Lahey 1992); Bigelow's reconstruction (Singer and Hilgard 1978; Zimbardo and Ruch 1979; Crider et al. 1983; Sdorow 1990; Lahey 1992); right parietal bone (Beaumont 1983); reversed printing of Harlow's illustration (Davison and Neale 1974; Bootzin and Acocella 1984; and Bootzin, Acocella, and Alloy 1993).

18. No particularity or vagueness: Suinn 1970; Davison and Neale 1974; Mowbray, Rodger, and Mellor 1979; Zimbardo and Ruch 1979; Lefrancois 1980; Groves and Schlesinger 1982; Fromkin and Rodman 1983; Bootzin and Acocella 1984; Bootzin, Acocella, and Alloy 1993; Coleman, Butcher, and Carson 1984; Rosenhan and Seligman 1984; Walsh 1985 (but plural in 1978); Dworetzky 1988; Sdorow 1990; Fromkin et al. 1990; Lahey 1992; R. E. Smith 1993; Kalat 1996 (but plural in 1981). Singularity: Rosenzweig and Leiman 1982; Crider et al. 1983; Bloom and Lazerson 1988; Plotnik 1996; Morris 1996 (but plural in 1988). Plurality: Luria [1962] 1966a; Treisman 1968; Eckstein 1970; Adey 1974; Brown 1976; Altrocchi 1980 (quoting Wooldridge 1963); Dimond 1980; McMahon and McMahon 1982; A. R. Damasio and Van Hoesen 1983; Stuss and Benson 1983; Beaumont 1983; Carlson 1994, 1995; Hockenbury and Hockenbury 1997; Tavris and Wade 1997; Myers 1998 (but singular in 1986). Qualification: extirpation of the anterior portion of frontal lobes (Brown 1976); near obliteration (Singer and Hilgard 1978); extensive damage to frontal lobes (Levitt 1981); both lobes almost completely removed (Atrens and Curthoys 1982); lobes removed (Kolb and Whishaw 1985); lobe blown away (Bloom and Lazerson 1988); massive damage (Myers 1998). Henderson and Gillesipie (1944) have only the prefrontal cortex damaged.

19. Convulsions: Suinn 1970; Restak 1984.

20. Hart 1975; Altrocchi 1980 (quoting Wooldridge 1963); Brown 1976; Treisman 1968; Kalat 1981; Kolb and Whishaw 1985; C. U. M. Smith 1970; and Rosenhan and Seligman 1984.

21. Levitt 1981 for the businessman. The other characteristics are in Suinn 1970; Plotnik 1996; Crider et al. 1983; A. Smith 1984, p. 248; Bloom and Lazerson 1988; Hockenbury and Hockenbury 1997; Groves and Schlesinger 1982; Tavris and Wade 1997; Altrocchi 1980; Mowbray, Rodger, and Mellor 1979; Kalat 1981; and Carlson 1994, 1995.

22. Sdorow 1990; Stevens 1971; Myers 1998; Lahey 1992; Atrens and Curthoys 1982; Ruch 1984; Vincent 1996; and Dimond 1980.

23. Levitt 1981; Luria [1962] 1966a; Bootzin and Acocella 1984; Bootzin, Acocella, and Alloy 1993; Eckstein 1970.

24. Mowbray, Rodger, and Mellor 1979; Bootzin and Acocella 1984; Bootzin, Acocella, and Alloy 1993; Altrocchi 1980 (quoting Woodridge 1963); Lefrancois 1980; and Kalat 1981.

25. Myers 1998; Shutts 1982; Crider et al. 1983; H. Damasio et al. 1994; Fulton 1949a; Stevens 1971; Bloom and Lazerson 1988; Plotnik 1996; and Vincent 1996.

26. Aitchison 1989; Kalat 1996; C. U. M. Smith 1970; Rosenzweig and Leiman 1982; Atrens and Curthoys 1982; Dimond 1980; Ruch 1984; A. Smith 1984, p. 248, and 1985, p. 337; Tavris and Wade 1997; Sdorow 1990; H. Damasio et al. 1994; A. R. Damasio 1994; and Blakeslee 1994.

27. Fromkin and Rodman 1983; Fromkin et al. 1990; Lahey 1992; Hockenbury and Hockenbury 1997; and McMahon and McMahon 1982.

28. Groves and Schlesinger 1982; Levitt 1981.

29. Tow 1955; Groves and Schlesinger 1982; Tavris and Wade 1997; Kalat 1981; Altrocchi 1980 (quoting Wooldridge 1963); Morris 1996; A. Smith 1985, p. 337; Lahey 1992; Hockenbury and Hockenbury 1997; Restak 1984; H. Damasio et al. 1994.

30. Ruch 1984; Myers 1998; Bloom and Lazerson 1988; Blakemore 1977; Crider et al. 1983; Brown 1976; A. R. Damasio and Van Hoesen 1983; Fromkin et al. 1990 (cf. Fromkin and Rodman 1983); H. Damasio et al. 1994 (cf. A. R. Damasio 1994, p. 22); and Hockenbury and Hockenbury 1997.

31. Luria [1962] 1966a, 1966b; Treisman 1968; and Atrens and Curthoys 1982.

32. Stuss and Benson 1983; Mowbray, Rodger, and Mellor 1979 (cf. Mowbray and Rodger 1963); Wooldridge 1963; Changeux [1983] 1985 (cf. Changeux and Connes [1989] 1995); Altrocchi 1980; Singer and Hilgard 1978; Walsh 1978; and Beaumont 1983.

33. Stuss and Benson 1983; Bloom and Lazerson 1988; Rosenhan and Seligman 1984; Sdorow 1990.

34. Weisfeld 1997; Plotnik 1996; Damasio 1994; Carlson 1994, 1995; Tavris and Wade 1997; and Myers 1998. See also Changeux and Connes [1989] 1995. According to Alford 1948, the emphasis given the moral aspects of the changes in Gage was natural given the New England milieu in which the accident occurred.

35. Beekman 1945; Steegmann 1962; Miller 1993. Compare Restak's (1984) quotation with the treatment by Treisman (1968); Suinn (1970); Harmatz (1978); Davison and Neale (1974); Blumer and Benson (1975); Zimbardo and Ruch (1979); D. Morgan (1981); Stuss and Benson (1983); Coleman, Butcher, and Carson (1984); Rosenhan and Seligman (1984); Bloom, Lazerson, and Hofstadter (1985); Fulton (1949a); and Walsh (1978 and 1985; cf. Kimble 1963, pp. 286–287).

36. Vincent 1996; Brickner 1934, 1936; Russell 1948 (see also Fulton 1949a); and Freeman and Watts 1950, pp. 175–179, 195.

37. Dimond 1980; Myers 1986; Crider et al. 1983; Beaumont 1983; and Fromkin et al. 1990.

38. Mettler includes slovenliness in his summary in Columbia-Greystone Associates 1949. Symptoms noticed by family in Zimbardo and Ruch 1979; Penfield and Evans 1934, 1935; and Rylander 1939. Lack of concern in Walsh 1978, Rosenzweig and Leiman 1982, and Kalat 1996. Brickner 1934, 1936 and his discussion in Ackerly and Benton 1948: Henderson and Gillesipie 1944, p. 512; Freeman and Watts 1950, p. 566.

39. Inability to plan in Lahey 1992; Bloom and Lazerson 1988; Kalat 1996; Carlson 1994, 1995; and Tavris and Wade 1997.

40. Treisman 1968; Fulton 1949a, 1949b; Elder and Miles 1902; Wilson 1879; Barker 1995; and Hughes 1897.

41. Beekman 1945; Restak 1984; and Steegmann 1962.

42. Weisfeld 1997. The direct effect is in Dimond 1980 and Beaumont 1983, and secondary psychological mechanisms are in Altrocchi 1980; Ruch 1984; Bloom, Lazerson, and Hofstadter 1985; Bloom and Lazerson 1988; Dworetzky 1988; and Sdorow 1990.

43. H. Damasio et al. 1994; A. R. Damasio 1994; and Hockenbury and Hockenbury 1997. For the movement debate, see Dupuy 1892. For language, see Marie 1906a, 1906b; and Moutier 1908.

15

The Hidden Portrait

... one of the oldest and most prominent physicians and surgeons of New England ...
—*New York Times*, 14 May 1907

Reaffirming the importance of Harlow's account of Phineas Gage as the basic source of our information about him is like recovering the truth represented in a portrait that has been distorted over the years by the work of enthusiastic but quite unskilled and amateur restorers. Just as proper real-life restorations often reveal traces of the portraits of other subjects under the main figure, so it is with Phineas Gage. The further we take our work of restoring him, the more intrigued we are by the figure we discern behind him: John Martyn Harlow. What can we make out about him?

The Harlow Family

Harlow's family was descended from Sgt. William Harlow, who came to the Americas in about 1630, and Rebecca Bartlett, granddaughter of the Richard Warren who arrived in Plymouth on the *Mayflower* in 1620. The first four generations of these Harlows lived Plymouth, Massachusetts. In the fifth generation, Isaac Harlow, the second of that name in the family, is recorded as being born in Sussex, New Jersey, and dying in Whitehall, New York. Isaac is described as an early settler in the Whitehall district, so it was presumably with him that the Harlows moved from Massachusetts.

Whitehall is a small town just south of Lake Champlain about five to ten miles west of New York's border with Vermont. Members of John Martyn's immediate family were farmers there, and it was there that

Ransom, his father and the son of Isaac, married Annis Martyn on 15 May 1805. John Martyn, the ninth of their twelve children to survive to maturity, was born in Whitehall on 25 November 1819. He was the fifth son and third-youngest child. According to Stone, all of Ransom's family were Baptists and very religious. Although Stone excepts "Dr. John" from the denominational aspect of his generalization, an obituary stated that "While a very young man he was leader of a choir in the local Baptist church in his native town" (i.e., Whitehall). Otherwise I know nothing of his early years, including his schooling.[1]

Fitting for College and Medicine

We can reconstruct the early part of John Martyn Harlow's higher education with some certainty. It was a rather less formal process in the United States during the early part of the nineteenth century than now. A student desirous of entering a profession typically attended an "academy" to be "fitted" or prepared for further study at a college (i.e., university). Attending an academy did not necessarily mean that one was graduated from it. Even those going into teaching, for example, might do as many or as few of the courses as an academy offered, and in their own time, before obtaining a position at a school.

Harlow's fitting began at Troy Conference Academy (previously the Methodist Collegiate Institute and now Green Mountain College) at West Pultney, Vermont. He, or rather a John Harlow of Whitehall, New York, is listed in the catalogue of the Troy Academy in the 1837–1838, Fall–Winter catalogue, is absent from the Spring–Summer edition, is found again in the fall of 1838, and is included as an M.D. in a list published in 1845 of those who had been members of the literary society known as the Young Men's Lyceum in 1839. An irregular attendance pattern like Harlow's was not unusual. Students often attended for a term, then absented themselves to help on the family farm, and returned at some later time. He was not graduated from Troy, because graduation was not instituted until 1844. Harlow completed the second phase of his fitting by attending the Ashby Academy in Ashby, Massachusetts, in 1840 at least, because he—or rather a "John J. Harlow, Whitehall, NY"—is listed among the students there at that time. After having been its Vice or Assistant Principal for a year, presumably after completing whatever courses he thought necessary there, he is said to have taught in private and public schools in Acton, Massachusetts, for several years.[2]

After being fitted, Harlow took the first step toward qualifying as a medical practitioner. At that time, those wishing to take up medicine worked with an established physician who acted as their "preceptor" or "instructor" (the term varied) in introducing them to medical practice. This experience usually lasted two years, after which the preceptors would recommend their charges to particular medical schools where they undertook at least two years of formal academic study. The curriculum of Jefferson Medical College in Philadelphia (now Thomas Jefferson University Medical School) is typical of the time: Physiology (and its applications to pathology, hygiene, and therapeutics), Materia Medica and General Therapeutics (the prescription and administration of medicines), Anatomy, The Practice of Medicine, The Practice of Surgery, Obstetrics and the Diseases of Women and Children, and Chemistry (in its application to Medicine), and the practical study of Anatomy (through dissection), and Clinical Instruction in Medicine and Surgery with in- and outpatients of the hospitals associated with the medical school. By modern standards, the courses were short; in each of the two years there were usually two terms each of four months (sixteen weeks). Teaching was, however, intensive in that each of the three lecture courses taken in each term occupied most of the daylight hours, Anatomy was apparently studied in the evenings of one of the months, and Clinical Instruction took up the Saturdays. At the end of the two years, students presented their theses for the degree of Doctor of Medicine.

Several published sources, some of which are based on information obtained from Harlow, aver that Harlow began his formal instruction in medicine and surgery at the Philadelphia School of Anatomy in 1840. Although this may have been so, it could have been only in the summer (March–November) term of that year, because the school did not then offer courses other than in that term. Further, the school offered neither degree nor diploma, so that its courses could only contribute toward degrees at other institutions. Within the period 1840–1844 we also find Harlow listed as a medical student in the *Catalogue* for the 1842 fall session of the Castleton Medical College, the oldest Vermont medical school and successor to the Vermont Academy of Medicine. Unfortunately, no detailed records of enrolment and academic progress now exist for either Philadelphia or Castleton. We know he was not graduated from Castleton because he is listed as a nongraduate in a history of the college that also gives the year of his enrollment as 1842.

Harlow attended Jefferson Medical College in 1843, the following year, where he is recorded then and only then in the list of students in the *Catalogue* for the 1843–1844 term. He was graduated M.D. on 20 March 1844 with a thesis (no longer extant) on "Counter-Irritation." Jefferson gave credit for courses taken elsewhere, so it is possible his time at Castleton and the otherwise undocumented course in 1840 at the Philadelphia School of Anatomy counted toward one of the two years Jefferson required. We have no details of his enrollment at Jefferson because not even Jefferson's Matriculation Book, which each student signed, recording his home address and preceptor, has survived from this period.[3]

The Castleton and Jefferson *Catalogues* give Harlow's residence as "Massachusetts," but his "instructor," Harris Cowdrey, M.D., is listed in only that for Castleton. Who Cowdrey (or Cowdry) was is instructive for the light it throws on the connection between Harlow's professional and personal life. Harris Cowdrey was born 27 September 1802 in Wakefield, Massachusetts, and was graduated M.D. in 1824 from the Berkshire Medical Institute in Pittsfield, Massachusetts. He commenced practice in Acton, Massachusetts, in October 1826. Nearly two years later, on 19 June 1828, Cowdrey married Abigail Davis (or Davies), daughter of Ebenezer and Abigail (Faulkner) Davis of Acton. Cowdrey was very interested in education and very active in Acton educational circles, serving as a Superintendent of Schools for sixteen years and was Chairman of the School Committee at the time of his death on 6 May 1875.

There is a reasonable possibility Harlow met or became more closely associated with Cowdrey when Harlow was working as a teacher. Harlow is said to have taught in Acton schools for "a number of years." Presumably this was after his year as Vice or Assistant Principal at Ashby and before commencing studies at Jefferson, that is, between 1841 and 1843. But for Cowdrey to be listed as his instructor at Castleton in 1842, Harlow must also have been "apprenticed" to him, formally or informally, late in 1840 or early in 1841. Whatever the precise dates were, the relation between Harlow and Cowdrey was close. It became much more so on 5 January 1843, when Harlow's marrying Charlotte Davis, Abigail's thirty-year-old sister, made him Harris Cowdrey's brother-in-law. There is a number of reasons for thinking they remained on good terms for the rest of their lives. Many of the children of the Cowdreys— Harlow's nephews and nieces—have "Harlow" as their second name;

Harlow willed $15,000 to Arthur Harris Cowdrey, Harris Cowdrey's son, and two amounts of $3,000 to Arthur's sons; and he appointed Arthur as one of the trustees of the share of his residuary estate left to his wife.[4]

Medicine and Phrenology in Cavendish and at Jefferson

We do not know what Harlow did immediately after being graduated. Some early sources have him beginning practice in Cavendish in 1844 or 1846, but he told the compiler of the official *Souvenir* of the Massachusetts State Government when he became a Massachusetts State Senator in 1885 that he commenced practice there in January 1845. When he began, the population of Cavendish was small, about 1,300, and he was young, only twenty-six-years-old. His house is the sixth building on the north side of Main Street, east of Depot Street on Hosea Doton's map. On the same map, the tavern or inn run by Joseph Adams on behalf of Samuel Dutton, where Phineas Gage lived, is the ninth building to the west of the intersection and marked as 'S. Dulton's [*sic*] Hotel' (figure 15.1; compare fig. 2.1). Harlow became a member of the Vermont Medical Association and was much involved in local Cavendish matters, especially in education, almost immediately on going there. Between 1847 and 1858, the entries for Windsor County in various editions of Walton's *Vermont Register* list him as "a" or "the" Superintendent of Schools for the town, and another source has him as Chairman of the School Committee for nine years.[5]

Apart from Gage, we know nothing of Harlow's medical work in Cavendish, but we do observe that what he says about Phineas Gage is couched in phrenological terms. Although Harlow's M.D. thesis was not on a phrenological topic ("Counter-Irritation"), it is impossible that he could have escaped the enormous impact that Gall's and Spurzheim's teaching exerted in the New England medical community at the time he was educated in it. Two of the eight members of Jefferson's faculty listed in the 1845 catalogue (Bache and Mitchell) had been signatories to the constitution of the first American Phrenological Society founded in Philadelphia in 1822, and active in it subsequently. A third (Meigs) was a notable opponent of phrenology, having translated Flourens's attack on Gall. Another (Dunglison) included much material on phrenology in his physiological textbook, insisting that the protagonists read the literature of the other side, but his own attitude has been characterized by Barker as one of "cautious interest."[6]

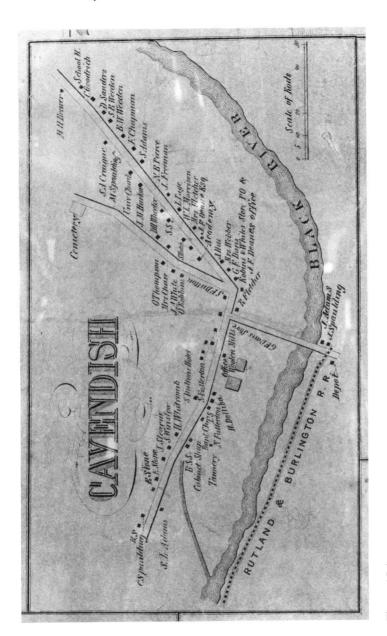

Figure 15.1

Hosea Doton's map of Cavendish, c. 1855

From Doton 1855. The map is one of twenty-eight village maps decorating the borders of Doton's cadastral wall map. Old Sturbridge Village photograph M1973.4 B29383 by Thomas Neil. Reproduced by kind permission of Old Sturbridge Village, Sturbridge, Maasachusetts.

When Harlow moved to Cavendish he had the opportunity of becoming acquainted with Charles French, who lived in Proctorsville, the next village, only two miles west of Cavendish. French was an enthusiast for the systems of phrenology and of Pitman shorthand that the Fowlers advocated. Of organizational and philosophical bent, French was secretary of the Phonological Society and prolific correspondent—in shorthand, of course—on questions of the law in relation to ethics and morality. Unfortunately no phrenological correspondence of his from the period 1848 to 1855 has survived, but it seems likely that he would have attended or even joined in sponsoring the phrenological lectures given by Nelson Sizer and Phineas Lyman Buell between 1839 and 1842. Their tour, mainly of New England, was an important factor in the growth of the Fowler and Wells phrenological organization, the main focus of popular interest in phrenology, in which Sizer was to become a central figure. He and Buell arrived in Duttonsville and were accommodated in Mr. Adams' hotel, and, to nobody's surprise, in "the very room" in which Phineas Gage, "the poor patient was quartered" in 1848.[7]

The influence of phrenology is obvious in much of Harlow's description of Gage. First there is his characterization of Gage's temperament as "nervo-bilious." Buell and Sizer fully described temperament of this type and the system to which it belonged in the book on phrenology they published in Woodstock, Vermont, in 1842. The system derived from that proposed by a French physician, Françoise Thomas de Troisvèvre, which Andrew Combe had introduced into phrenology. Thomas proposed that temperaments should be based on the functions of the three major systems of organs: those of the nervous system, mainly in the brain, located in the cranium; those responsible for the circulation and the purification of the blood, the heart and lungs, located in the thorax; and those that converted food into energy and disposed of bodily wastes, mainly the stomach, liver, spleen, and bowels, located in the abdominal cavity. There were thus cranial, thoracic, and abdominal temperaments.

Two things about Thomas's theory especially appealed to Andrew Combe. The first was that it seemed to provide a physical basis for the venerable Hippocratic humeral theory of temperaments. The second was that in Thomas's system, the relative size of the groups of organs determined basic temperamental characteristics. There was therefore a match between Thomas's principle and the "universal law" of the phrenologists that, other things being equal, the size of a cerebral organ indexed its functional power. Although many other phrenologists were similarly impressed, they did not adopt Thomas's particular grouping of organs or they substituted their names for his. A number of hybrids of the four Hippocratic temperaments eventually resulted, with names based on the organ systems that various phrenologists identified as important.

All three of George Combe, Andrew's brother, and the leading figure in phrenology in the British isles, Caspar Spurzheim, Gall's erstwhile disciple, and the Fowlers seem to have been responsible for developing the four temperaments most commonly mentioned in the American phrenological literature up to about 1850. Under the Fowlers's direction, determining the temperament of the subject became a necessary preliminary to a phrenological reading. The types together with the organ groups determining them were

1. The *nervous* temperament, based on the brain and nerves. It determined the excitability and activity of the mental powers, and the capacity of the individual for vivid and rapid mental action. In a large and well-proportioned brain the result was an intellect of great activity and strength.

2. The *bilious* (sometimes still called the *choleric*), deriving from the activity of the muscles and bones. It imparted energy and strength to mind and body, allowing the endurance of great mental and physical labor.

3. The *lymphatic* (sometimes *phlegmatic*), resulting from the glands and the digestive–eliminative organs. It provided for coolness of passion, a liking for inactivity, and slow, languid, and feeble action.

4. The *sanguine* temperament, based on the heart and lungs. It provided for bodily activity, freshness, animation, zeal, and ardor.

Thomas's original system had allowed for three combinations of his three basic types as well as what he called a mixed temperament.

One basic combination Thomas allowed for was the cranial-thoracic (or encephalo-thoracic) temperament characterized by great moral and physical force. George Combe and the American phrenologists recognized the same type in their nervo-bilious temperament. As George Combe described it, "the great energy of passion, sentiment, and intellect" deriving from the development of the nervous system was joined to a thoracically based constitution that "fits a man for fatigue and labour."

We have seen Harlow attributed this temperament to Gage in 1868. Usually the excitable and active mental powers the "nervo" component implied were allied with physical weakness (Edgar Allen Poe being a favorite and willing phrenological example) but, in Gage's case, the "bilious" portion contributed the athletic frame that imparted energy and strength to mind and body and made possible the endurance of great mental and physical labor.[8]

Harlow, Phrenology, and Gage

From Nelson Sizer we also learn of the possibility of a relation between Harlow and phrenology that was closer than an intellectual one. Sizer and Buell's 1842 Duttonsville lectures were organized by a local committee of which Sizer wrote "Dr. Harlow ... then a young physician assisted as a member." Between the end of October and 20 November 1845, they were in Vermont once more where they again met Harlow, whom Sizer now described as "our excellent friend." After the 1848 account of Gage's accident was published they met Harlow and "conversed on the subject" with him.

I am still unable to resolve the difficulties about accepting Sizer's account in its entirety. Since 'discovering' his role, to which I drew attention in 1986, I have found weak confirmation of his story in that some of the dates and places Sizer gives are also found in contemporaneous accounts of the lectures in the *American Phrenological Journal*. There are no specific reports there or elsewhere of lectures in Cavendish or visits to it by Sizer and Buell. There are two problems with Sizer's story. First, the dates. Sizer and Buell could not have seen a "Dr." Harlow in 1842 because Harlow was not graduated until 1844, but they could have seen him in Duttonsville in 1845 because he was in practice there by then. Both the date of 1844, given by one source, and Harlow's own of January 1845 for commencing his practice are early enough (an 1846 date given by another source seems to be of his purchasing Chamberlain's practice). Second, as to places, Harlow's schooling has him at Ashby in 1840, teaching in Acton around 1842, perhaps also beginning his medical tutelage under Harris Cowdrey, and enrolled at Castleton then. It therefore seems unlikely that Sizer and Buell could have seen Harlow in Duttonsville in 1842.

On the other hand, Sizer and Buell did conduct lecture tours of New England in 1842 and 1845. In their book they say that they first covered the Connecticut Valley between "Windsor, Conn., and Windsor, Vt." From the book and the irregular reports of their travels that appeared in the *American Phrenological Journal*, we know they lectured in many places and examined many subjects in the Valley. Although the date is a little uncertain, it seems that in Duttonsville on the 1842 tour they examined a young man blinded in one eye from infancy (in whom they found marked differences between the organs of Size and Colour on the two sides of his head). At that time they also published their book on phrenology in Woodstock, Vermont, about twenty miles to the northeast of Duttonsville. By 1845, when they undertook a second tour, the *Journal* noted how much interest already existed in an area of Massachusetts that began about twenty five to thirty miles to the northwest of Boston, with the towns of Chelmsford, Littleton, and Westford, and extended westerly to Fitchburg and Leominster. If that interest was partly the result of the first tour in 1842, Harlow had then been living and working in an area much traveled by Sizer and Buell: Acton is about five to ten miles from each of the first three of these towns, and Ashby about the same distance from the last two. Possibly Harlow helped arrange the 1842 lectures of Sizer and Buell in one or other of the Massachusetts towns in which he lived, but it could not have been in Duttonsville or as a "Doctor" but only as an apprentice physician or a teacher. A source of Sizer's misattribution consistent with this latter possibility is suggested by an alteration to the Acton town record of Harlow's marriage: the "Mr." in front of his name has been crossed out and "Dr." substituted. If the alteration was made before 1844, he could have been known as "Dr. Harlow" before he was graduated.

In his recollections, Sizer described the change in Gage as follows:

The man had a good constitution, and recovered; but during the course of his illness he was profane, irreverent, disrespectful, extremely coarse and vulgar in his remarks, so much so, that persons of delicacy, especially women, found it impossible to endure his presence. These traits had not been manifested by him previously.

Now compare Sizer with this sentence from the 1851 description in *The American Phrenological Journal*, mentioned briefly in chapter 6, and reproduced here as figure 15.2:

after the man recovered, and while recovering, he was gross, profane, coarse, and vulgar, to such a degree that his society was intolerable to decent people. Before the injury he was quiet and respectful.

Note the similarities. First, both appear to say that the change was evident during the recovery period, not simply after it, and both also mention his effect upon others. Neither of these points was made by Harlow

"A MOST REMARKABLE CASE.—The *Journal of American Medical Science* contains an account of an injury to the brain and recovery of the man, which draws considerably upon one's faith to credit. The story in brief is that the person injured was engaged in blasting, and was tamping in the charge, when it exploded, and the tamping-iron, three feet seven inches in length, and an inch and a quarter in diameter, weighing thirteen and a quarter pounds, passed through the left cheek, just behind and below the mouth, ascended into the brain behind the left eye, passed from the skull, which it shattered and raised up, "like an inverted funnel," for a distance of about two inches in every direction around the wound, flew through the air, and was picked up by the workmen, "covered with blood and brains," several rods behind where he stood. The man was placed in a cart and was carried three-quarters of a mile. He got out of the cart himself, walked up stairs, and in ten weeks was nearly well, and though he lost a considerable portion of his brains he exhibited no difference in mental perceptions and power than before the accident. This case occurred in Vermont, upon the line of the Rutland and Burlington Railroad, in September, 1848, in the practice of Dr. J. M. Harlow, of Cavendish, Vt. The physician, in commenting on the case, says it is unparalleled in the annals of surgery, and that its leading feature is its improbability."—*Phila. Ledger.*

We are well acquainted with several of the leading men in the village where the above occurrence took place, and have been assured by them that the statement relative to the wound and recovery is correct. But that there was no difference in his mental manifestations after the recovery, is, however, *not* true.

We have been informed by the best authority that after the man recovered, and while recovering, he was gross, profane, coarse, and vulgar, to such a degree that his society was intolerable to decent people. Before the injury he was quiet and respectful. If we remember correctly, the iron passed through the regions of the organs of BENEVOLENCE and VENERATION, which left these organs without influence in his character, hence his profanity, and want of respect and kindness; giving the animal propensities absolute control in the character. The above report probably alludes to *Intellectual* "perceptions," while it erroneously uses the word *mental,* which involves all the faculties, the feelings as well as the intellect.

Figure 15.2
Facsimile of *American Phrenological Journal* comment on Bigelow's report From *American Phrenological Journal* 1951, 13: 89, col. 3.

in 1848, nor, of course, by Bigelow, and neither appears anywhere else. Second, three of the six adjectives are identical and a fourth is expressed as an opposite (respectful vs. disrespectful).

Sizer's explanation of the change derived from phrenological principles. The tamping iron had gone in

under the cheek bone ... passing behind the eye, cutting off the optic nerve, and passing out at the top of the head, about two inches back from where the hair commences to grow, in the neighborhood of Benevolence and the front part of Veneration.

Sizer believed that Gage's

organ of Veneration seemed to have been injured, and the profanity was the probable result.

The *Journal* description was also followed by a phrenological explanation:

The iron passed through the regions of the organs of BENEVOLENCE and VENERATION ... hence his profanity, and want of respect and kindness.

Perhaps the evident similarity between Sizer's and this other account merely reflects what we might call the reliability of phrenological diagnosis. But one more point made in the *Journal* description has an almost too familiar sound: the destruction of the organs gave "the animal propensities absolute control in the character." Sizer does not say anything like this. Only Harlow, in 1868, had referred to the balance between Gage's intellectual faculties and his animal propensities being destroyed and, peculiarly enough, this second account also refers to the intellectual faculties. Harlow had intimated in his 1848 paper that there was to be a later communication covering what he termed the "mental manifestations," a phrase that also recurs in this second and obviously phrenological context. True, other people sometimes used terms like "intellectual faculties," "animal propensities," "intellectual capacity," "mental manifestations," and "animal passions," but phrenologists did so much more frequently. Harlow's use points to phrenology.

Whence this second description? It is also in the unattributed comment on Bigelow's 1850 paper mentioned in chapter 6 (fig. 15.2). It begins:

We are well acquainted with several of the leading men in the village ... and have been assured by them that the statement [in the report of Bigelow's paper] relative to the wound and recovery is correct. But that there was no difference in his mental manifestations after the recovery, is, however, not true.

The source of such a flat denial? The comment answers:

We have been informed by the best authority that after the man recovered, and while recovering, he was gross, profane, coarse, and vulgar ...

Who could that authority—note the singular—have been if not Harlow? Already reasonably certain that the description came to the *Journal* from Sizer, we can now be reasonably certain that Harlow provided it to him. It therefore seems to me extremely likely that Harlow was not only markedly influenced by Gall's system but was very probably a follower of it.[9]

Life in Woburn

If what we know of Harlow's life and work in Cavendish is sketchy, and the details of his relation to phrenology somewhat uncertain, we have a more rounded picture of Harlow in Woburn, Massachusetts. He gave up his Cavendish practice in 1857 because of poor health and spent three years traveling and studying in Minnesota (where he had relatives) and Philadelphia, before setting up again in 1861 in Woburn, a town some twenty kilometers (twelve miles) northwest of Boston. That he came with a high reputation is evident from an unsigned short commendation, presumably written by the editor, that appeared in the *Middlesex Journal* of 9 November, 1861. The article gave an interesting ground for recommending him:

DR. J. M. HARLOW, of Cavendish, Vt., has taken up his residence in Woburn, for the purpose of practicing as a Physician and Surgeon. Dr. H. is a graduate of Jefferson College, Philadelphia, and has enjoyed a reputation and position in Cavendish of the highest order. His patients were among the first circles, and speak of his abilities in the best terms. Perhaps some of our readers may remember the celebrated case of a Mr. Gage who "had an iron bar four feet in length and one and one fourth inches in diameter, shot through his head, while blasting rocks at the building of the Rutland and Burlington Railroad." It was Dr. Harlow, we learn from the Bellows Falls Times, who attended him and brought him through his troubles. Dr. Harlow possesses recommendations from some of the first practitioners in New England, with some of whom he has been connected in the treatment of many difficult cases. The following, from Professor Phelps, speaks much in his favor as a physician:

"DARTMOUTH COLLEGE,
Hanover, N.H., Sept. 23d, '61.

To whom it may concern—
I take great pleasure in giving my testimony most decidedly in favour of Dr. J. M. Harlow, for many years my professional neighbor.

As a practitioner of medicine, I have ever considered him one of the most valuable that a community could possess; uniting as he does a most untiring devotion to his patients, with an amount of accurate and extensive medical knowledge, as well as a sound judgment, such as few are endowed with.

EDW. E. PHELPS, M.D., LL.D., &C,
Prof. Theor. and Pract. of Medicine in Dartmouth College"

We refer our readers to Dr. Harlow's advertisement, which can be found under our Special Notice head

The Special Notice read:

DR. J. M. HARLOW
Formerly of Cavendish, Vermont, respectfully tenders his professional services in the practice of MEDICINE and SURGERY to the people of Woburn and vicinity, and hopes after an extensive and varied professional experience during the last 18 years in the successful practice of his profession, to deserve and receive the patronage of this community.
Office for the present at the CENTRAL HOUSE.
Dr. H. refers to the following gentlemen:—Hon Richard Fletcher, Boston; Ed. E. Phelps, M.D., LL.D., Windsor, Vt.; John W. Graves, M.D., Lowell, Mass.; Alfred Hitchcock, M.D., Fitchburg; A. A. Ranney, Esq., 35 Court St., Boston; Hon. B. F. White, Boston; Ex-Gov. Ryland Fletcher, Otis Robbins, Esq., and Rev. Jos. Freeman, Cavendish, Vt.; and the people of Cavendish and vicinity generally.

The same Notice had appeared in the *Woburn Journal* the day before. There, the editor's commendation, although shorter and failing to mention Harlow's connections with "the first circles" or his treatment of Gage, was no less warm. Fortuitously, perhaps, that editor placed his paragraph directly under a report of the Annual Meeting of the Middlesex East District Medical Society.

The minutes of the Middlesex East District Medical Society show that Harlow passed the examination for membership in the Massachusetts Medical Society a month later:

Woburn Dec 17th 1861
The Board of Censors met in the P M at Woburn with the secretary.
Present Drs. Chapin Toothaker & E. Cutter
Dr Chapin was elected Chairman.
Upon examination
Dr. John. M. Harlow
of Woburn was admitted to the Massachusetts Medical Society.
Dr Harlow signed the form of Subscription at the same time and place.

Ephraim Cutter
Secy ex officio

Harlow now involved himself thoroughly in the medical and general life of Woburn, a life much influenced by the War of the Rebellion, then some eight months old.[10]

A member of the Republican Party from its foundation in 1856, Harlow had, it was said when his eighty-seventh birthday was celebrated in 1906, "all along ... not only advocated and voted to sustain Republican doctrine, but on any proper call for aid was never known to be backward in thrusting his hand deep down into his pocket for the necessary wherewithal to respond to it." One assumes he shared the strong antislavery feeling of most Republicans, a sentiment Harris Cowdrey certainly held very strongly. During the War of the Rebellion, Harlow volunteered his services as a "gratuitous and patriotic offering" to Governor Andrew as a Special Examining Surgeon of Recruits. In that unpaid capacity he examined Albert Ballard Lovejoy on 27 August, 1862. Lovejoy was a thirty-one-year-old currier from Brentwood, New Hampshire, then resident in Woburn who had volunteered four days earlier for nine month's service in the Union Army. Harlow found Lovejoy's major systems and organs to be "sound," and found him not a drinker or to have had the "horrors," not to have had fits or a head injury, not to be subject to piles or have difficulty in urinating. As one "authorized to make conclusive examinations," Harlow accepted Lovejoy into the Union army.

Albert Lovejoy's rendezvous was Camp Lander, about ten miles northeast of Woburn at Wenham. There, on 16 September, he was mustered into G Company as a private in the Fifth Massachusetts Infantry. After training, his regiment joined with other Massachusetts, Rhode Island, and New York units to form a mixed force of 11,000 infantry, cavalry, and artillery that was sent in late October to North Carolina. After first taking part in the Williamstown expedition, his regiment joined the Goldsboro expedition, participating in the battles there and at Whitehall and New Bern, was twice involved in raising the siege of Washington, North Carolina, and finally joined the Gun Swamp expedition. On 22 June 1863, after ten months arduous service, Lovejoy's regiment began the journey back to Boston. Lucky not to be among the 11 percent casualties suffered by the regiment, Lovejoy was mustered out at Camp Lander on 2 July 1863. Before enlisting he was already married with one child. After the war, he and his wife had two more children. It is not known when and where he died.[11]

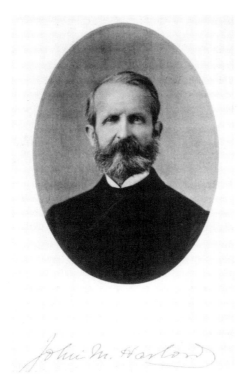

Figure 15.3
John Martyn Harlow as State Senator in 1885
From Government of the Commonwealth of Massachusetts 1885, facing p. 128.
Reproduced by kind permission of the State Library of Massachusetts.

Harlow did not see active service in the war but was made a member of Burbank Post No. 33, Grand Army of the Republic [G.A.R.] after it. He remained staunchly Republican. When the Democrat and Conservative forces of Woburn were marshaling for the postwar elections, Harlow helped found a Grant Club to oppose them, holding office as one of its vice-presidents. This interest in politics eventually led him to the first of what was to be four forays into the political life of Massachusetts (fig. 15.3). In November 1884 he stood for the Massachusetts State Senate and was elected for the 1885 term with slightly more than 54 percent of the votes counted. A year later he was successful for the 1886 term with nearly 56 percent. In the Senate he was a member of the committees on Education and Metropolitan Drainage and Chairman of the committee on Public Health. Ten years later, as the 1894 Republican candidate, he was successful in the first of two successive elections for the Governor's Executive Council, being elected with some 60 percent of the vote both times. Over the two terms he served in 1895 and 1896, he chaired two of the council's committees and served on a number of others. He was, an obituary note said, "endowed naturally with a large amount of executive ability, which displayed itself more publicly than ever before in his life" during his work on the council. At the end of his second term, when he retired from politics, he was seventy-six.

Harlow was heavily involved in Woburn's educational and civic affairs. He served on the School Committee, was a member of the Board of Selectmen, was on the first commission to establish a pure water supply, and was Chairman of the Board of Sinking Fund Commissioners. He was a Trustee of the Woburn Public Library and used his Senate position to secure the act for its incorporation. In their memorandum of condolences to Mrs. Harlow, the Trustees of the Library said that this had safeguarded the Library's trust funds from "the vicissitudes of local political changes" and went on to characterize him as one who had given the Board

the benefit of his bright mind, his business acumen and his strong individuality. He was a shrewd man of affairs, a careful administrator of the public and private trusts committed to his care, and a public-spirited citizen, always active in civic life. His marked individuality has left a permanent impress on this community.

At his funeral, the Rev. Stephen A. Norton said that to all the offices Harlow held in Woburn and Massachusetts, Harlow gave

the careful attention which his nature and character called for; and in them all he was the man of dependence and strength. Dr. Harlow will be regarded in the years to come as one of the large, broad-minded and forceful makers of this city, and of wide influence in this state.

Every comment about his public life echoes these sentiments. As the *Woburn Journal* said in a public notice of his eighty-seventh birthday, "No citizen of Woburn is more highly respected, or thought more of, than Dr. or Hon., John M. Harlow."[12]

Medical Practice and Medical Politics
Medicine was the dominant focus of Harlow's activity. Soon after arriving in Woburn his "agreeable manners and skill" made him a competitor of the five leading physicians in the town where his forty-six-year-residence led to "a very extensive medical practice." Of his practice it was said:

In skill he was much more than an ordinary practitioner, and his standing in the estimation of the public furnishes the highest tribute to his character, tact, sympathy and personal worth. In numberless homes he has shown a kindliness and friendship which will not be forgotten by the different generations of our citizens who have known and respected him as a man of high mind, and self-sacrificing, kind-hearted and true. These will preserve while they live anecdotes of his prowess in combating disease, and reminiscences of his wit and cases of his generosity which have been in these long years not a few.

Some of what we know of Harlow's everyday practice can be gleaned from occasional newspaper reports of local accidents. Thus in the period close to finalizing his work on Gage, he was called on to treat the extensive fractures to Miss Sarah Hart's ankle, leg and peloric bone, and the severe contusions to her lower body suffered when she was crushed between the platform and ceiling of a steam elevator; the concussion and serious injuries to the head and face of Mrs. Stephen Dow, who was thrown from her carriage when the horse drawing it bolted; and the scalp of young Master Noyes "torn in a frightful manner" when he fell under the wheels of the local hose carriage while chasing it on its way to a fire. In 1897, Harlow requested the attendance of Drs. Blake of Woburn, Cowdry of Stoneham, and Warren of Boston when he fractured both bones of his left leg below the knee. He had been thrown from a horse-drawn sleigh while being driven home from the Central House, where he had his practice. He was then nearly seventy-eight years of age.[13]

The records of the Middlesex East District Medical Society show that between 1869 and 1891 Harlow mentioned briefly his own cases of aphasia in an eight-year-old boy, and the convulsions and death of a fourteen-year-old girl who had eaten green chestnuts. He presented such pathological specimens as a tumor of the cerebellum, an ulcerated duodenum, a reef knot in an umbilical cord, and an eight-foot-long tapeworm that he had removed from a Harvard student by administering an emulsion of pumpkin seed (*cucurbita pepo*) followed some hours later by castor oil and turpentine. (In the discussion, Dr. Holmes said that one of his patients who had been treated in much the same way complained that he preferred the disease to this part of the remedy.) Harlow also contributed to discussions on "narcotic poisoning"—the inadvertent administration of an overdose of morphia—in treating various conditions, including angina. Here he stressed the value of galvanism and artificial respiration.[14]

Manuscripts of the four longer contributions Harlow made to the monthly meetings of the society during that period are included in appendix F. Dealing with more complex medical problems, they allow an evaluation of Harlow's medical knowledge and skill.

Case 1: Placenta praevia. The case was that of a mother aged forty-two-years with a history of a previous miscarriage and a threatened miscarriage in the fourth month of the present pregnancy. About a week prior to her delivery, Harlow found the placenta over the os, and he ordered rest. A week later she was delivered of a boy weighing six and a half pounds after which Harlow's examination revealed what turned out to be another placenta. It signaled the presence of a twin, a girl weighing five pounds, who was born by breech ten minutes after her brother. Both babies and the mother survived.

Case 2: Imperforate hymen. A fourteen-year-old girl fell from a hammock, striking the ground with her left hip. Soon after she developed periodically incapacitating pain in that hip, down her left leg, and in her back. Harlow was called about four weeks later when, in addition to those symptoms, he was told by the girl's mother that during the previous year she had also suffered rectal pain and attacks of bleeding from internal piles. She "had never menstruated nor given any indication of doing so." Harlow's remedies seemed to work but three weeks later, her mother asked Harlow for a suppository of opium and belladonna because of an exacerbation of her piles. Three weeks later again, Harlow was called because the girl had had another and severe attack of rectal pain. Harlow therefore examined her more formally. His rectal examination found no evidence of piles, but it did cause vaginal pain. He was unable to examine her vagina because it was closed by a firm inelastic membrane. This suggestion of an imperforate hymen was confirmed during a full examination under ether the following afternoon. The hymen was then punctured, thirty fluid ounces of a dark viscous fluid drawn off, and the opening then enlarged. No internal abnormality was revealed. Despite transitory symptoms of "nervous shock," she had recovered five days later after a daily regime of washing the vagina, initially with a weak solution of carbolic acid and later with permanganate of potash.

Case 3: Pain and inflammation in the ilio-caecal region. The patient, a thirty-five-year-old Irishman, had been attacked five days earlier with severe pain in the ilio-caecal region (the region of the vermiform appendix) and inflammation that had soon extended over the whole abdomen. Harlow immediately gave a hypodermic injection of morphia and prescribed a pill containing opium, calomel (a purgative), and ipecac (a combined emetic and purgative) to be given every four hours for twenty-four hours. Before that time elapsed, "the bowels moved freely after having been confined eight days." A small piece of what Harlow supposed to be a fragment of intestine was found in the feces. The patient recovered rapidly. At the onset of the attack, self-administered cathartics had had no effect. There was considerable enteritis, but the peritoneum was not much affected, and Harlow concluded that the trouble was at the ilio-caecal valve.

The minutes are ambiguous as to whether Harlow used the diagnostic term "typhlitis" (discussed below) in presenting this case, but he and others certainly did so in the discussion that followed. Several other cases of the condition were mentioned, all of which had recovered. Harlow also mentioned that he had seen five chronic cases, and elaborated slightly on three of them. He believed it took years for full recovery.

Case 4:   Placenta lateralis.   In about the seventh or eight month of her pregnancy, a woman seemed to go into labor and Harlow was called. He found the os undilated and he remained for about an hour because of hemorrhaging. He then prescribed morphia and "perfect rest in bed" in the hope of the child's being carried to term. About twenty-four hours later he was called again. The patient was clearly worse and his examination located the placenta covering the os. Dr. Morse, a colleague whom he called in, seems to have confirmed the diagnosis and decided on a forceps delivery. This was carried out under ether but the child was dead. Harlow stayed with the patient giving brandy "in teaspoon doses all night." Despite her weakness, loss of blood, and dependence on neighbors for assistance, she had recovered within two weeks.

Dr. Ian Cope, a notable Australian surgeon and obstetrician and gynecologist, who has added the history of nineteenth-century medicine to his specialities, examined the manuscripts of Harlow's papers and case reports for me in order to evaluate Harlow's medical knowledge and skill against the standards of the times. He concludes that Harlow's management of cases 1, 2, and 4 was appropriate, and that of 1 and 4 showed expertise for the times. Dr. Cope thought case 3 was most likely one of appendicitis, and that Harlow's understanding of it was also in keeping with that of the time. "Typhlitis" and related morbid conditions of the vermiform appendix were not properly understood until the 1886 paper by Reginald Fitz, of Boston, two years after Harlow's report. (Fitz's work was discussed at the October 1886 meeting of the society.) In his summary, Dr. Cope concluded that "Harlow's medical knowledge for the times was good and his level of skill appears to be above average" (appendix F).

At various times in the "political" side of medical life we find Harlow as President of the Middlesex East District Medical Society, Vice-President of the Massachusetts Medical Society (1886–1887), and Councillor of the State Medical Society. Although I have only scanty details about the periods for which he held these offices, when they are mentioned the words most often used are that they were for many or several years or terms. As a member of the Committee of the Council of the State Medical Society and the State Board of Health, Lunacy and Charity, Harlow did much to establish the Massachusetts State Board of Health, the first such separate body in the United States. Presumably it was because of his involvement in the state's medical life that Governor Walcott appointed him a trustee of the Massachusetts General Hospital. Neither is it surprising that after his death his brother physicians summed up these activities by saying that since he had joined their society he had been "ever zealous in all its labor & activities, always faithful & loyal to its interests, friendly & helpful to its individual members & to the medical profession at large & so adding to its efficiency and success."[15]

Riches, Religion, and Reputation

When Harlow came to Woburn, "he already possessed a considerable fortune" which "he largely but modestly increased during the remainder of his life." In fact, he showed more than a little talent for financial matters, becoming President and Director of the Woburn National Bank and the Woburn Gas Light Company, Director of the later Woburn National Bank, manager of vast or large estates, and he was known "very generally as a man of excellent judgement and ability in financial affairs." At his funeral, the Rev. Norton said, "Men of large business ability recognized and consulted his wisdom. I have heard it said, by those whose experience made them qualified to speak, that had he cared to make financial affairs his special field he must have attained to great eminence as a financier." The *New York Times* reported his death as a special notice and characterized him as one of the "most prominent surgeons of New England." The notice, although small, was about twice as large as that for a "financier" and former President and current Director of a railroad, and three to four times the size of a notice for "one of the wealthiest men" in the State of New York who was "one of the best known American exporters of cattle." The *Times* went on to say that Harlow "was the wealthiest man in Woburn."

Harlow is buried in Lot 129 of the Woburn cemetery. In his will he left $150,700 in cash to various relatives and friends, including $60,000 to his widow, and a total of $21,000 to Arthur Harris Cowdrey and his daughters. The rest of his estate was put into trust for his widow, with Cowdrey as one of the trustees. On Mrs. Harlow's death, this residuary estate was to be divided into fortieths, of which twenty-nine were to be disposed of according to his wishes, and eleven according to hers. In 1913, when she died, each these fortieths were worth between $4,500 and $5,000 (different recipients give different values). Consequently, the value of this part of the residuary estate amounted to between $407,000 and $428,000—real estate, some shares, and the horses, carriage, and a 1912 model Cadillac motor car being excluded. The two groups to benefit most from the bequests were the medical and medical-charitable, with forty-five percent (Massachusetts General Hospital alone being left 25 percent of the total), and 27.5 percent left to bodies in the educational and library spheres (the Woburn Public Library being left 17.5 percent).[16]

The way in which John Martyn Harlow and his wife disposed of their property illustrates the importance to both of religious and moral values in everyday life. In its obituary, the *Woburn Journal* stressed this aspect of Harlow

In conformity with the ideas of his Puritan ancestry, Dr. Harlow held some positive opinions. He could never forgive Count Rumford—our eminent Woburn native—for fighting against the Americans in the ranks of the British army, more than a century ago; and he had an old-fashioned integrity which had no patience with those who practised crooked methods of finance or who used their advantages in public life for their own private gain.

In his own note, the editor added, "In his long residence and extensive practice in Woburn, in sickness and in trouble, he served the rich and poor alike."

At Harlow's funeral, the Rev. Norton stressed that Harlow had

inherited character ... and the blood of Pilgrim and Puritan lived in his veins. In all his long life and manifold relations and many responsibilities he was the soul of honor. He scorned ways that are dark and questionable. Nobody ever accused him, I think, of owning a penny that was not justly his own.

Nor, he confirmed, did Harlow help only in medical and public matters

People came to him for advice in their personal affairs, and he gave them freely of his time and of his wisdom.... And many were the poor people whose need was deeper than advice could meet, who went from his door with the more substantial and immediate relief. These things were not blazoned abroad.

Harlow's religious values do not seem to have been associated with his adhering to a particular religion. We have seen that he sang in the Baptist choir but did not follow the Baptist tradition of his own family. Similarly, according to Norton, when the church to which he had belonged became extinct, he "took in all the churches in his sympathies, and did not limit himself to one as a place to help." Apparently the Woburn First Congregational (Trinitarian) Church was not the one that had disappeared, even though it was the church he regularly attended and on whose Parish Committee he served. It was alive enough for him to leave it $5,000 and two-fortieths of his residuary estate. He also left two-fortieths to the Evangelical Society of Acton (in memory of his first wife), one-fortieth to the Woburn Baptist Church (in memory of his parents "who were of that faith"), and one-fortieth to each of the Woburn Methodist and Trinity Churches, the Burlington Church of Christ, and the North Woburn Congregational Society.[17]

Medicine was however the dominant focus. The Middlesex East District Medical Society recognized this aspect and Harlow's contribution to the profession in January 1899 when they appointed him as chairman of the committee to organize the Semi-Centennial celebration of the society. His committee planned the celebrations for 23 October 1900, the society having been founded in that month in 1850. By April the following year an afternoon program of speakers had been organized, an orchestra employed to play during it, a dinner arranged, and tickets put on sale. The following is from the official record of "the order of exercises" that resulted:

Informal reception at the hall at 2.30 P.M. to members and invited guests.
Call to order by the President at 3.00.
Address by the President.
Historical Sketch of the Society by Dr. S. W. Abbott.
Music by the Highland Orchestra.
Poem by Rev. Daniel March, D.D.
Dinner in the Banqueting Hall at 4.15 P.M.
Address by Dr. J. M. Harlow, Chairman.
Prayer by Rev. Dr. March.
Addresses by Mayor W. F. Davis, W. B. Stevens, Esq., Rev. Dr. March, Dr. J. S. Clark, Dr. H. P. Walcott, Dr. F. W. Draper and Dr. E. Cutter
Music during the dinner by the Highland Orchestra.

In the course of his historical sketch, Dr. Abbott singled Harlow out for the following special mention:

Some recent observations have shown that the average duration of human life in our own State has increased several years during the half-century now closing; and if, as I believe, this result is due in any measure to human agency, our noble profession may justly claim a lion's share of the credit.

One case is recorded in full in our records which deserves special attention, since it has become conspicuous in the annals so far as the recovery or the preservation of human life is concerned. The case occurred in another State, but was very properly reported at one of our meetings by one of our members who has been for many years an honored member of this Society—Dr. J. M. Harlow of Woburn. I refer to the case of Mr. P. Gage, of Cavendish, Vt., who was injured in 1850 [sic] by the passage through his skull of an iron bar weighing thirteen pounds, carrying with it a considerable portion of the substance of the brain. This man recovered and lived for twelve years afterward, and was enabled to attend to his duties as a stage driver. When we reflect that a missile of only 1-3000th part of the size and weight of this projectile (a 22-100th inch pistol ball) constitutes a very frequent cause of death, we can only consider this remarkable case as little less than miraculous.

Later in the afternoon Harlow, acting as toastmaster "contributed in a very graceful and happy manner to the success of the occasion." After calling upon Rev. Dr. March to invoke the divine blessing, and doing ample justice to the dinner, Harlow then addressed the Society:

Members of the Middlesex East District Medical Society, Invited Guests, and our Lady Friends:
Fifty years of the life of this Society marks an interesting epoch of its existence, and you are invited here to erect the milestone which shall mark the period. In acting the part assigned to me, it is my pleasant duty to bid you welcome, one and all, to the festivities of this occasion.

I congratulate you, ladies and gentlemen, upon having lived in the most interesting period of the nineteenth century, and not alone of the nineteenth century, but the most interesting period in the history of the world. Wallace, in his recent book, entitled 'The Wonderful Century,' draws a striking comparison between the achievements of human endeavor in the nineteenth century and in all preceding ages. He finds twenty-four important discoveries in the nineteenth century, while he has found but fifteen discoveries of similar magnitude in all past times. To consider these in detail is not my purpose, as the brief time allotted to this opening, would render such attempt a dismal failure.

I can only make mere mention of some of the more important which especially concern the medical and surgical professions. In the words of our own Cabot, "In no realm of human thought has this recent advance been more rapid than in that of medicine, and in none other has it been of such wide and lasting benefit to humanity."

When we mention surgical ansthesia [*sic*] cellular physiology and pathology, antiseptic surgery and sepsis in its application to both medicine and surgery, and the germ theory of disease, the discovery of antitoxin and its application, we have an array of gifts for which the human race may well feel grateful to the medical men of the nineteenth century. Added to these we may mention the illumination of the cavities of the body by electricity and the uses of the Rontgen rays in surgical investigation of the solids, the cell theory in embryology, the germ theory in zymotic diseases and the discovery of the nature and function of the white blood corpuscles. In aid of this wonderful forward movement in the discovery of many of the first principles in the domain of physiology and pathology, and without which much of the work of investigators would have been impossible, I may mention the discovery and the development of the compound microscope, which was but a crude affair of a single lens first given to the world near the close of the fifteenth century, and which has now grown to be an instrument of great precision and power.

In conclusion, permit me to congratulate you again upon this forward movement in medicine and upon the fact of its rapid emergence already taking place (and well nigh accomplished) from the domain of speculation, based upon theory and idealism, into the domain of realism founded upon demonstrable facts.

I detain you no longer, knowing full well that you came here, not to hang upon words of mine, but to listen to those who come after me and who will rightly be preferred before me.

Harlow retained his place in the memory and sentiments of the society for many years.[18]

The commemorative Centennial publication of 1950 noted

The case of the "Crowbar Skull," reported by Dr. J. M. Harlow of Woburn in 1867 [*sic*], attracted world-wide attention. The patient, a Mr. Gage of Vermont, suffered an injury from the passage through his skull of an iron bar weighing thirteen pounds as a result of a premature explosion of dynamite [*sic*]. He survived, living for twelve years, although exhibiting definite personality changes. This skull may now be seen in the Anatomical Museum of the Harvard Medical School. Dr. Harlow later presented to the society the plates for the illustrations in his publication of the case.

Elsewhere the commemorative booklet recorded that "In 1865 Dr. John M. Harlow of Woburn became President of the Society. In 1869 [*sic*] he published in the 'Medical and Surgical Journal' [*sic*] the celebrated 'crowbar skull' case." After repeating some of the detail about Gage, and before citing the whole of the section of Harlow's will about the bequest to the society, the article remarked that "He was very active in the affairs of the society and demonstrated his interest in it in a very commendable manner."[19]

Harlow had willed one-fortieth of his residuary estate to the Middlesex East District Medical Society to be invested for the purpose of "defraying the ordinary expenses of the Middlesex East District Medical Society, including therein the expense of their Annual Dinner." The annual dinner seems always to have been held under Harlow's name, sometimes with his portrait and abbreviated CV printed on the menu. The bequest was so used until 1991, when the $9,000 remaining in the fund was absorbed into the general funds of the Middlesex District Medical Society (formed by a merger in 1990 of the East and South district societies). In 1998, the successor society donated $2,000 to help defray the costs of the bronze plaque erected at Cavendish to commemorate the 150th. Anniversary of the accident to Phineas Gage. On the plaque, both the donation and Harlow's role in treating Gage were fully acknowledged.

Harlow's memory has not always been so kept alive. Thus I have been unable to locate any record of purchases from the one-fortieth of her estate that Frances willed to the Boston Medical Library to be invested for the purchase of books "to be marked Purchased from Funds given by Dr. John Martyn Harlow." More significantly, Harlow has no memorial at the Massachusetts General Hospital. He left seven-fortieths of his residuary estate to the hospital, to which Frances added three-fortieths of hers, "to be used in erecting a ward in said Hospital to be known as the John Martyn Harlow Ward." On her death in 1917 those bequests were together worth between $50,000 and $60,000. However, there seems to be no record of them being used in any way to mark Harlow's work on behalf of either the profession to which he belonged or the hospital of which he had been a Trustee.[20]

The Obscure Country Physician

In 1868 Harlow referred to himself as having been, in 1848, "an obscure country physician." There may once have been some basis for this self-depreciatory characterization. However, the skill with which John Martyn Harlow treated Phineas Gage, the clarity of his analysis of its medical and psychological features, the cadence and beautiful simplicity of the language with which he reported his findings, and the many contributions he made to the public, medical, and political life of Woburn and Massachusetts ensured that this was not true at the end of his life in 1907.

Notes

1. For the Harlow genealogy, see appendix G. The religion of the immediate family is in Stone 1901, pp. 244–246, and the choir is in *Woburn Journal* (Massachusetts), 17 May 1907.

2. Ruth-Ann Knieriemen, Archivist, Green Mountain College, the successor of the Methodist Collegiate Institute and the Troy Conference Academy, provided information and catalogues listing Harlow (Troy Conference Academy, 1838a and 1838b). Nothing is now known in Ashby or Fitchburg about the Ashby Academy; however, the American Antiquarian Society holds a copy of the 1840 catalogue (Ashby Academy, 1840). Harlow does not seem to be listed in any Acton Town school records nor mentioned in the collections of local newspapers held by the public libraries and historical societies of Acton and of Fitchburg.

3. Curriculum is from Jefferson Medical College 1843. Harlow is in Castleton Medical College 1842, pp. 3–4; Waite 1949, p. 251; and Jefferson Medical College 1844, 1845.

4. Cowdrey is in Hurd 1890, p. 298. For Harlow's marriage on 5 January 1843 to Charlotte Davis see *Vital Records* 1923. In Acton, Charlotte had belonged to a group opposed to Unitarian ideas and broke from the Congregational Church to form the Evangelical Society, now the Acton Congregational Church (Acton Historical Commission survey quoted by Susan Paju, Acton Memorial Library reference librarian, in a letter to me of 17 December 1997). Charlotte's obituary noted how her work and charity in Woburn "happily blended" with the professional life of her husband. She was described as of strong character, having "an intimate acquaintance with the profoundest subjects of enquiry, and the aid she has been to her husband in making his career, were the materials of a rare womanhood." She died on 5 July 1886 after having "borne physical pain for many years" (*Woburn Journal* [Massachusetts], 11 July 1886). Two years after Charlotte's death, on 2 August 1888, Harlow married Frances Kimball Ames, a Woburn native. Educated at the Abbot (Female) Academy in Andover, Frances was well known as a teacher in Woburn, Westfield, and Roxbury, and at the Abbot Academy. She survived John Martyn, dying of diabetes on 2 May 1914 (*Woburn Telegram* [Massachusetts], 2 May 1914). There were no children from either marriage.

5. Dates for Harlow in Cavendish: Bridgman 1895 and 1896, pp. 117–118 in both (cf. Atkinson 1880, p. 394; and Kelly 1912, p. 385); and Government of the Commonwealth of Massachusetts 1885. Harlow purchased Oliver Chamberlain's medical practice in 1846 (Aldrich and Holmes 1891, p. 513). The map of Cavendish is Doton 1855 and Adams can be identified as the keeper of "S. Dulton's [*sic*] Inn," that is, Samuel Dutton's Inn, from Wriston 1991, pp. 178–179. The offices Harlow held are in Walton 1846, 1847, 1857, and 1858, and in the *Woburn Journal* (Massachusetts) 17 May 1907.

6. Harlow's thesis is from Jefferson Medical College 1845. Walsh 1976a, 1976b for New England medical phrenology; Miegs's translation is Flourens 1846; and

see Barker 1995 for Dunglison. Mütter and Pancoast do not seem to have expressed an opinion about phrenology.

7. Mrs. Barbara Gammon of Springfield, Vermont, kindly allowed me to examine her collection of French's papers and shorthand correspondence. The only letters from the 1848–1850 period that I could identify seemed to contain nothing about Gage. The phrenological visits are in Buell and Sizer 1842 and Sizer 1882.

8. Thomas 1826 for his theory of temperament. Reviews and discussion of the theory are in A. Combe 1827; G. Combe 1830; Kennedy 1829; Fowler 1839; and Caldwell 1839. Stern 1971 for Poe and temperament as a necessary part of a Fowler reading.

9. Sizer's discussion of Harlow and Gage is in Sizer 1882, pp. 105–106, 193–196. Particular places in Vermont and Massachusetts in which Sizer and Buell lectured or where phrenology was especially popular are mentioned in Buell and Sizer 1842, pp. 13–16, 151–152, and the *American Phrenological Journal* 1843, 5, pp. 285–286; 1845, 7, p. 344; 1846, 8, pp. 58–60; 1851, 13, p. 22, and Davies, [1955] 1971, pp. 20–35, 59–61. The comment on Gage is "A most remarkable case" 1851. William Windsor a phrenologist who may have known Sizer personally, says that Sizer was "intimately acquainted with Dr. Harlow" (Windsor 1921, p. 571).

10. *Middlesex Journal* commendation and Special Notice in issue of 9 November, 1861, p. 2, col. 3 and p. 3 col. 3 respectively; corresponding *Woburn Journal* material on 8 November. Minutes of the Middlesex East District Medical Society are held by the Woburn Public Library.

11. Harlow's politics are from *Woburn Journal* (Massachusetts), 30 November 1906, and Cowdrey's antislavery feelings are in Hurd 1890. Cowdrey's son, Arthur Harris Cowdrey, who was graduated M.D. from Harvard in 1857, also shared these feelings. At the outbreak of the War of the Rebellion he served as Assistant Surgeon in the Seventh Regiment, Massachusetts Volunteer Infantry. He was eventually promoted to Major in the Thirty-seventh U.S. Colored Infantry. Harlow's record of Lovejoy's examination is on a "Form for Examining a Recruit" lying loose among the records and papers of the Middlesex East District Medical Society held by the Woburn Public Library. I have to thank Nancy Daddona, of Prospect, Connecticut, a distant Lovejoy relative, for Albert's family details and for finding his service history from the Civil War Research and Genealogy Database.

12. Harlow and the Grant Club are in *Woburn Journal* (Massachusetts), 6 June 1868, p. 2, col. 2. Eva Murphy, Fingold Library, Massachusetts State House has been unable to document Harlow's membership in Burbank Post 33, G.A.R. Senate election results are from Fingold Library, State House, Boston, Massachusetts; Woburn offices are in Bridgman 1895, 1896 and the *Woburn Journal*, 17 May 1907; Library Board condolences are from Board of Trustees, Woburn Public Library, 4 June 1907; the funeral address is Norton 1907, pp. 7–8; the birthday appreciation is in the *Woburn Journal*, 30 November 1906.

13. Harlow's practice in the *Woburn Journal* (Massachusetts), 17 May 1907. In sequence the cases are from the *Woburn Journal* 2 November 1867, p. 2, col. 3; 4 January 1868, p. 2, col. 3; 25 July 1868, p. 2, col. 4. Harlow's fractured leg is from the *Woburn Journal* 5 February 1897, p. 2, col. 4.

14. Cases, specimens, and discussions are in the Record Books of the Middlesex East District Medical Society as follows: aphasia, the green chestnut death, vol. 1, 17 November 1869, p. 241; the cerebellar tumor and the ulcerated duodenum, vol. 2, 13 November 1878, p. 169; the umbilical reef knot, vol. 3, 6 August 1884, p. 149; the tapeworm, vol. 3, 4 November 1884, pp. 162–163; and narcotic poisoning, vol. 3, 15 September 1886, p. 207. Some of these cases are also in appendix F of this book.

15. Some documentation of Harlow's medical "political" work is in Burrage 1923, p. 172, and in the manuscript in the Woburn Public Library of the draft resolution put to a regular meeting of the Middlesex East District Medical Society, 23 October 1907.

16. Financial acumen is in the *Woburn Journal* (Massachusetts) obituary of 17 May 1907; in the funeral address by Norton 1907, p. 7; and in the *New York Times*, 14 May 1907, p. 11, col. 6. Wills of John Martyn Harlow (74709) and Frances Kimball Harlow (100187) are at the Middlesex County Probate Office. Horses, carriages, and stable furniture are mentioned in the inventories of both wills, but the Cadillac, a 1912 model, is only in Frances's. Medical and medical charitable beneficiaries were the Massachusetts General Hospital, which received seven-fortieths from him and three-fortieths from her; the Woburn Charitable Association, four-fortieths from her to erect a surgical building at the local Charles Choate Memorial Hospital; the Home for Aged Women in Woburn, two-fortieths from him; the Boston Medical Library, one-fortieth from her; and the Middlesex East District Medical Society, one-fortieth from him. The educational and library beneficiaries were the Woburn Public Library, with seven-fortieths from him; the Woburn School for a High School Library, one-fortieth from him; and three-fortieths from her to the Abbot [Female] Academy, now the Philips Academy, in Andover, Massachusetts, where she had been educated.

17. Obituary in *Woburn Journal* (Massachusetts), 17 May 1907; remarks at the funeral are Norton 1907, pp. 9, 10; details of the wills of John Martyn and Frances Harlow are in note 16.

18. The "exercises" for the semi-centennial, Abbot's appreciation of Harlow, and Harlow's address are from Middlesex East District Medical Society 1900.

19. The centennial references to Harlow are from Middlesex East District Medical Society 1950.

20. The distribution of the remainder of the trust fund set up under Harlow's Will to the merged societies is from the petition and Trial Docket 74709 of the Department of the Trial Court of the Probate and Family Court, Commonwealth of Massachusetts, dated 3 July 1991; the 1941 dinner menu is loose among the papers of the Middlesex East District Medical Society held by the Woburn Public Library; details of the wills of John Martyn and Frances Harlow are in Note 16.

16

A Realistic Conclusion

What do we make of our oddly famous patient? First, what is the source of his fame? We note that Phineas Gage's accident made no headlines— literally or figuratively. As will be remembered from figure 2.1, the simple italicized side heading with which the Ludlow *Free Soil Union* introduced the first newspaper report of his injury was close in size to that of the text. At a guess, it would rank at the lowest level of what passed for a 'headline' in newspapers from the middle of the nineteenth century. Although that report was printed within twenty-four hours of the accident, it was almost swamped by items about more mundane death and injury. Most of the other reports of Phineas's accident were based on that of the *Free Soil Union* and their placement and sub or copyediting style shows that of the *Free Soil Union* to be typical. None stood out to any greater extent. Neither were the few early reports widely reprinted. Figuratively speaking, if all the ink needed for printing those 'headlines' were to be poured into one container, there would not be enough to print a single banner headline in one of today's newspapers.

Gage Achieves Fame

How then did Phineas Gage achieve fame? Next to nothing is known about his birth, his education, his personality characteristics, and his working life before and after the accident that thrust him into fame. Phineas was supposed to have begged on the steps of the medical school building in Boston, to have carried his tamping iron with him as he exhibited himself in the larger cities of New England, and to have spent time as an exhibit with Barnum's Museum in New York. Seemingly he did all this without anyone noticing him. During the year and a half he worked for Currier at the Dartmouth Inn in Hanover no one from among the medical faculty or students at the nearby medical school, or from among the local medical practitioners, left a record of seeing him. The South American years are even more of a mystery: we do not know the means by which Phineas Gage traveled to Chile, exactly what he was employed at, and whether he was settled in his work or not. We know nothing of the illness that caused him to go to San Francisco, until 1986 we did not know that 1860 was the true year of his death, and we cannot be certain of the date his body was exhumed.

Medicine, Localization, and Ignorance

If those who saw and talked about Phineas Gage did not make him famous—and he himself certainly did not—who or what did? His fame came only from the attention he attracted in the narrow, twinned medical fields of the treatment of injuries of the brain and the study of the functions localized in it. In medicine he was of course unambiguously famous as a survivor. Harlow's treatment of him was explicitly compared with that of others, as Noyes and Kemper did with the treatment of their patients (chapter 4). Sometimes the comparison was with Phineas's symptoms and was direct. At other times it was implicit, as when Ferrier's *Gulstonian Lectures* rather than Harlow's reports were drawn on. For example, T. Smith compared his patient's transitory symptoms with the summary made by Ferrier. Following his unsuccessful attempt at suicide by shooting himself in the frontal lobes, Smith's patient's temperament changed and he became violent and overbearing but was sometimes lethargic and irritable.

Some fame accrued to Phineas through more tenuous links, as when he was connected explicitly, but usually vaguely, with lobotomy. Although I considered the specific literature in chapter 11, Goonetilleke provides an unusual individual example. At autopsy, the brain of Goonetilleke's sixty one-year old patient was found to have a large 4 cm. diameter cylindrical defect through both frontal lobes. It had been caused by the almost horizontal passage of a bullet entering the right temple and emerging from the left. Although there was no record of the circumstances of the shooting, which had taken place thirty-four years earlier, nor of personality change after the injury, Goonetilleke assumed that it had probably been a suicide attempt during an episode of depression. Then, after discussing Gage as the first recorded case showing personality changes after frontal injury and outlining the effects of lobotomy, Goonetilleke interpreted his patient's subsequent "normal married life" as the consequence of a lobotomy she had carried out on herself. Other accruals were even more tenuous, especially from the literature on mental illness. Cases of dual personality as well as delusions of being possessed by another being were attributed to the two hemispheres being functionally disconnected. Explanations based on disconnection were supported by the assertion that Gage's recovery could be attributed to the functions of the left hemisphere being taken over the right, that is, that the hemispheres functioned vicariously.[1]

In the field of localization proper Phineas's fame was more clearly ambiguous. At the time of Harlow's first report in 1848 medical sentiment was antilocalization. Partly this was because of the threat that notions of localization seemed to pose to conservative ideological, philosophical, and political doctrines. But it was also partly due to the paucity of cogent physiological evidence. Harlow's failure to produce the "future communication" in which he was to remark Gage's deleterious "mental manifestations" effectively granted Gage complete psychological recovery. Meshing with that failure, Henry Jacob Bigelow's further authoritative pronouncement of Gage's recovery gave Phineas a paradoxical pride of place in the antilocalization camp. His case seemed to deny the brain any substantial functions. In that context, the small voices raised by the occasional phrenologist or writer to such committees as that of the American Medical Association on surgery were simply not heard.

By the time of Harlow's 1868 report, medical sentiment had changed considerably. There was then much sympathy for the notion that the brain functioned in a reflex manner. On the basis of data collected by Broca, the Daxes, and others a language function had been tentatively localized in the left frontal lobe. Hughlings Jackson was also close to announcing that processes representing movement were localized in the cortex. Given that encouraging shift, it may seem surprising so little attention was paid Harlow's description of the ways in which Gage had changed. There was, however, a very good reason for the neglect: hardly anyone knew about his report. As Mrs. Hanks from the History of Medicine Division of the National Library of Medicine suggested to me in 1986, the *Publications of the Massachusetts Medical Society,* in which Harlow's 1868 report appeared, circulated to society members and tended not to be acquired by libraries. My subsequent searches of various library databases, the last in February of 1999, as well as earlier searches of the *National Union Catalogue, Pre-1956 Imprints* and the *Index of National Library Medical Serial Titles,* located only ten copies of the

Publications and eleven of the pamphlet form of Harlow's paper in US libraries. From personal knowledge of holdings other than these, I know this total to be an underestimate, but it does not seem to be a gross one.

When Ferrier's *Gulstonian Lectures* rescued Gage from what life was left him in the obscurity of the *Publications of the Massachusetts Medical Society*, other factors conspired to maintain the ambiguity about his fame. Undoubtedly one was that the lectures had been given in England. The news about Gage was thus publicized in a place where the case was not well known and from which it failed to reach the place where it was somewhat better known. The conservatism of the medical profession also played a role. The editor of Kirkes's textbook actively resisted displaying a true picture of Gage, and a similar motivation probably lay behind some of those summaries of Ferrier's lectures that failed to mention the changes. Then there was the ubiquitous and conservative influence of Henry Jacob Bigelow. The *Boston Medical and Surgical Journal*'s bibliographical review of Harlow's 1869 pamphlet devoted so much space to Bigelow's role that one could have been excused for thinking that Phineas had come under Bigelow's care rather than Harlow's, and it was Bigelow's opinion that counted.

Mental Changes in the Sensory-Motor Framework

Many physiologists and medical practitioners also had problems with the mental phenomena. Changes seemed to be present in only between one third and one half of cases of frontal damage and tumor. That fact limited what could be made of the Gage case for diagnosis and in brain surgery. The changes were also difficult to conceptualize. From Ferrier and Starr to Dandy and Brickner we saw how this problem posed itself as the vagueness of terms like "mental degradation," "mental symptoms," and "little mental peculiarities" and the like. Those who accepted Gage had changed, had difficulty in describing the symptoms in a meaningful way. There was also the related problem of fitting the changes into the kind of physiology and psychology provided by the sensory-motor framework. Ferrier's gallant effort to base an explanation on the loss of an inhibitory-motor mechanism so stretched the sensory-motor framework that that hypothetical mechanism had only the shortest of lives. And there was no alternative explanatory framework. Those who like Starr or Elder and Miles drew on inhibition were appealing to a process better understood metaphorically than physiologically.[2]

Nearly ninety years after Gage's death, Teuber introduced his analysis of the problems posed by the modern versions of sensory-motor physiology and psychology by saying, "It is hardly an accident that the frontal lobes have continued to pose such insuperable difficulties to interpretations in traditional stimulus-response terms." As an example he noted that the deficits on the delayed-response task that had proved so difficult for Becky and Lucy could not be explained as an inability to overcome response preferences. Clearly Teuber was not impressed by Brickner's thirty-year-earlier explanation that the fundamental problem from which Joe A. suffered was his inability to form complex associations from simple ones. Nor do I think he would have found Brickner's concept of restraint more than a sidestepping of the issues posed by the very general way Ferrier and others had used the concepts of inhibition and attention. Those who accepted the changes did not possess a framework from which they could generate an adequate explanation of what had caused the alterations.

Representations and Misrepresentations of Gage

At the end of the nineteenth century Gage's case had achieved its premier position among those of recovery from serious brain injury. But even by then the outlines of the misrepresentations evident in chapters 13 and 14 had already been sketched. For example, in 1905 A. W. Campbell the Australian histologist who first revealed the structural differences between the prefrontal and frontal areas, listed the symptoms of what he called "a peculiar form of mental disturbance" seen in a majority of instances of extensive left-sided frontal lesions. They were a low sense of humor, a delight in causing annoyance, violence when waywardness was opposed, a lack of gratitude, and an inefficient control of animal passions. There was, he said, no better illustration of this pattern of symptoms than Phineas Gage. The tamping iron, the passage of which he described accurately, had turned Gage from "an intelligent and industrious artisan into an altogether depraved being." In much the same way as the textbook authors considered in chapter 14, Campbell represented the changes in Phineas's behavior as different from what they were.[3]

Misinterpretations of specific cases similar to Gage's are also still not infrequent. Thus, nearly thirty-five years ago, Brenda Milner felt impelled to insist that K. M., the patient reported on by Hebb and Penfield, did not show the same kind of frontal syndrome as the other patients with whom he was commonly classed. The victim of a frontal head injury at age twenty, K. M. had become subject to epileptic convulsions, frequently having several major seizures each week. In 1938 Penfield controlled this otherwise intractable epilepsy by removing about one third of each of K. M.'s frontal lobes. After the operation his personality changed for the better in that he was polite and considerate, rather than violent and aggressive. His seizures were so successfully controlled by medication that he joined the US army in 1942, being discharged only after he had had a convulsion while off medication. When Milner saw K. M. in 1962 he had not been able to hold down a job for more than twenty years, and was being cared for by his family, with whom he lived. Milner's psychological investigation showed little cognitive intellectual impairment but K. M.'s performance on some tests was typical of patients with frontal damage. Despite this deficit, despite his not working, and despite his social dependence, Milner emphasized that K. M. had "a pension, and he uses this pension apparently quite wisely." He paid some money for his keep and otherwise contributed to the household. Nevertheless, K. M. is still often cited in the frontal lobe literature as being unable to plan or organize future activity. Milner's considerable reservation is not mentioned.[4]

Already by 1900 what little Harlow had recorded about Gage was also not being considered fully or was being ignored. Thus, in his 1900 work on brain in relation to mind, Christison was content to rely mostly on Bigelow's account. Because he claimed that Gage had lived for twelve years, Christison must have known more. But it was not much more: Gage, he said, had earned his living as a coachman and barn hand. In the early 1920s, Tilney and Riley cited the Gage case as the first to throw light on the functions of the so-called silent areas. Although they said that many later cases confirmed those functions, they described the tamping iron as entering Gage's skull through the left eye. As late as the eve of the one hundredth anniversary of the accident, Mettler and Mettler based what they said about Gage in their note on the history of the development of knowledge of the effects of cranial trauma on Bigelow rather than Harlow.

Franz said in 1905 that during the previous four years, he had found terms like apathetic, dull, stolid, restless, nervous, and deficient in intellect inadequate to encompass the changes in human cases with frontal lobe damage. He called for careful analyses of the mental condition following frontal lobe damage rather than the casual observations that dominated clinical reports. Evidently Franz placed little weight upon what Harlow had said because he referred to Gage as showing only mental deterioration. Gage's imperfect pre and post history led Wood Jones and Porteus to put the Gage case aside explicitly and completely in their related judgement of 1928. Fifty years later Fuster also stressed that it was of limited value, however colorful and disturbing it might be. The "irregularities of the injury, probable damage outside the frontal cortex, and subsequent foci of irritation" curtailed what could be learned from it. Fuster did not mention that it was equally limited on the psychological and behavioral sides.[5]

Harlow: Discourse, Monologue, or Fact?

We know that Harlow is the source of almost all of the little we know about Phineas Gage's behavior before and after his accident. How much faith can we place in what he tells us? Is what he says true? We know the language Harlow used to describe Phineas's temperament, the disturbance of the balance between his intellectual faculties, and the quantitative alteration in his mental operations reflected his phrenological views. They may also have affected his judgement of the lack of damage to the right hemisphere. His phrenological and other preconceptions may also have affected what he passed on from Phineas's family, especially from his mother. Read carefully, one sees that Harlow's combination of direct quotation and paraphrases about Gage's working in the weeks prior to his death tell us only part of what he learned from Phineas's mother. What was omitted there may not be important but it could be different from what he passes on to us. There could be other gaps. We know that Harlow held back on reporting the mental manifestations in 1848, but we do not know why. Perhaps his medical ethics made him unwilling to describe the still-living Phineas so negatively. Or was it tactfulness or some other kind of self-imposed censorship? All we do know is that Harlow did not tell his medical audience in 1848 all he knew about Gage.

There may also have been gaps in what Phineas's mother passed on to Harlow. Mothers are notoriously defensive about the behavior of their children and perhaps Mrs. Gage did not tell Harlow about the less desirable aspects of her son's behavior. Suppose he was violent and aggressive, or sexually promiscuous, or drank too much. Would she have told Harlow everything about these things? That she may have hidden facts like these is suggested by what we discern in the relation between the year given for Phineas's death as 1861 and the age of thirty six years, zero months and zero days recorded on his interment record. The year 1861 and an age at death of exactly thirty six years gives Phineas a birth date some ten months after the documented date of the marriage of Hannah Trusell Swetland and Jesse Eaton Gage on 27 April 1823. But Phineas's birth date is given in C. V. Gage's genealogy as 9 July 1823, about thirteen weeks after the marriage. If this otherwise undocumented birth date is correct, and Phineas's mother was the source of the information about his death, is it possible she was concealing the time that had elapsed between her son's conception and her marriage to Jesse? If she misled Harlow and others on this point, might not she have hidden other things about her son?

Nevertheless, with all their limitations, many of the things we know about Phineas Gage are facts existing independently of any particular individual observer or speaker. True, we have no records of his childhood or schooling and we know nothing of his employment before becoming a foreman with the contractors of that part of the Rutland and Burlington Rail Road being built at Cavendish. Nor do we know precisely what caused the explosion, and we know little of the detail of the damage done to his brain by the tamping iron. We know almost nothing about where he traveled and very little about how he was employed before his death. On the other hand, we know the identity of his mother and a number of other members of his family and within a few months and miles we can be certain when and where he was born. We know the place, date and general circumstances of the accident that befell him. We also have the instrument that caused his injury, his skull and the permanent record of the bony damage done it. We know exactly where and when he died, and we have a record of the cause of his death. Rather than constructions or discursive domains created by the words of those who have spoken and written about Phineas, we do have some quite definite facts about him.

Factual status can also be accorded many of the inferences we can draw from what we know existed independently of any particular observer. For example, Gage was the foreman of a gang working on a cutting outside Cavendish. From what we know of the work of such foremen, a good deal of what we can infer about Gage's cognitive, planning, and social skills can be treated as fact. Had he been sub-contractor we would be able to make more inferences. Other inferences have less certain status as facts. Gage is said to have driven a stagecoach. If he had, we could make certain inferences about his foresight, judgement and

perceptual-motor skills from what we know of the duties and responsibilities of stagecoach drivers.

Facts established in this way may be important but they are only a little
more revealing than knowing that one cannot live except by work or
that Napoleon died on 5 May 1821. What we need to know is the status
of what Harlow tells us about Gage's behavior before and after the
accident. Is it also factual? The opinion of his family, conveyed by the
American Medical Association's *Report of the Standing Committee on
Surgery* in April 1850 is consistent with what Harlow did say and might
be taken as based on independent observation of the same behaviors. But
it is too general to count much toward what we want to know: Gage's
mental powers were greatly impaired, the degenerative process was still
going on, and the deficiency of his mental faculties was more marked
than his loss of bodily powers. Although the short *American Phrenological Journal* comment of 1851 almost exactly matches Harlow's
description, its status may have to be discounted, not because it was
limited, but because Harlow probably supplied it. If he did not, and
the description was independent of him, the agreement may have been
because both descriptions were interpretations of the same facts from a
phrenological perspective.

More generally, because so much of what we know about Gage's
behavior comes from Harlow, is Harlow's only another discourse, possibly even a monologue? Should the fabrications I scrutinized, especially
those in chapters 5, 6, and 14, be regarded as equivalent to Harlow's
account? Are they merely different ways of talking about the same thing?
It is just because Harlow is the source of almost all that we do know that
we can answer no to all of these questions. Not one of them is based on
anything other than Harlow's few words. None of the constructors produces independent evidence that things were different from what Harlow
says. Not only are these constructions not equivalent; pretty evidently
they cannot be true. Thus, because Harlow is virtually the only source, we
can say that these constructions are not true representations of Gage.

My opening thesis was that when we speak or write about some thing,
that thing exists independently of our thinking, writing, and speaking
about it. We do not build or construct the thing itself, only an idea of it.
What did Harlow, Mrs. Gage and others construct? What they observed
directly about Phineas were the real changes brought about by the accident. But because all perception is selective to some degree, they almost
certainly attended to different aspects of his behavior. To take a small

example, Harlow seems to have been struck by defects in Phineas's ability to calculate, his family by the effects on his memory. Perhaps his family interpreted his inability to attend to or concentrate on tasks as the memory defect they told J. B. S. Jackson about. Interpretation, or the attribution of meaning to a perception according to one's preconceptions, may well have colored what they reported to Harlow. We can also be sure that preconceptions affected what others saw. For example, because of the combined effect of the sensory-motor framework and his antiphrenological stance, Bigelow denied that Gage had changed at all. That Harlow also interpreted what he saw in the light of his preconceptions is also certain, but we cannot be sure what effect they had on the picture he constructed of Phineas Gage. It does not seem to be as gross as with Bigelow. What Harlow tells us about Gage is confirmed very broadly by what has been observed in other cases of similar damage. What made its way into print about Phineas Gage constitutes more than a figurative corpus of facts for those who wrote about him later. It is also a corpus of facts that approximates the reality of how Phineas changed.

Phineas Gage 150 Years On

Vivid though Harlow's description of Gage is, it is far from providing the detail we need for a full analysis of Phineas's behavior before and after the accident. That lack, together with the slightness of our knowledge of the specific locale and extent of the damage to his brain, provides too meager a foundation on which to base hypotheses of the relation between the frontal lobes and their psychological functions. Is Phineas Gage now fit to be remembered only by such things as the plaque on Cavendish Town Green unveiled on 13 September 1998 to commemorate the 150th anniversary of his accident? What has to be remembered is that his was the first case to point to a relation between brain and personality functions. That is its lasting importance.

Appreciated properly, Harlow's story, that is, the story as he wrote it, enables us to see how little substance there is in the many exaggerations and misrepresentations of the changes in Phineas supposedly brought about by the tamping iron. Harlow's words and the representations of figure 16.1 give us a clear if limited picture. Until further facts are discovered, Harlow probably lets us see Phineas Gage as clearly as we ever will.

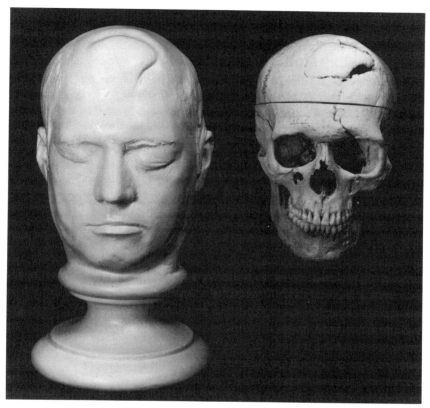

Figure 16.1
Phineas Gage's life mask (probably made for Henry Jacob Bigelow in late 1849) and skull (body probably exhumed in late 1867)
Reproduced by courtesy of the Warren Anatomical Museum, Harvard University.

Notes

1. T. Smith 1879 compares his patient's transitory symptoms with Ferrier's summary; the lobotomy comparison is in Goonetilleke 1979; and C. H. Hughes 1875 provides an example of the duality argument.

2. The Kirkes's story is in chapter 14 and The *Boston Medical and Surgical Journal*'s notice is "Bibliographical Notices" 1869. Ferrier, Starr, Dandy, and Elder and Miles are in chapter 10; Brickner is in chapter 11.

3. Teuber 1964; Campbell 1905.

4. K. M. was originally described in Hebb and Penfield 1940; his later status is described by Jasper 1995 and Milner 1995; and Milner's comment is in Ackerly 1964. A. R. Damasio 1994 provides an illustration of the way K. M. is cited in the contemporary literature.

5. Christison 1900; Tilney and Riley 1921; Mettler and Mettler 1945; Franz 1906; Wood Jones and Porteus 1928; Fuster 1980. After making his criticism, Franz described the method he had developed in 1901 to train monkeys and cats on specific tasks before observing the effects of selectively ablating different parts of the brain on those tasks. It was the method later used by Jacobsen and Fulton.

Appendix A

Facsimiles of the Gage Papers

Introduction

Because the source papers on Gage are so difficult to find and, partly as a consequence, so little read, I thought their reproduction in facsimile would be a useful addition to my text. They also provide a standard against which the reader can judge for him- or herself the accuracy of the many stories about Gage that I have mentioned or analyzed, including my own.

The papers included are

A1. (p. 383) John Martyn Harlow's original report of 1848 describing the accident and the stormy nature of Gage's recovery.

A2. (p. 388) Harlow's short letter of 3 January 1849 describing what he had found on visiting Gage in Lebanon two days earlier.

A3. (p. 390) Henry Jacob Bigelow's 1850 paper containing (a) the testimony of three of those who had seen Gage within minutes of the accident, (b) his own demonstration that the tamping iron could have passed through a skull in the way Harlow had described, and (c) his estimate of the damage to Gage's skull and brain.

A4. (p. 401) Harlow's follow-up report of 1868 in which (a) he described the changes in Gage's behavior to a medical audience for the first time, (b) he set out the only account of Gage's subsequent history, (c) he displayed the skull and described the injury, and (d) he gave an estimate of the brain damage.

A5. (p. 423) J. B. S. Jackson's entries about Gage from the *Warren Museum Catalogue* of 1870. Although Jackson does not seem to have made an independent study of Gage, he had a great deal of interest in his case, as his visit to Lebanon in August 1849 shows. That had been undertaken with the intention of examining Gage, but Phineas was in Montpelier. Jackson's Preface and the catalogue entries themselves show how he judged the case, and more important, contain details about Gage that neither Harlow nor Bigelow reports.

I am grateful to the following individuals and libraries for helping me find or obtain copies of these source documents: Ms. Hilde Heilemann of Lane Medical Library, Stanford University; Carole Hughes, Dana Medical Library, University of Vermont; Dr. Russell Johnson and the Young Special Collection Library of the

University of California at Los Angeles; Dr. Arthur P. Shimamura, Department of Psychology, and the library of the University of California at Berkeley; Mrs. Jacintha Silver of the Brownless Medical Library of the University of Melbourne; and Ms. Donna Webber, Countway Library, Harvard University. The copies actually used come from the Brownless Medical Library of the University of Melbourne and the Lane Medical Library of Stanford University.

THE

BOSTON MEDICAL AND SURGICAL JOURNAL.

Vol. XXXIX.   Wednesday, December 13, 1848.   No. 20.

PASSAGE OF AN IRON ROD THROUGH THE HEAD.

To the Editor of the Boston Medical and Surgical Journal.

Dear Sir,—Having been interested in the reading of the cases of " Injuries of the Head," reported in your Journal by Professor Shipman, of Cortlandville, N. Y., I am induced to offer you the notes of a very severe, singular, and, so far as the result is taken into account, hitherto unparalleled case, of that class of injuries, which has recently fallen under my own care. The accident happened in this town, upon the line of the Rutland and Burlington Rail Road, on the 13th of Sept. last, at 4½ o'clock, P. M. The subject of it is Phineas P. Gage, a foreman, engaged in building the road, 25 years of age, of middle stature, vigorous physical organization, temperate habits, and possessed of considerable energy of character.

It appears from his own account, and that of the by-standers, that he was engaged in charging a hole, preparatory to blasting. He had turned in the powder, and was in the act of tamping it slightly before pouring on the sand. He had struck the powder, and while about to strike it again, turned his head to look after his men (who were working within a few feet of him), when the tamping iron came in contact with the rock, and the powder exploded, driving the iron against the left side of the face, immediately anterior to the angle of the inferior maxillary bone. Taking a direction upward and backward toward the median line, it penetrated the integuments, the masseter and temporal muscles, passed under the zygomatic arch, and (probably) fracturing the temporal portion of the sphenoid bone, and the floor of the orbit of the left eye, entered the cranium, passing through the anterior left lobe of the cerebrum, and made its exit in the median line, at the junction of the coronal and sagittal sutures, lacerating the longitudinal sinus, fracturing the parietal and frontal bones extensively, breaking up considerable portions of brain, and protruding the globe of the left eye from its socket, by nearly one half its diameter. The tamping iron is round, and rendered comparatively smooth by use. It is pointed at the end which entered first, and is three feet, seven inches in length, one and one quarter inch in diameter, and weighs 13¼ pounds. I am informed that the patient was thrown upon his back, and gave a few convulsive motions of the extremities, but spoke in a few minutes. His men (with whom he was a great favorite) took him in their arms and carried him to the road, only a few rods distant, and sat him into an ox cart, in which he rode, sitting erect, full three quarters of a mile, to the hotel of Mr. Joseph Adams, in this village. He got out of the cart himself, and with a little assistance walked up a long flight of stairs, into the hall, where he was dressed.

Being absent, I did not arrive at the scene of the accident until near 6 o'clock, P. M. You will excuse me for remarking here, that the picture presented was, to one unaccustomed to military surgery, truly terrific ; but the patient bore his sufferings with the most heroic firmness. He recognized me at once, and said he hoped he was not much hurt. He seemed to be perfectly conscious, but was getting exhausted from the hemorrhage, which was very profuse both exterally and internally, the blood finding its way into the stomach, which rejected it as often as every 15 or 20 minutes. Pulse 60, and regular. His person, and the bed on which he was laid, were literally one gore of blood. Assisted by my friend, Dr. Williams, of Proctorsville, who was first called to the patient, we proceeded to dress the wounds. From their appearance, the fragments of bone being uplifted and the brain protruding, it was evident that the fracture was occasioned by some force acting from below upward. The scalp was shaven, the coagula removed, together with three small triangular pieces of the cranium, and in searching to ascertain if there were other foreign bodies there, I passed in the index finger its whole length, without the least resistance, in the direction of the wound in the cheek, which received the other finger in like manner. A portion of the anterior superior angle of each parietal bone, and a semi-circular piece of the frontal bone, were fractured, leaving a circular opening of about $3\frac{1}{2}$ inches in diameter. This examination, and the appearance of the iron which was found some rods distant, smeared with brain, together with the testimony of the workmen, and of the patient himself, who was still sufficiently conscious to say that " the iron struck his head and passed through," was considered at the time sufficiently conclusive to show not only the nature of the accident, but the manner in which it occurred.

I have been asked why I did not pass a probe through the entire extent of the wound at the time. I think no surgeon of discretion would have upheld me in the trial of such a foolhardy experiment, in the risk of disturbing lacerated vessels, from which the hemorrhage was near being staunched, and thereby rupturing the attenuated thread, by which the sufferer still held to life. You will excuse me for being thus particular, inasmuch as I am aware that the nature of the injury has been seriously questioned by many medical men for whom I entertain a very high respect.

The spiculæ of bone having been taken away, a portion of the brain, which hung by a pedicle, was removed, the larger pieces of bone replaced, the lacerated scalp was brought together as nearly as possible, and retained by adhesive straps, excepting at the posterior angle, and over this a simple dressing—compress, night-cap and roller. The wound in the face was left patulous, covered only by a simple dressing. The hands and fore arms were both deeply burned nearly to the elbows, which were dressed, and the patient was left with the head elevated, and the attendants requested to keep him in that position.

10, P. M., same evening.—The dressings are saturated with blood, but the hemorrhage appears to be abating. Has vomited twice only since being dressed. Sensorial powers remain as yet unimpaired. Says he does not wish to see his friends, as he shall be at work in a day or two. Tells where they live, their names, &c. Pulse 65; constant agitation of the lower extremities.

14th, 7, A. M.—Has slept some; appears to be in pain; speaks with difficulty; tumefaction of face considerable, and increasing; pulse 70; knows his friends, and is rational. Asks who is foreman in his pit. Hemorrhage internally continues slightly. Has not vomited since 12, M.

15th, 9, A. M.—Has slept well half the night. Sees objects indistinctly with the left eye, when the lids are separated. Hemorrhage has ceased. Pulse 75.

8, P. M., same day.—Restless and delirious; talks much, but disconnected and incoherent. Pulse 84, and full. Prescribed vin. colchicum, ℥ss. every six hours, until it purges him. Removed the night-cap.

16th, 8, A. M.—Patient appears more quiet. Pulse 70. Dressed the wounds, which in the head have a fœtid sero-purulent discharge, with particles of brain intermingled. No discharge from bowels. Ordered sulph. magnesia, ℥j., repeated every four hours until it operates. Iced water to the head and eye. A fungus appears at the external canthus of the left eye. Says "the left side of his head is banked up."

17th, 8, A. M.—Pulse 84. Purged freely. Rational, and knows his friends. Discharge from the brain profuse, very fœtid and sanious. Wound in face healing.

18th, 9, A. M.—Slept well all night, and lies upon his right side. Pulse 72; tongue red and dry; breath fœtid. Removed the dressings, and passed a probe to the base of the cranium, without giving pain. Ordered a cathartic, which operated freely. Cold to the head. Patient says he shall recover. He is delirious, with lucid intervals.

19th, 8, P. M.—Has been very restless during the day; skin hot and dry; tongue red; excessive thirst; delirious, talking incoherently with himself, and directing his men.

20th and 21st.—Has remained much the same.

22d, 8, A. M.—Patient has had a very restless night. Throws his hands and feet about, and tries to get out of bed. Head hot. Says "he shall not live long so." Ordered a cathartic of calomel and rhubarb, to be followed by castor oil, if it does not operate in six hours.

4, P. M., same day.—Purged freely twice, and inclines to sleep.

23d.—Rested well most of the night, and appears stronger and more rational. Pulse 80. Shaved the scalp a second time, and brought the edges of the wound in position, the previous edges having sloughed away. Discharge less in quantity and less fœtid. Loss of vision of left eye.

392   *Passage of an Iron Rod through the Head.*

From this time until the 3d of October, he lay in a semi-comatose state, seldom speaking unless spoken to, and then answering only in monosyllables. During this period, fungi started from the brain, and increased rapidly from the orbit. To these was applied nitrate of silver cryst., and cold to the head generally. The dressings were renewed three times in every twenty-four hours ; and in addition to this, laxatives, combined with an occasional dose of calomel, constituted the treatment. The pulse varied from 70 to 96—generally very soft. During this time an abscess formed under the frontalis muscle, which was opened on the 27th, and has been very difficult to heal. Discharged nearly ℥ viij. at the time it was punctured.

Oct. 5th and 6th.—Patient improving. Discharge from the wound and sinus, laudable pus. Calls for his pants and wishes to get out of bed, though he is unable to raise his head from the pillow.

7th.—Has succeeded in raising himself up, and took one step to his chair, and sat about five minutes.

11th.—Pulse 72. Intellectual faculties brightening. When I asked him how long since he was injured, he replied, " four weeks this afternoon, at 4½ o'clock." Relates the manner in which it occurred, and how he came to the house. He keeps the day of the week and time of day, in his mind. Says he knows more than half of those who inquire after him. Does not estimate size or money accurately, though he has memory as perfect as ever. He would not take $1000 for a few pebbles which he took from an ancient river bed where he was at work. The fungus is giving way under the use of the crys. nitrate of silver. During all of this time there has been a discharge of pus into the fauces, a part of which passed into the stomach, the remainder being ejected from the mouth.

20th.—Improving. Gets out and into bed with but little assistance. Sits up thirty minutes twice in twenty-four hours. Is very childish ; wishes to go home to Lebanon, N. H. The wound in the scalp is healing rapidly.

Nov. 8th.—Improving in every particular, and sits up most of the time during the day. Appetite good, though he is still kept upon a low diet. Pulse 65. Sleeps well, and says he has no pain in the head. Food digests easily, bowels regular, and nutrition is going on well. The sinus under the frontalis muscle has nearly healed. He walks up and down stairs, and about the house, into the piazza, and I am informed this evening that he has been in the street to-day.—I leave him for a week, with strict injunctions to avoid excitement and exposure.

15th.—I learn, on inquiry, that Gage has been in the street every day except Sunday, during my absence. His desire to be out and to go home to Lebanon has been uncontrollable by his friends, and he has been making arrangements to that effect. Yesterday he walked half a mile, and purchased some small articles at the store. The atmosphere was cold and damp, the ground wet, and he went without an overcoat, and with thin boots. He got wet feet and a chill. I find him in bed, depressed and very irritable. Hot and dry skin ; thirst ; tongue coated ; pulse

110 ; lancinating pain in left side of head and face ; rigors, and bowels constipated. Ordered cold to the head and face, and a black dose to be repeated in six hours, if it does not operate. He has had spiculæ of bone pass into the fauces, which he expelled from the mouth within a few days.

16th, A. M.—No better. Cathartic has operated freely. Pulse 120 ; skin hot and dry ; thirst and pain remain the same. Has been very restless during the night. Venesection f ℥ xvj. Ordered calomel, grs. x., and ipecac. grs. ij., followed in four hours by castor oil.

8, P. M., same day.—Purged freely ; pulse less frequent ; pain in head moderated ; skin moist. R. Antim. et potassa tart., grs. iij. ; syr. simplex, f ℥ vj. Dose a dessert spoonful every four hours.

17th.—Improving. Expresses himself as " feeling better in every respect ;" has no pain in the head.

18th.—Is walking about house again ; says he feels no pain in the head, and appears to be in a way of recovering if he can be controlled.

At this date I shall leave the case at present. The result, and a few remarks of a practical nature, together with the mental manifestations of the patient, I reserve for a future communication. I think the case presents one fact of great interest to the practical surgeon, and, taken as a whole, is exceedingly interesting to the enlightened physiologist and intellectual philosopher. In my effort to be brief, which I fear you will think an utter failure, I have omitted much in my notes that might interest some readers. Allow me to say here, that I have seen a communication in " The Reflector and Watchman," stating that " there is a piece of bone loose in the top of his head, as large as a dollar, which will have to be removed, should he live." The fractured portions of bone, excepting those which were removed at the first dressing, have united firmly, and the above remark was made unadvisedly. Should you think these notes of sufficient importance to deserve a place in your Journal, they are at your service. Yours, very respectfully,

Cavendish, Vt., Nov. 27, 1848. J. M. HARLOW.

FITCH'S BOOK ON CONSUMPTION.

[Communicated for the Boston Medical and Surgical Journal.—Concluded from p. 323.]

IN the introductory article in his book, the author arrogates to himself the discovery of the " grand uses of the lungs," as before alluded to. He there also asserts that, by this discovery, he was able to lay the foundation of a " certain method of elucidating and treating their diseases." I propose now to inquire into this discovery, in order that we may fully understand what it is, that due appreciation in return may be rendered. At page 28, we have the following account of what led to the discovery—as well as the discovery itself. He there states, that while pursuing some investigations upon " Nervous Influence," he made the discovery of the " grand uses of the lungs ;" to use his own words,

506   *Medical Intelligence.*

who consider education of the first importance in a medical practitioner.
At Cleveland there was a regularly chartered school, well organized, which
was transferred to Columbus—but whether any fragment of it remains in
Cleveland, cannot be ascertained at the moment of writing. Not far from
Cleveland there is still another ; and lastly, at the seat of government, the
Starling College has been so richly endowed by the man whose name it
bears, that should it fail to meet the expectations of the community, the
fault must be charged in after years to the course of instruction. In this
school, the youngest in the series, Frederick Merrick, M.D., is the professor of Botany and Chemistry. On him it devolved to open the present
session, in behalf of the faculty. That he accomplished the undertaking
satisfactorily, is abundantly evident by the complimentary attention of the
class in requesting the manuscript for publication. A prominent item of
instruction in this off-hand, pleasant lecture, is this : Be careful in medicine to discriminate between what is true and what is false. Aye, there's
the rub. When Dr. Merrick can clearly demonstrate an unerring method
of ascertaining a point so desirable, he will have discovered the philosopher's stone. To the end of time, the schools will disagree in doctrine, and
theorists, like locusts, will forever abound, to the disturbance of students,
and to the injury of inductive medicine. Dr. Merrick has a disciplined
mind, large benevolence, an ardent love for truth, which he would have
always take the homely name of facts, and by their indications he would
be influenced.

The Scalpel.—A new Journal of health, designed, according to the title,
for popular as well as professional reading, edited by Edward H. Dixon,
M.D., of New York. has been commenced, and without having specific
days of publication, is to be issued at such times as may appear expedient.
No annual subscribers are solicited, as the editor expresses his intention of
discontinuing the Scalpel whenever he may judge proper. It is beautifully printed, and certainly has a large amount of purely original matter.
Dr. Dixon has been a frequent contributor to our Journal in years past,
and few have exhibited more ingenuity, as many of our readers are aware,
in the practice of surgery. A variety of apparatus for relieving the sufferings of surgical patients, have been devised by Dr. Dixon, and are favorably known to the profession ; and he has been equally happy in operations, and in the practice of a branch for which he evidently has a decided
predilection. He is a vigorous, fearless, independent writer, capable of
expressing himself clearly on all subjects, and we wish him good success
in his new enterprise.

Washington Co. (N. Y.) Medical Society.—The anniversary meeting
of the Washington County Medical Society was held on the last Tuesday
of June, 1848. The following are its officers. Dr. Henry C. Gray, *President ;* Dr. Simeon F. Crandall, *Vice President ;* Dr. Wm. A. Collins,
Recording Secretary ; Dr. P. V. S. Morris, *Corresponding Secretary ;*
Dr. James Savage, *Treasurer ;* Drs. S. F. Crandall, Cornelius Holmes,
Hiram Corliss, *Censors.* Dr. H. C. Gray, Delegate to the American Medical Association. Dr. Hiram Corliss, Delegate to the State Med. Society.

Medical Miscellany.—Twenty cases of scarlet fever existed among the
children of the Female Orphan Asylum, in this city, on Sunday last.—

Medical Miscellany.

507

Drs. Hitchcock & French, of Ashby, Mass., have recently removed a fibrous tumor of the uterus in a patient 38 years of age. The operation was performed by ligature through means of Gooch's canula. From extreme anemia and emaciation, caused by years of hemorrhage and pain, she has rapidly regained flesh, strength and life.—At the last meeting of the Paris Institute, M. Bernard and M. Bareswell presented a sample of alcohol which they had obtained from the fermentation of sugar extracted from the human liver.—In Montreal, on the 28th of December, an inquest was held on the body of Sarah Griffith, 18 years old, who died suddenly. A *post-mortem* examination of the body was had, from which it appeared that she died thus suddenly in consequence of tight lacing, which affected the heart and other internal organs.—A Singapore paper relates a marvellous tale, to the effect that, after a violent earthquake at Chantibun, the roads, the fields, and the markets, were strewed with hairs, which exactly resembled human hair, and which, when burned, emitted the usual smell of burning hair.—A dentist of Durham has lately used gutta percha for the manufacture of sets of gums for artificial teeth.—Mr. J. Murray, the eminent chemist, in a letter, recommends the introduction of electricity into hospitals and infirmaries as a therapeutic agent.—Mr. Webb, of Balsam, Eng., has operated successfully on several animals affected with lockjaw. —A cholera quarantine is in force at Kingston, Jamaica.—In Northampton, Mass., there were 80 deaths in 1848, of which 9 were between 80 and 90. The marriages were only 30.—In the Canadian Insane Asylum, two lunatics were put in the same apartment, and the result was, one of them was horribly mutilated.—In Boston, $12.599 35, was paid for hospital money during 1848. It came out of sailors. who pay 20 cents each, a month, for the support of marine hospitals.—A note, dated Jan. 3d. from Dr. Harlow, of Cavendish, Vt., the medical attendant of Mr. Gage, who had an iron rod shot through his head, as lately reported in the Journal, says the patient is now at Lebanon, N. H., " walking about the house, and riding out, improving both mentally and physically."—A woman in Illinois has had 18 children in 10 years.—A bill for the establishment of an asylum for the insane is before the Legislature of North Carolina.—The latest accounts from New Orleans show that the cholera has much abated in that city. Cases have occurred at numerous places up the Mississippi river, at Cincinnati, and at Mobile. At New York it has censed to exist. In London, the fatal cases for the week ending Dec. 20th, were 31, against 29 for the previous week. The total number of cases in England from the first appearance of the malady was, to Dec. 20th, 3737, whereof 1772 had proved fatal, 505 had recovered, and 1400 were under treatment, or the result not recorded. The cases in Scotland have been no fewer than 2922, whereof 1356 have perished.

MARRIED,—In Providence, R. I., Dr. W. H. Smith to Miss R. M. Stillman.

DIED,—In England, Dr. Samuel Cooper, the celebrated surgeon.

Report of Deaths in Boston—for the week ending Jan. 13th, 62.—Males, 28—females. 34.— Of consumption. 18—scarlet fever, 9—lung fever. 3—dropsy, 1—dropsy on the brain, 3—disease of the heart, 5—disease of the hip, 1—pleurisy, 1—diabetes, 1—infantile, 4—inflammation of the lungs, 2—canker, 1—accidental, 2—scrofula, 1—rheumatism, 1—croup, 2—measles, 1— child-bed, 2—apoplexy, 1—old age, 1—smallpox, 1—paralysis, 1.
Under 5 years, 22—between 5 and 20 years 6—between 20 and 40 years, 20—between 40 and 60 years, 8—over 60 years. 6.

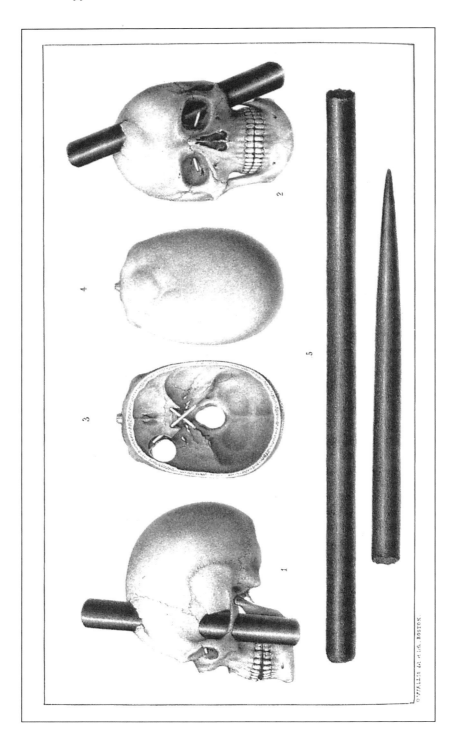

THE

AMERICAN JOURNAL

OF THE MEDICAL SCIENCES

FOR JULY 1850.

ART. I.—*Dr. Harlow's Case of Recovery from the passage of an Iron Bar through the Head.* By HENRY J. BIGELOW, M. D., Professor of Surgery in Harvard University. (With a plate.)

THE following case, perhaps unparalleled in the annals of surgery, and of which some interesting details have already been published, occurred in the practice of Dr. J. M. Harlow, of Cavendish, Vermont. Having received a verbal account of the accident, a few days after its occurrence, from a medical gentleman who had examined the patient, I thus became incidentally interested in it; and having since had an opportunity, through the politeness of Dr. Harlow, of observing the patient, who remained in Boston a number of weeks under my charge, I have been able to satisfy myself as well of the occurrence and extent of the injury as of the manner of its infliction. I am also indebted to the same gentleman for procuring at my request the testimony of a number of persons who were cognizant of the accident or its sequel.

Those who are skeptical in admitting the co-existence of a lesion so grave, with an inconsiderable disturbance of function, will be interested in further details connected with the case ; while it is due to science that a more complete record should be made of the history of so remarkable an injury.

The accident occurred upon the line of the Rutland and Burlington Railroad, on the 13th of September, 1848. The subject of it, Phineas P. Gage, is of middle stature, twenty-five years of age, shrewd and intelligent. According to his own statement, he was charging with powder a hole drilled in a rock, for the purpose of blasting. It appears that it is customary in filling the hole to cover the powder with sand. In this case, the charge having been adjusted, Mr. Gage directed his assistant to pour in the sand; and at the interval of a few seconds, his head being averted, and supposing the sand to have been properly placed, he dropped the head of the iron as usual upon the charge, to consolidate or "*tamp it in.*" The assistant had failed to obey the order, and the iron striking fire upon the rock, the uncovered powder was ignited and the explosion took place. Mr. Gage was at this time standing above the hole, leaning forward, with his face slightly averted ; and the bar of iron was projected directly upwards in a line of its axis, passing completely through his head and high into the air. The wound thus received, and which is more fully described in the sequel, was oblique, traversing the cranium in a straight line from the angle of the lower jaw on one side to the centre of the frontal bone above, near the sagittal suture, where the missile emerged ; and the iron thus forcibly thrown into the air was picked up at a distance of some rods from the patient, smeared with brains and blood.

From this extraordinary lesion, the patient has quite recovered in his faculties of body and mind, with the loss only of the sight of the injured eye.

The iron which thus traversed the skull weighs thirteen and a quarter pounds. It is three feet seven inches in length, and one and a quarter inches in diameter. The end which entered first is pointed ; the taper being seven inches long, and the diameter of the point one quarter of an inch ; circumstances to which the patient perhaps owes his life. The iron is unlike any other, and was made by a neighbouring blacksmith to please the fancy of the owner.

Dr. Harlow, in the graphic account above alluded to, states that "immediately after the explosion the patient was thrown upon his back, and gave a few convulsive motions of the extremities, but spoke in a few minutes. His men (with whom he was a great favourite) took him in their arms and carried him to the road, only a few rods distant, and sat him into an ox cart, in which he rode, sitting erect, full three quarters of a mile, to the hotel of Mr. Joseph Adams, in this village. He got out of the cart himself, and with a little assistance walked up a long flight of stairs, into the hall, where he was dressed."

Mr. Joseph Adams, here spoken of, has furnished the following interesting statement :—

This is to certify that P. P. Gage had boarded in my house for several weeks previous to his being injured upon the railroad, and that I saw him and conversed with him soon after the accident, and am of opinion that he was perfectly conscious of what was passing around him. He rode to the house, three-quarters of a mile, sitting in a cart, and walked from the cart into the piazza, and thence up stairs, with but little assistance. I noticed the state of the left eye, and know, from experiment, that he could see with it for several days, though not distinctly. In regard to the elevated appearance of the wound, and the introduction of the finger into it, I can fully confirm the certificate of my nephew, Washington Adams, and others, and would add that I repeatedly saw him eject matter from the mouth similar in appearance to that discharged from the head. The morning subsequent to the accident I went in quest of the bar, and found it at a smith's shop, near the pit in which he was engaged.

The men in his pit asserted that "they found the iron, covered with blood and brains," several rods behind where Mr. Gage stood, and that they washed it in the brook, and returned it with the other tools; which representation was fully corroborated by the greasy feel and look of the iron, and the *fragments* of *brain* which I SAW upon the rock where it fell.

(Signed)   JOSEPH ADAMS,

CAVENDISH, *Dec.* 14, 1849.   *Justice of the Peace.*

The Rev. Joseph Freeman, whose letter follows, informed himself of the circumstances soon after the accident.

CAVENDISH, *Dec.* 5, 1849.

DEAR SIR—I was at home on the day Mr. Gage was hurt; and seeing an Irishman ride rapidly up to your door, I stepped over to ascertain the cause, and then went immediately to meet those who I was informed were bringing him to our village.

I found him in a cart, sitting up without aid, with his back against the fore-board. When we reached his quarters, he rose to his feet without aid, and walked quick, though with an unsteady step, to the hind end of the cart, when two of his men came forward and aided him out, and walked with him, supporting him to the house.

I then asked his men how he came to be hurt? The reply was, "The blast went off when he was tamping it, and the tamping-iron passed through his head." I said, "That is impossible."

Soon after this, I went to the place where the accident happened. I found upon the rocks, where I supposed he had fallen, a small quantity of brains. There being no person at this place, I passed on to a blacksmith's shop a few rods beyond, in and about which a number of Irishmen were collected. As I came up to them, they pointed me to the iron, which has since attracted so much attention, standing outside the shop-door. They said they found it covered with brains and dirt, and had washed it in the brook. The *appearance* of the iron corresponded with this story. It had a greasy appearance, and was so to the touch.

After hearing their statement, as there was no assignable motive for misrepresentation, and finding the appearance of the iron to agree with it, I was compelled to believe, though the result of your examination of the wound was not then known to me.

I think of nothing further relating to this affair which cannot be more minutely stated by others.

Very respectfully, yours,
(Signed)   JOSEPH FREEMAN.

Dr. J. M. HARLOW.

Dr. WILLIAMS first saw the patient, and makes the following statement in relation to the circumstances :—

NORTHFIELD, *Vermont, Dec.* 4, 1849.

Dr. BIGELOW: Dear Sir—Dr. Harlow having requested me to transmit to you a description of the appearance of Mr. Gage at the time I first saw him after the accident, which happened to him in September, 1848, I now hasten to do so with pleasure.

Dr. Harlow being absent at the time of the accident, I was sent for, and was the first physician who saw Mr. G., some twenty-five or thirty minutes after he received the injury; he at that time was sitting in a chair upon the piazza of Mr. Adams's hotel, in Cavendish. When I drove up, he said, "Doctor, here is business enough for you." I first noticed the wound upon the head before I alighted from my carriage, the pulsations of the brain being very distinct; there was also an appearance which, before I examined the head, I could not account for: the top of the head appeared somewhat like an inverted funnel; this was owing, I discovered, to the bone being fractured about the opening for a distance of about two inches in every direction. I ought to have mentioned above that the opening through the skull and integuments was not far from one and a half inch in diameter; the edges of this opening were everted, and the whole wound appeared as if some wedge-shaped body had passed from below upward. Mr. Gage, during the time I was examining this wound, was relating the manner in which he was injured to the bystanders; he talked so rationally and was so willing to answer questions, that I directed my inquiries to him in preference to the men who were with him at the time of the accident, and who were standing about at this time. Mr. G. then related to me some of the circumstances, as he has since done; and I can safely say that neither at that time nor on any subsequent occasion, save once, did I consider him to be other than perfectly rational. The one time to which I allude was about a fortnight after the accident, and then he persisted in calling me John Kirwin; yet he answered all my questions correctly.

I did not believe Mr. Gage's statement at that time, but thought he was deceived; I asked him where the bar entered, and he pointed to the wound on his cheek, which I had not before discovered; this was a slit running from the angle of the jaw forward about one and a half inch; it was very much stretched laterally, and was discoloured by powder and iron rust, or at least appeared so. Mr. Gage persisted in saying that the bar went through his head: an Irishman standing by said, "Sure it was so, sir, for the bar is lying in the road below, all blood and brains." The man also said he would have brought it up with him, but he thought there would be an inquest, and it would not do.

About this time, Mr. G. got up and vomited a large quantity of blood, together with some of his food; the effort of vomiting pressed out about half a teacupful of the brain, which fell upon the floor, together with the blood, which was forced out at the same time. The left eye appeared more dull and glassy than the right. Mr. G. said he could merely distinguish light with it.

Soon after Dr. Harlow arrived, Mr. Gage walked up stairs, with little or no assistance, and laid down upon a bed, when Dr. H. made a thorough examination of the wounds, passing the whole length of his forefinger into the superior opening without difficulty; and my impression is that he did the same with the inferior one, but of that I am not absolutely certain: after this we proceeded to dress the wounds in the manner described by Dr. H. in the Journal. During the time occupied in dressing, Mr. G. vomited two or three times fully as freely as before. All of this time Mr. G. was perfectly conscious, answering all questions, and calling his friends by name as they came into the room.

I did not see the bar that night, but saw it the next day after it was washed. Hoping you will excuse this hasty sketch, I remain yours, &c.

Dr. Harlow's account of his first visit to the patient, and of the subsequent symptoms, is here appended.

"Being absent, I did not arrive at the scene of the accident until near 6 o'clock, P. M. You will excuse me for remarking here that the picture presented was, to one unaccustomed to military surgery, truly terrific; but the patient bore his sufferings with the most heroic firmness. He recognized me at once, and said he hoped he was not much hurt. He seemed to be perfectly conscious, but was getting exhausted from the hemorrhage, which was very profuse both externally and internally, the blood finding its way into the stomach, which rejected it as often as every fifteen or twenty minutes. Pulse 60, and regular. His person and the bed on which he was laid were literally one gore of blood. Assisted by my friend, Dr. Williams, of Proctors-ville, who was first called to the patient, we proceeded to dress the wounds. From their appearance, the fragments of bone being uplifted and the brain protruding, it was evident that the fracture was occasioned by some force acting from below upward. The scalp was shaven, the coagula removed, together with three small triangular pieces of the cranium, and in searching to ascertain if there were other foreign bodies there, I passed in the index finger its whole length, without the least resistance, in the direction of the wound in the cheek, which received the other finger in like manner. A portion of the anterior superior angle of each parietal bone, and a semicircular piece of the frontal bone, were fractured, leaving a circular opening of about three and a half inches in diameter. This examination, and the appearance of the iron which was found some rods distant, smeared with brain, together with the testimony of the workmen, and of the patient himself, who was still suffi-ciently conscious to say that 'the iron struck his head and passed through,' was considered at the time sufficiently conclusive to show not only the nature of the accident, but the manner in which it occurred.

"I have been asked why I did not pass a probe through the entire extent of the wound at the time. I think no surgeon of discretion would have up-held me in the trial of such a foolhardy experiment, in the risk of disturbing lacerated vessels, from which the hemorrhage was near being staunched, and thereby rupturing the attenuated thread, by which the sufferer still held to life. You will excuse me for being thus particular, inasmuch as I am aware that the nature of the injury has been seriously questioned by many medical men for whom I entertain a very high respect.

"The spiculæ of bone having been taken away, a portion of the brain, which hung by a pedicle, was removed, the larger pieces of bone replaced, the lacerated scalp was brought together as nearly as possible, and retained by adhesive straps, excepting at the posterior angle, and over this a simple dressing—compress, nightcap and roller. The wound in the face was left patulous, covered only by a simple dressing. The hands and forearms were both deeply burned nearly to the elbows, which were dressed, and the patient was left with the head elevated, and the attendants requested to keep him in that position.

"10 P. M., same evening. The dressings are saturated with blood, but the hemorrhage appears to be abating. Has vomited twice only since being dressed. Sensorial powers remain as yet unimpaired. Says he does not wish to see his friends, as he shall be at work in a day or two. Tells where they live, their names, &c. Pulse 65; constant agitation of the lower extremities.

"14*th*, 7 A. M. Has slept some; appears to be in pain; speaks with dif-ficulty; tumefaction of face considerable, and increasing; pulse 70; knows his friends, and is rational. Asks who is foreman in his pit. Hemorrhage

"15*th*, 9 A. M. Has slept well half the night. Sees objects indistinctly with the left eye, when the lids are separated. Hemorrhage has ceased. Pulse 75. 8 P. M., Restless and delirious; talks much, but disconnected and incoherent. Pulse 84, and full. Prescribed vin. colchicum, f℥ss every six hours, until it purges him. Removed the night-cap.

"16*th*, 8 A. M. Patient appears more quiet. Pulse 70. Dressed the wounds, which in the head have a fetid sero-purulent discharge, with particles of brain intermingled. No discharge from bowels. Ordered sulph. magnesia, ℥ j, repeated every four hours until it operates. Iced water to the head and eye. A fungus appears at the external canthus of the left eye. Says 'the left side of his head is banked up.'

"17*th*, 8 A. M. Pulse 84. Purged freely. Rational, and knows his friends. Discharge from the brain profuse, very fetid and sanious. Wounds in face healing.

"18*th*, 9 A. M. Slept well all night, and lies upon his right side. Pulse 72; tongue red and dry; breath fetid. Removed the dressings, and passed a probe to the base of the cranium, without giving pain. Ordered a cathartic, which operated freely. Cold to the head. Patient says he shall recover. He is delirious, with lucid intervals.

"19*th*, 8 P. M. Has been very restless during the day; skin hot and dry; tongue red; excessive thirst; delirious, talking incoherently with himself, and directing his men.

"20*th* and 21*st*. Has remained much the same.

"22*d*, 8 A. M. Patient has had a very restless night. Throws his hands and feet about, and tries to get out of bed. Head hot. Says 'he shall not live long so.' Ordered a cathartic of calomel and rhubarb, to be followed by castor oil, if it does not operate in six hours. 4 P. M. Purged freely twice, and inclines to sleep.

"23*d*. Rested well most of the night, and appears stronger and more rational. Pulse 80. Shaved the scalp a second time, and brought the edges of the wound in position, the previous edges having sloughed away. Discharge less in quantity and less fetid. Loss of vision of left eye.

"From this time until the 3d of October, he lay in a semi-comatose state, seldom speaking unless spoken to, and then answering only in monosyllables. During this period, fungi started from the brain, and increased rapidly from the orbit. To these was applied nitrate of silver cryst., and cold to the head generally. The dressings were renewed three times in every twenty-four hours; and in addition to this, laxatives, combined with an occasional dose of calomel, constituted the treatment. The pulse varied from 70 to 96—generally very soft. During this time an abscess formed under the frontalis muscle, which was opened on the 27th, and has been very difficult to heal. Discharged nearly ℥viij at the time it was punctured.

"*Oct.* 5*th* and 6*th*. Patient improving. Discharge from the wound and sinus, laudable pus. Calls for his pants, and wishes to get out of bed, though he is unable to raise his head from the pillow.

"7*th*. Has succeeded in raising himself up, and took one step to his chair, and sat about five minutes.

"11*th*. Pulse 72. Intellectual faculties brightening. When I asked him how long since he was injured, he replied, 'four weeks this afternoon, at half past four o'clock.' Relates the manner in which it occurred, and how he came to the house. He keeps the day of the week and time of day in his mind. Says he knows more than half of those who inquire after him. Does not estimate size or money accurately, though he has memory as perfect as ever. He would not take one thousand dollars for a few pebbles which he took from an ancient river bed where he was at work. The fungus is giving way under the use of the cryst. nitrate of silver. During all of this time there has been a discharge of pus into the fauces, a part of which passed into the stomach, the remainder being ejected from the mouth.

"*20th.* Improving. Gets out and into bed with but little assistance. Sits up thirty minutes twice in twenty-four hours. Is very childish ; wishes to go home to Lebanon, N. H. The wound in the scalp is healing rapidly.

"*Nov. 8th.* Improving in every particular, and sits up most of the time during the day. Appetite good, though he is still kept upon a low diet. Pulse 65. Sleeps well, and says he has no pain in the head. Food digests easily, bowels regular, and nutrition is going on well. The sinus under the frontalis muscle has nearly healed. He walks up and down stairs, and about the house, into the piazza, and I am informed this evening that he has been in the street to-day.—I leave him for a week, with strict injunctions to avoid excitement and exposure.

"*15th.* I learn, on inquiry, that Gage has been in the street every day except Sunday, during my absence. His desire to be out and to go home to Lebanon has been uncontrollable by his friends, and he has been making arrangements to that effect. Yesterday he walked half a mile, and purchased some small articles at the store. The atmosphere was cold and damp, the ground wet, and he went without an overcoat, and with thin boots. He got wet feet and a chill. I find him in bed, depressed and very irritable. Hot and dry skin ; thirst, tongue coated ; pulse 110 : lancinating pain in left side of head and face ; rigors, and bowels constipated. Ordered cold to the head and face, and a black dose to be repeated in six hours, if it does not operate. He has had spiculæ of bone pass into the fauces, which he expelled from the mouth within a few days.

"*16th,* A. M. No better. Cathartic has operated freely. Pulse 120 ; skin hot and dry ; thirst and pain remain the same. Has been very restless during the night. Venesection f$\overline{3}$xvj. Ordered calomel, gr. x, and ipecac. gr. ij, followed in four hours by castor oil.

"8 P. M., same day. Purged freely ; pulse less frequent ; pain in head moderated ; skin moist. R. Antim. et potassa tart., gr. iij ; syr. simplex, f$\overline{3}$vj. Dose a dessertspoonful every four hours.

"*17th.* Improving. Expresses himself as 'feeling better in every respect;' has no pain in the head.

"*18th.* Is walking about the house again ; says he feels no pain in the head, and appears to be in a way of recovering if he can be controlled."

Remarks.—The leading feature of this case is its improbability. A physician who holds in his hand a crowbar, three feet and a half long, and more than thirteen pounds in weight, will not readily believe that it has been driven with a crash through the brain of a man who is still able to walk off, talking with composure and equanimity of the hole in his head. This is the sort of accident that happens in the pantomime at the theatre, but not elsewhere. Yet there is every reason for supposing it in this case literally true. Being at first wholly skeptical, I have been personally convinced ; and this has been the experience of many medical gentlemen who, having first heard of the circumstances, have had a subsequent opportunity to examine the evidence.

This evidence is comprised in the testimony of individuals, and in the anatomical and physiological character of the lesion itself.

The above accounts from different individuals, concur in assigning to the accident a common cause. They are selected as the most complete among about a dozen of similar documents forwarded to me by Dr. Harlow, who was kind enough to procure them at my request; and which bear the signature of many respectable persons in and about the town of Cavendish, and all corroborative of the circumstances as here detailed. The accident occurred in open day, in a quarry in which a considerable number of men were at work, many of whom were witnesses of it, and all of whom were attracted by it. Suffice it to say, that in a thickly populated country neighbourhood, to which all the facts were matter of daily discussion at the time of their occurrence, there is no difference of belief, nor has there been at any time doubt that the iron was actually driven through the brain. A considerable number of medical gentlemen also visited the case at various times to satisfy their incredulity.

Assuming the point that the wound was the result of a missile projected from below upwards, it may be asked whether the wound might not have been made by a stone, while the bar was at the same moment thrown into the air. It may be replied in answer, that the rock was not split, nor, as far as could be learned, disintegrated. Besides, an angular bit of stone wouldhave been likely to have produced quite as much laceration as the bar of iron; and it is in fact possible that the tapering point of the latter divided and repelled the soft parts, especially the brain, in a way that enabled the smooth surface of the iron to glide through with less injury. And assuming the only possible hypothesis, that the round bar followed exactly the direction of its axis, the missile may be considered as a sphere of one and a quarter inches diameter, preceded by a conical and polished wedge.

The patient visited Boston in January, 1850, and remained some time under my observation, during which he was presented at a meeting of the Boston Society for Medical Improvement, and also to the medical class at the hospital. His head, now perfectly healed, exhibits the following appearances.

A linear cicatrix of an inch in length occupies the left ramus of the jaw near its angle. A little thickening of the soft tissues is discovered about the corresponding malar bone. The eyelid of this side is shut, and the patient unable to open it. The eye considerably more prominent than the other, offers a singular confirmation of the points illustrated by the prepared skull described below. It will be there seen that the parts of the orbit necessarily cut away are those occupied by the levator palpebræ superioris, the levator oculi, and the abducens muscles. In addition to a ptosis of the lid, the eye is found to be incapable of executing either the outward or upward motion; while the other muscles animated by the motor communis are unimpaired. Upon the head, and covered by hair, is a large unequal depression and elevation. A portrait of the cast of the shaved head is given in the plate; and it will be there seen that a piece of cranuim of about the size of the palm of the hand, its posterior border lying near the coronal suture, its anterior edge low upon the forehead, was raised upon the latter as a hinge to allow the egress of the bar; and that it still remains raised and prominent. Behind it is an irregular and deep sulcus several inches in length, beneath which the pulsations of the brain can be perceived.

In order to ascertain how far it might be possible for this bar of an inch and a quarter diameter to traverse the skull in the track assigned to it, I procured a common skull, in which the zygomatic arches are barely visible from above; and having entered a drill near the left angle of the lower jaw, passed it obliquely upwards to the median line of the cranium just in front of the junction of the sagittal and coronal sutures. This aperture was then enlarged until it allowed the passage of the bar in question, and the loss of substance strikingly corresponds with the lesion said to have been received by the patient. From the coronoid process of the lower jaw is removed a fragment measuring about three-quarters of an inch in length. This fragment in the patient's case might have been fractured and subsequently reunited.

The hole now enters obliquely beneath the zygomatic arch, encroaching equally upon all its walls. In fact, it entirely occupies this cavity; the posterior wall of the antrum being partially excavated at the front of the hole, the whole orbitar portion of the sphenoid bone being removed behind, as also the anterior part of the squamous portion of the temporal bone, and the internal surface of the zygoma and malar bone laterally. In the orbit, the sphenoid bone, part of the superior maxillary below, and a large part of the frontal above, are cut away, and with these fragments much of the spheno-maxillary fissure; leaving, however, the optic foramen intact about a quarter of an inch to the inside of the track of the bar.

The base of the skull upon the inside of the cranium presents a cylindrical hole of an inch and a quarter diameter, and such as may be described by a pair of compasses, one leg of which is placed upon the lesser wing of the sphenoid bone at an eighth of an inch from its extremity, cutting the frontal, temporal and sphenoid bones; the other, half an inch outside the internal optic foramen.

The calvaria is traversed by a hole, two-thirds of which is upon the left, and one-third upon the right of the median line, its posterior border being quite near the coronal suture. The iron freely traverses the oblique hole thus described.

It is obvious that a considerable portion of the brain must have been carried away; that while a portion of its lateral substance may have remained intact, the whole central part of the left anterior lobe, and the front of the sphenoidal or middle lobe must have been lacerated and destroyed. This loss of substance would also lay open the anterior extremity of the left lateral ventricle; and the iron, in emerging from above must have largely impinged upon the right cerebral lobe, lacerating the falx and the longitudinal sinus.

Yet the optic nerve remained unbroken in the narrow interval between the iron and the inner wall of the orbit. The eye, forcibly thrust forward at the moment of the passage, might have again receded into its socket, from which it was again somewhat protruded during the subsequent inflammation.

It is fair to suppose that the polished conical extremity of the iron which first entered the cavity of the cranium prepared the passage for the thick cylindrical bar which followed; and that the point, in reaching and largely breaking open the vault of the cranium, afforded an ample egress for the cerebral substance, thus preventing compression of the remainder.

Yet it is difficult to admit that the aperture could have been thus violently forced through without a certain comminution of the base of the cranium driven inwards upon the cerebral cavity.

Little need be said of the physiological possibility of this history. It is well known that a considerable portion of the brain has been in some cases abstracted without impairing its functions. Atrophy of an entire cerebral hemisphere has also been recorded.

But the remarkable features of the present case lie not only in the loss of cerebral substance, but also in the singular chance which exempted the brain from either concussion or compression; which guided the enormous missile exactly in the direction of its axis, and which averted the dangers of subsequent inflammation. An entire lung is often disabled by disease; but I believe there is no parallel to the case in the Hunterian collection of a lung and thorax violently transfixed by the shaft of a carriage.

Taking all the circumstances into consideration, it may be doubted whether the present is not the most remarkable history of injury to the brain which has been recorded.*

REFERENCE TO PLATE.

1. Lateral view of a prepared cranium, representing the iron bar in the act of traversing its cavity.

2. Front view of ditto.

3. Plan of the base seen from within. (In these three figures the optic foramina are seen to be intact, and occupied by small white rods. In the first two figures, no attempt has been made to represent the elevation of the large anterior fragment, which must have been more considerable than is here shown.)

4. Cast taken from the shaved head of the patient, and representing the present appearance of the fracture; the anterior fragment being considerably elevated in the profile view.

5. The iron bar of the length and diameter proportioned to the size of the other figures.

* The iron bar has been deposited in the museum of the Massachusetts Medical College, where it may be seen, together with a cast of the patient's head.

PUBLICATIONS

OF THE

MASSACHUSETTS MEDICAL SOCIETY.

VOLUME II.

—————

BOSTON:

PRINTED BY DAVID CLAPP & SON.....334 WASHINGTON ST.

MEDICAL AND SURGICAL JOURNAL OFFICE.

1 8 6 8 .

THE expense of printing the "Publications of the Massachusetts Medical Society" is defrayed by a Fund devised to the Society by the late Dr. GEORGE C. SHATTUCK.

RECOVERY

FROM THE

PASSAGE OF AN IRON BAR THROUGH THE HEAD.

By JOHN M. HARLOW, M.D.,

OF WOBURN.

(With a Plate.)

READ JUNE 3, 1868.

43

RECOVERY AFTER SEVERE INJURY TO THE HEAD.

Mr. President and Fellows of the
Massachusetts Medical Society:

I have the pleasure of being able to present to you, to-day, the history and sequel of a case of severe injury of the head, followed by recovery, which, so far as I know, remains without a parallel in the annals of surgery. The case occurred nearly twenty years ago, in an obscure country town (Cavendish, Vt.), was attended and reported by an obscure country physician, and was received by the Metropolitan Doctors with several grains of caution, insomuch that many utterly refused to believe that the man had risen, until they had thrust their fingers into the hole in his head, and even then they required of the Country Doctor attested statements, from clergymen and lawyers, before they *could* or *would* believe—many eminent surgeons regarding such an occurrence as a physiological impossibility; the appearances presented by the subject being variously explained away.

It is due to science, that a case so grave, and succeeded by such remarkable results, should not be lost sight of ; that its subsequent history, termination, and pathological evidences, in detail, should have a permanent record. My desire to lay before the profession the sequel of this case, has not permitted me to remain altogether oblivious as to the whereabouts of my patient, and after tracing him in his wanderings over

330　　　　RECOVERY AFTER

the greater part of this continent, I am able to present to
you indubitable evidence that my report of the case, in the
Boston Medical and Surgical Journal, was no fiction. You
will find the report in Vol. 39, No. 20, page 389, of the
Journal; also a subsequent report, with comments, by Prof.
Henry J. Bigelow, in the American Journal of the Medical
Sciences for July, 1850.*

The accident occurred in Cavendish, Vt., on the line of
the Rutland & Burlington Railroad, at that time being built,
on the 13th of September, 1848, and was occasioned by
the premature explosion of a blast, when this iron, known
to blasters as a tamping iron, and which I now show you,
was shot through the face and head.

The subject of it was Phin. P. Gage, a perfectly healthy,
strong and active young man, twenty-five years of age, nervo-
bilious temperament, five feet six inches in height, average
weight one hundred and fifty pounds, possessing an iron will
as well as an iron frame; muscular system unusually well
developed—having had scarcely a day's illness from his childhood to the date of this injury. Gage was foreman of a
gang of men employed in excavating rock, for the road way.
The circumstances were briefly as follows:—

He was engaged in charging a hole drilled in the rock,
for the purpose of blasting, sitting at the time upon a shelf
of rock above the hole. His men were engaged in the pit,

* Soon after the publication of this case in the Boston Medical and Surgical
Journal, in November, 1848, I received a letter from Henry J. Bigelow, Professor
of Surgery in the Medical Department of Harvard University, requesting me to
send Gage to Boston, generously proposing to defray his expenses and compen-
sate him for loss of time. Gage being quite well, and the hole in the top of his
head entirely closed, accepted this proposition, and remained in Boston, under
the observation of Prof. Bigelow, eight or nine weeks, where he was examined
by many medical men, Prof. Bigelow being thoroughly convinced, at a time
when the accident had very few believers either in the medical profession or out
of it, that the lesion was as represented—that the iron had traversed the cranium
and brain as stated. With my concurrence he reported the case, with illustrations, in the American Journal of the Medical Sciences for July, 1850.

a few feet behind him, loading rock upon a platform car, with a derrick.   The powder and fuse had been adjusted in the hole, and he was in the act of "tamping it in," as it is called, previous to pouring in the sand.   While doing this, his attention was attracted by his men in the pit behind him. Averting his head and looking over his right shoulder, at the same instant dropping the iron upon the charge, it struck fire upon the rock, and the explosion followed, which projected the iron obliquely upwards, in a line of its axis, passing completely through his head, and high into the air, falling to the ground several rods behind him, where it was afterwards picked up by his men, smeared with blood and brain.   The missile entered by its pointed end, the left side of the face, immediately anterior to the angle of the lower jaw, and passing obliquely upwards, and obliquely backwards, emerged in the median line, at the back part of the frontal bone, near the coronal suture.   The wound thus occasioned will be demonstrated and fully described to you hereafter.   The iron which thus traversed the head, is known with blasters as a "tamping iron," is round and rendered comparatively smooth by use, and is three feet seven inches in length, one and one-fourth inches in its largest diameter, and weighs thirteen and one-fourth pounds. The end which entered first is pointed, the taper being about twelve inches long, and the diameter of the point one-fourth of an inch.

The patient was thrown upon his back by the explosion, and gave a few convulsive motions of the extremities, but spoke in a few minutes.   His men (with whom he was a great favorite) took him in their arms and carried him to the road, only a few rods distant, and put him into an ox cart, in which he rode, supported in a sitting posture, fully three-quarters of a mile to his hotel.   He got out of the cart himself, with a little assistance from his men, and an hour

RECOVERY AFTER

afterwards (with what I could aid him by taking hold of his left arm) walked up a long flight of stairs, and got upon the bed in the room where he was dressed. He seemed perfectly conscious, but was becoming exhausted from the hæmorrhage, which, by this time, was quite profuse, the blood pouring from the lacerated sinus in the top of his head, and also finding its way into the stomach, which ejected it as often as every fifteen or twenty minutes. He bore his sufferings with firmness, and directed my attention to the hole in his cheek, saying, " the iron entered there and passed through my head." Pulse at this time 60, soft and regular. He recognized me at once, and said " he hoped he was not much hurt." His person, and the bed on which he lay, was one gore of blood. Assisted by my friend Dr. Williams, who was first called to the patient in my absence, we proceeded to examine and dress his wounds. From the appearance of the wound in the top of the head, the fragments of bone being lifted up, the brain protruding from the opening and hanging in shreds upon the hair, it was evident that the opening in the skull was occasioned by some force acting from below, upward, having very much the shape of an inverted funnel, the edges of the scalp everted and the frontal bone extensively fractured, leaving an irregular oblong opening in the skull of two by three and one-half inches. The globe of the left eye was protruded from its orbit by one-half its diameter, and the left side of the face was more prominent than the right side. The pulsations of the brain were distinctly seen and felt.

The scalp was shaven, the coagula removed, with three small triangular pieces of the frontal bone, and in searching to ascertain if there were foreign bodies in the brain, I passed the index finger of the right hand into the opening its entire length, in the direction of the wound in the cheek, which received the left index finger in like manner, the introduction of the finger into the brain being scarcely felt. Aside from the triangular pieces already alluded to as removed, there were two other pieces detached from the frontal bone, the anterior being two and one-half by two inches, and the posterior one and one-half by two inches in size, leaving the antero-posterior diameter of the opening in the skull fully three and one-half inches.

This examination, and the appearance of the iron which was found some rods distant smeared with blood and brain, together with the testimony of the workmen and of the patient himself, who was sufficiently conscious to say that the iron "struck his head and passed through," was considered at the time as sufficiently conclusive, not only of the nature of the accident, but the manner in which it occurred. The small pieces of bone having been taken away, a portion of the brain, an ounce or more, which protruded, was removed, the larger pieces of bone replaced, the edges of the soft parts approximated as nearly as possible, and over all a wet compress, night cap and roller. The face, hands and arms were deeply burned. The wound in the cheek was left open, the hands and arms were dressed, and the patient was left with the head elevated, and the attendants directed to keep him in that position. This was at 7½ o'clock, P.M. At 10, P.M., same evening, the dressings are saturated with blood, but the hæmorrhage is abating. Has vomited twice only, since being dressed. Mind clear. Says he "does not care to see his friends, as he shall be at work in a few days." Gives the names and residence of his relatives in Lebanon, N. H. Pulse 65. Constant agitation of his legs, being alternately retracted and extended like the shafts of a fulling mill.

At 7, A.M., the 14th, has slept some during the night; appears to be in pain; speaks with difficulty; tumefaction of face considerable, and increasing. Recognizes his mother and uncle. Bleeding into mouth continues. Asks who is foreman in his pit. Has not vomited since midnight.

On the following day, the 15th, the hæmorrhage entirely ceased. Slept well half of the night, and could see objects indistinctly with the left eye.

For a detailed and daily record of the progress of the case, I will refer you to the Boston Medical and Surgical Journal of Dec. 13, 1848. It is sufficient for my present purpose to call your attention to a brief abstract of some of the most important features of the case which followed.

On the 15th Sept., two days after the accident, the patient lost control of his mind, and became decidedly delirious, with occasional lucid intervals. On that day a metallic probe was passed into the opening in the top of the head, and down until it reached the base of the skull, without resistance or pain, the brain not being sensitive.

16th, there began an abundant fœtid, sanious discharge from the head with particles of brain intermingled, finding its way out from the opening in the top of the head, and also from the one in the base of the skull into the mouth. On the 18th, he slept well nearly all night, but was as incoherent as ever in the morning. 22d, at 8, A.M., I learn that he has had a very restless night. Throws his hands and feet about, tries to get out of bed. Head very hot. Says " he shall not live long so." 23d, I find he has rested and been quiet most of the night. Appears stronger and more rational. Pulse, which has varied from 60 to 84 since the injury, I find at 80. The scalp was reshaven and the edges of the wound brought into apposition as nearly as possible, the edges having sloughed away. The discharge less in quantity and less fœtid.

At this date, ten days after the injury, vision of the left eye, though quite indistinct before, was totally lost. Up to this time it had not occurred to me that it was *possible* for

Gage to recover. The head had been dressed by myself three times every day; ice water kept on the head and face; the discharges carefully cleaned off, externally, while the attendants washed the mouth and fauces as often as necessary, with water and disinfecting solutions. The opening in the top of the head was always carefully covered with oiled silk underneath the wet compresses. To-day he appears stronger and more rational than before; calls for food.

Sept. 24th, 9, A.M. I find in my notes, taken at the time, that he has a pulse at 84; vision with right eye, and hearing with both ears, normal; bowels confined; can tell the day of the week and time of day; remembers persons who have visited him and incidents which have transpired since his injury. This improvement, however, was of short duration, though the discharge from the wounds had abated. I learned that in the night following he became stupid, did not speak unless aroused, and then only with difficulty; the integuments between the lower edge of the fracture in frontal bone and left nasal protuberance, swollen, hot and red, something like an erysipelatous blush. Pulse 96, soft. Failing strength. Is supported with food and stimulants. During the three succeeding days the coma deepened; the globe of the left eye became more protuberant, with fungus pushing out rapidly from the internal canthus. This fungus first made its appearance on the 19th, six days after the injury; also large fungi pushing up rapidly from the wounded brain, and coming out at the opening in the top of the head. On the 27th, the swelling upon the forehead fluctuated. The exhalations from the mouth and head horribly fœtid. Pulse 84. Comatose, but will answer in monosyllables when aroused. Will not take nourishment unless strongly urged. Calls for nothing. Surface and extremities incline to be cool. Discharge from the wound scanty, its exit being interfered with by the fungi. The friends and attendants are in hourly expectancy

44

336   RECOVERY AFTER

of his death, and have his coffin and clothes in readiness to remove his remains immediately to his native place in New Hampshire. One of the attendants implored me not to do anything more for him, as it would only prolong his sufferings—that if I would only keep away and let him alone, he would die. She said he appeared like "water on the brain." I said it is not water, but matter that is killing the man—so with a pair of curved scissors I cut off the fungi which were sprouting out from the top of the brain and filling the opening, and made free application of caustic to them. With a scalpel I laid open the integuments, between the opening and the roots of the nose, and immediately there were discharged eight ounces of ill-conditioned pus, with blood, and excessively fœtid. Tumefaction of left side of face increased. Globe of left eye very prominent.

From this date, Sept. 28th, to Oct. 6th, the discharge from the openings was very profuse and fœtid. Erysipelatous blush on skin of left side of face and head. Pulse ranging from 80 to 96. Speaks only when spoken to. Swallows well, and takes considerable nourishment, with brandy and milk; says he has no pain.

Oct. 6th—twenty-three days after the injury—I find entered in my note book as follows:—General appearance somewhat improved; pulse 90, and regular; more wakeful; swelling of left side of face abating; erysipelas gone; openings discharging laudable pus profusely; calls for his pants, and desires to be helped out of bed, though when lying upon his back cannot raise his head from the pillow. By turning to one side he succeeded in rising, and sat upon the edge of the bed about four minutes. Says he feels comfortable. Appears demented, or in a state of mental hebetude.

Oct. 11th—twenty-eighth day.—Very clear in his mind; states how long he has been upon his bed, how he was injured, the particulars of the explosion, and the time in the day when it occurred.

Oct. 15th—thirty-second day.—Progressing favorably. Fungi disappearing; discharging laudable pus from openings. Takes more food, sleeps well, and says he shall soon go home. Remembers passing and past events correctly, as well before as since the injury. Intellectual manifestations feeble, being exceedingly capricious and childish, but with a will as indomitable as ever; is particularly obstinate; will not yield to restraint when it conflicts with his desires.

Oct. 20th—thirty-seventh day.—Improving; gets out of and into bed with but little assistance; eats and sleeps well. Sensorial powers improving, and mind somewhat clearer, but very childish. The fungi have disappeared. The opening in the top of the head is closing up rapidly, with a firm membranous tissue.

Nov. 8th—fifty-sixth day.—Improving in every respect. Sits up most of the time during the day. Appetite good, though he is not allowed a full diet. Pulse 65. Sleeps well, and says he has not any pain in his head. He walks down stairs, about the house and into the piazza, and I am informed that he has been in the street to-day. I leave him to-day, with strict injunctions to avoid excitement and exposure.

Nov. 15th—sixty-fourth day.—Returned last evening, and learn that Gage has been in the street every day during my absence, excepting Sunday. Is impatient of restraint, and could not be controlled by his friends. Making arrangements to go home. Yesterday he walked half a mile, purchased some articles at the store, inquired the price, and paid the money with his habitual accuracy; did not appear to be particular as to price, provided he had money to meet it. The atmosphere was cold and damp, the ground wet, and he went without an overcoat, and with thin boots; got wet feet and a chill. I find him in bed, depressed and very irritable; hot and dry skin; thirst; tongue coated; pulse

110; lancinating pain in left side of head and face; rigors, and bowels constipated. Ordered cold to the head and face, and a cathartic, to be taken and repeated if it does not operate in six hours.

Nov. 16th, A.M.—No better. Cathartic has operated freely. Pulse 120; has passed a sleepless night; skin hot and dry; pain and thirst unabated. Was bled from the arm ℥ xvi., and got: ℞. Hydrarg. chloridi, gr. x.; ipecac, gr. ij. M.

8, P.M., same day.—Pulse falling; heat and pain moderated. Took a solution of ant. pot. tart. during night, and slept well.

17th, A.M.—Much improved. Has been purged freely during night, and says he feels better every way. Has no pain in head.

18th.—Is walking about house again, free from pain in head, and appears to be in a way of recovering, if he can be controlled. Has recently had several pieces of bone pass into the fauces, which he expelled from the mouth. The discharge from the head very slight, and the opening steadily closing up.

On the 25th he was taken, in a close carriage, a distance of thirty miles, to Lebanon, N. H., his home, where I saw him the succeeding week, and found him going on well. He continued to improve steadily, until on Jan. 1, 1849, the opening in the top of his head was entirely closed, and the brain shut out from view, though every pulsation could be distinctly seen and felt. Gage passed the succeeding winter months in his own house and vicinity, improving in flesh and strength, and in the following April returned to Cavendish, bringing his "iron" with him.

He visited me at that time, and presented something like the following appearances. General appearance good; stands quite erect, with his head inclined slightly towards the right side; his gait in walking is steady; his movements rapid, and easily executed. The left side of the face is wider than the right side, the left malar bone being more prominent than its fellow. There is a linear cicatrix near the angle of the lower jaw, an inch in length. Ptosis of the left eyelid; the globe considerably more prominent than its fellow, but not as large as when I last saw him. Can adduct and depress the globe, but cannot move it in other directions; vision lost. A linear cicatrix, length two and one-half inches, from the nasal protuberance to the anterior edge of the raised fragment of the frontal bone, is quite unsightly. Upon the top of the head, and covered with hair, is a large unequal depression and elevation—a quadrangular fragment of bone, which was entirely detached from the frontal and extending low down upon the forehead, being still raised and quite prominent. Behind this is a deep depression, two inches by one and one-half inches wide, beneath which the pulsations of the brain can be perceived. Partial paralysis of left side of face. His physical health is good, and I am inclined to say that he has recovered. Has no pain in head, but says it has a queer feeling which he is not able to describe. Applied for his situation as foreman, but is undecided whether to work or travel. His contractors, who regarded him as the most efficient and capable foreman in their employ previous to his injury, considered the change in his mind so marked that they could not give him his place again. The equilibrium or balance, so to speak, between his intellectual faculties and animal propensities, seems to have been destroyed. He is fitful, irreverent, indulging at times in the grossest profanity (which was not previously his custom), manifesting but little deference for his fellows, impatient of restraint or advice when it conflicts with his desires, at times pertinaciously obstinate, yet capricious and vacillating, devising many plans of future operation, which are no sooner arranged than they are abandoned in turn for others appearing more feasible.   A child in his intellectual capacity and manifestations, he has the animal passions of a strong man.   Previous to his injury, though untrained in the schools, he possessed a well-balanced mind, and was looked upon by those who knew him as a shrewd, smart business man, very energetic and persistent in executing all his plans of operation.   In this regard his mind was radically changed, so decidedly that his friends and acquaintances said he was " no longer Gage."

His mother, a most excellent lady, now seventy years of age, informs me that Phineas was accustomed to entertain his little nephews and nieces with the most fabulous recitals of his wonderful feats and hair-breadth escapes, without any foundation except in his fancy.   He conceived a great fondness for pets and souvenirs, especially for children, horses and dogs—only exceeded by his attachment for his tamping iron, which was his constant companion during the remainder of his life.   He took to travelling, and visited Boston, most of the larger New England towns, and New York, remaining awhile in the latter place at Barnum's, with his iron.   In 1851 he engaged with Mr. Jonathan Currier, of Hanover, New Hampshire, to work in his livery stable.   He remained there, without any interruption from ill health, for nearly or quite a year and a half.

In August, 1852, nearly four years after his injury, he turned his back upon New England, never to return.   He engaged with a man who was going to Chili, in South America, to establish a line of coaches at Valparaiso.   He remained in Chili until July, 1860, nearly eight years, in the vicinity of Valparaiso and Santiago, occupied in caring for horses, and often driving a coach heavily laden and drawn by six horses.   In 1859 and '60 his health began to fail, and in the beginning of the latter year he had a long illness, the precise nature of which, I have never been able to learn. Not recovering fully, he decided to try a change of climate, and in June, 1860, left Valparaiso for San Francisco, where his mother and sister resided. The former writes that " he arrived in San Francisco on or about July 1st, in a feeble condition, having failed very much since he left New Hampshire. He suffered much from seasickness on his passage out from Boston to Chili. Had many ill turns while in Valparaiso, especially during the last year, and suffered much from hardship and exposure."

After leaving South America, I lost all trace of him, and had well nigh abandoned all expectation of ever hearing from him again. As good fortune would have it, however, in July, 1866, I was able to learn the address of his mother, and very soon commenced a correspondence with her and her excellent son-in-law, D. D. Shattuck, Esq., a leading merchant in San Francisco. From them I learned that Gage was dead—that after he arrived in San Francisco his health improved, and being anxious to work, he engaged with a farmer at Santa Clara, but did not remain there long. In February, 1861, while sitting at dinner, he fell in a fit, and soon after had two or three fits in succession. He had no premonition of these attacks, or any subsequent ill feeling. " Had been ploughing the day before he had the first attack; got better in a few days, and continued to work in *various places;*" could not do much, *changing often,* " and always finding something which did not suit him in every place he tried." On the 18th of May, 1861, three days before his death, he left Santa Clara and went home to his mother. At 5 o'clock, A.M., on the 20th, he had a severe convulsion. The family physician was called in, and bled him. The convulsions were repeated frequently during the succeeding day and night, and he expired at 10, P.M., May 21, 1861— twelve years, six months and eight days after the date of his injury. These convulsions were unquestionably epileptic. It is regretted that an autopsy could not have been had, so that the precise condition of the encephalon at the time of his death might have been known. In consideration of this important omission, the mother and friends, waiving the claims of personal and private affection, with a magnanimity more than praiseworthy, at my request have cheerfully placed this skull (which I now show you) in my hands, for the benefit of science.*

I desire, here, to express gratefully my obligations, and those of the Profession, to D. D. Shattuck, Esq., brother-in-law of the deceased; to Dr. Coon, Mayor of San Francisco, and to Dr. J. D. B. Stillman, for their kind coöperation in executing my plans for obtaining the head and tamping iron, and for their fidelity in personally superintending the opening of the grave and forwarding what we so much desired to see.

The missile entered, as previously stated, immediately anterior and external to the angle of the inferior maxillary bone, proceeding obliquely upwards in the line of its axis, passed under the junction of the superior maxillary and malar bones, comminuting the posterior wall of the antrum, entered the base of the skull at a point, the centre of which is one and one-fourth inches to the left of the median line, in the junction of the lesser wing of the sphenoid with the orbitar process of the frontal bone—comminuting and removing the entire lesser wing, with one-half of the greater wing of the sphenoid bone—also fracturing and carrying away a large portion of the orbitar process of the frontal bone, leaving an opening in the base of the cranium, after the natural efforts at repair by the deposit of new bone, of one inch in its lateral, by two inches in its antero-posterior

---

* The skull and iron have been deposited, by the writer, in the Museum of the Medical Department of Harvard University, in Boston.

diameters, with a line of fracture or fissure leading anteriorly through the orbitar plate of the frontal bone, the anterior
fossa, and deflecting laterally, towards the median line,
divides the left frontal sinus, at the supra-orbitar notch, and
ascends the forehead along the left margin of the ridge, for
the attachment of the falx major.   Inferiorly the line of
separation begins at the infra-orbitar foramen and the malar
process of the supra-maxillary from the body of the bone,
terminating at a point upon the superior maxillary opposite
the last molar tooth.—The bones implicated in its passage
were the superior maxillary, malar, sphenoid and frontal.
The iron, as you will perceive, entered the left cerebrum, at
the fissure of Sylvius, possibly puncturing the cornu of the
left lateral ventricle, and in its passage and exit must have
produced serious lesion of the brain substance—the anterior
and middle left lobes of the cerebrum—disintegrating and
pulpifying it, drawing out a considerable quantity of it at
the opening in the top of the head, and lacerating unquestionably the upper aspect of the falx major and the superior
longitudinal sinus.   As the iron emerged from the head, it
comminuted the central portion of the frontal bone, leaving
an irregular oblong opening in the bone of three and one-
half inches in its antero-posterior, by two inches in its lateral
diameter.   Two of these fragments, as you will see from
the specimens before you, were re-united.*

* See plates at the end of this article, showing the direction of the passage of
the bar, lines of fracture in the skull, and the comparative size of the iron and
head.

45

Remarks.

I.   No attempt will be made by me to cite analogous cases, as after ransacking the literature of surgery in quest of such, I learn that all, or nearly all soon came to a fatal result.   Hence I conclude to leave that task to those who have more taste for it.   This case is chiefly interesting to me, as serving to show the wonderful resources of the system in enduring the shock and in overcoming the effects of so frightful a lesion, and as a beautiful display of the recuperative powers of nature.   It has been said, and perhaps justly, that "the leading feature of this case is its improbability." (BIGELOW.)   This may be so, but I trust, after what has been shown you to-day, that the most skeptical among you have been convinced of its actual occurrence—that it was no "Yankee invention," as a distinguished Professor of Surgery in a distant city was pleased to call it.   Moreover, it would seem, when we take into account all the *favoring circumstances*, that we may not only regard partial recovery as possible, but exceedingly probable.   These I will name briefly.

1st.   The subject was the man for the case.   His physique, will, and capacity of endurance, could scarcely be excelled.

2d.   The shape of the missile—being pointed, round and comparatively smooth, not leaving behind it prolonged concussion or compression.

3d.   The point of entrance outside of the superior maxillary bone—the bolt did little injury until it reached the floor of the cranium, when, at the same time that it did irreparable mischief, it opened up its way of escape, as without this opening in the base of the skull, for drainage, recovery would have been impossible.

4th.   The portion of the brain traversed, was, for several reasons, the best fitted of any part of the cerebral substance to sustain the injury.

II.   This case has been cited as one of complete recovery, it being often said that a very considerable portion of the left cerebrum was lost, without any impairment to the intellect.   I think you have been shown that the subsequent history and progress of the case only warrant us in saying that, physically, the recovery was quite complete during the four years immediately succeeding the injury, but we learn from the sequel that ultimately the patient probably succumbed to progressive disease of the brain.   Mentally the recovery certainly was only partial, his intellectual faculties being decidedly impaired, but not totally lost; nothing like dementia, but they were enfeebled in their manifestations, his mental operations being perfect in kind, but not in degree or quantity.   This may perhaps be satisfactorily accounted for in the fact that while the anterior and a part of the middle lobes of the left cerebrum must have been destroyed as to function, its functions suspended, its fellow was left intact, and conducted its operations singly and feebly.

III.   Little has been said in the foregoing account as to the treatment or conduct of this case, this being regarded as quite unnecessary.   The initiatory treatment, received from the iron, though it might not be well received in this presence, you will permit me to say, was decidedly antiphlogistic, a very large amount of blood having been lost.   May we not infer that this prepared the system for the trying ordeal through which it was about to pass?   The recovery is attributed chiefly to the *vis vitæ, vis conservatrix*, or, if you like it better, to the *vis medicatrix naturæ*, of which this case is a striking examplification.

I desire to call your attention, in passing, to two critical periods in the progress of the case, when what was done undoubtedly changed the tendency to a fatal result.   The first was on the fourteenth day, when the large abscess, which probably communicated with the left lateral ventricle,

346   SEVERE INJURY TO THE HEAD.

was opened, followed by a marked improvement in all the symptoms. The second was on the sixty-fourth day, at which time he was bled sixteen ounces.

I indulge the hope, that surely but *little* if anything was done to retard the progress of the case, or to interfere with the natural recuperative powers. Nature is certainly greater than art. Some one has wisely said, that vain is learning without wit. So may we say, vain is art without nature. For what surgeon, the most skilful, with all the blandishments of his art, has the world ever known, who could presume to take one of his fellows who has had so formidable a missile hurled through his brain, with a crash, and bring him, without the aid of this *vis conservatrix*, so that, on the fifty-sixth day thereafter, he would have been walking in the streets again? I can only say, in conclusion, with good old Ambrose Paré, I dressed him, God healed him.

Fig. 1.

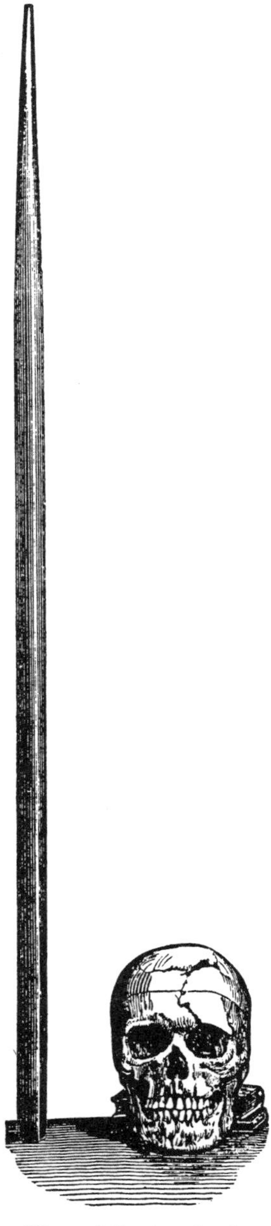

Fig. 2.

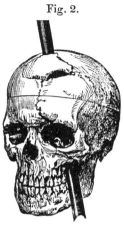

Front and lateral view of the cranium, representing the direction in which the iron traversed its cavity; the present appearance of the line of fracture, and also the large anterior fragment of the frontal bone, which was entirely detached, replaced, and partially re-united.

Fig. 3.

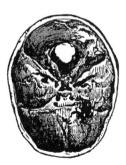

View of the base of the skull from within; the orifice caused by the passage of the iron having been partially closed by the deposit of new bone.

View of the tamping iron, and front view of the cranium, showing their *comparative* size.

HARVARD UNIVERSITY

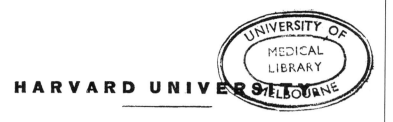

A

DESCRIPTIVE CATALOGUE

OF THE

WARREN ANATOMICAL MUSEUM.

BY

J. B. S. JACKSON, M.D.,

CURATOR OF THE MUSEUM; AND SHATTUCK PROFESSOR
OF MORBID ANATOMY.

BOSTON:

A. WILLIAMS AND COMPANY.

1870.

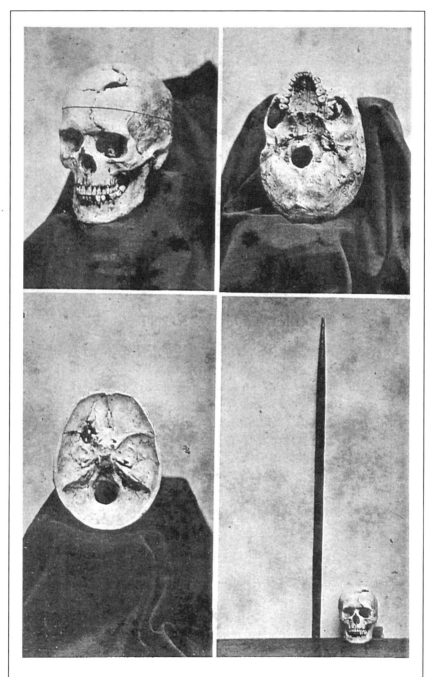

SEE NOS. 949, 3106.

INTRODUCTION.

THE Medical Department of Harvard University was established in the year 1782. In 1808 Dr. John C. Warren was appointed Adjunct Professor of Anatomy and Surgery; and, when that chair was vacated, in the year 1815, by the death of his father, Dr. W. was appointed to fill his place. How faithfully and honorably to himself, and to the College, he performed the duties of his office, and during a long period of years, is well known to the profession. The zeal with which he pursued his favorite studies, and with which he improved the opportunities that a very extensive professional practice afforded him, led to the collection of a great number of pathological and other specimens; and, on resigning his professorship, in 1847, the greater part of this collection was presented to the College, and with it the sum of $6,000, for its preservation and increase. In acknowledgment of so valuable a donation, the Corporation of the University voted that the Museum should be called by the name of its founder. Unfortunately, Dr. W.'s time was so fully occupied by his professional practice, that but little was left to him for those records, or even references, upon which the value of the pathological portion of a museum so much depends. Before the transfer, however, was made to the College, Dr. W. had a record made of the specimens, from his dictation; but it was, for the most part, and excepting a few references, a mere enumeration. The tendency to preserve interesting specimens is very strong in so devoted an anatomist and surgeon as Dr. W. always had been; and the consequence was, that he collected a large number of what might essentially be called duplicates. Pathological specimens that resemble each other very closely are often preserved in reference to their clinical history; and the diver-

3

sity in regard to the symptoms, and the progress of two cases, when the anatomical appearances are nearly similar, is often a very interesting pathological fact. If, however, the history is wanting, and the duplicate must be preserved in spirit, it is an undesirable one ; and accordingly many such were removed, after the collection came into the possession of the College.

Since Dr. Warren made his donation, the collection has steadily increased from year to year ; and it still continues to, as shown in part by the number of specimens that has been added since the printing of the catalogue was commenced last August, and that could not be introduced in their proper place ; many others having been added, and that were so introduced. It would be impossible to enumerate the many individuals who have shown an active interest in the Museum, and to whom the College is greatly indebted ; specimens having often been sent in from the country, and even from distant parts of the country, as well as from our immediate neighborhood. Some of our contributors, however, deserve especial notice. The late Dr. George Hayward, who occupied the chair of Surgery and Clinical Surgery, for a period of ten years (1840–50), made a collection of Thibert's models when he was in Europe, and for the illustration of his lectures. They amounted altogether to one hundred and sixty specimens, and in 1847 he presented them to the College. The late Dr. John Ware, also, Professor of the Theory and Practice of Medicine, collected ninety-one models by the same artist, and for the same purpose ; and these he presented to the College in 1849. Prof. O. W. Holmes has made a great many valuable preparations, to illustrate his department of healthy anatomy ; and he has also, independently of the Museum, a large number of microscopical preparations, either made by himself, or obtained by correspondence, and that he uses annually in a special course to the medical class. Prof. H. J. Bigelow has collected a large number of specimens in the course of his surgical practice, and many of them are of very great practical and scientific value. A series of colored lithographs, illustrative of diseased structures, is very fine, and ought especially to be mentioned. They form a small portion of a large number of lithographs, that Prof. B. had taken many years ago, in connection with a proposed work on tumors, but which unfortunately was never

INTRODUCTION.   v

completed. Very exquisite drawings were made in water
colors by a foreign artist, and from typical and recent specimens; these were then lithographed, and the copies that are
shown in the Museum were colored by the same artist, after
the originals. A collection of enlarged drawings in water
colors, by the same artist, suitable for the lecture-room, and
illustrative of surgical anatomy and pathology, may also be
alluded to, though independent of the Museum. In this collection there are four hundred and twenty-six plates, and
altogether nine hundred and sixty-seven figures; many of the
drawings being from recent specimens, and showing the microscopic as well as the gross appearances. Some of the other
departments are, also, illustrated more or less fully. Prof.
R. M. Hodges has always shown a most active interest in the
Museum since he was connected with the College as a student,
and the large practice in which he has been engaged of late
years has enabled him to secure for it very many specimens,
and some of them of the greatest interest. His anatomical
preparations, also, are very fine, and could hardly be surpassed
for the freedom and beauty of the dissections. The most valuable specimen that has ever been added to the Museum, and
probably ever will be, was given two years ago by Dr. John M.
Harlow, of Woburn. It was the skull of the man through
whose head a large iron bar passed, and who essentially recovered from the accident. For the professional zeal and the
energy that Dr. H. showed, in getting possession of this remarkable specimen, he deserves the warmest thanks of the
profession, and still more, from the College, for his donation.
Unfortunately, and notwithstanding the evidence that Dr. H.
has furnished, the case seems, generally, to those who have not
seen the skull, too much for human belief.

The whole number of specimens now in the Museum amounts
to three thousand six hundred and eighty-nine. The last specimen   *6*
is numbered 3681; but thirteen were accidentally omitted, and
afterwards added as the volume was being printed; and five   *&*
were repeated. Of these, one thousand one hundred and sixteen specimens were given by Dr. Warren, including three
hundred and thirteen phrenological casts; and one hundred
and twenty-three specimens were paid for from the Museum
Fund. The number of specimens preserved in spirit is nine

hundred and four; and of these, seven hundred and seven, with one or two exceptions, are separately displayed in glass jars. The rest, after being numbered and classified, are preserved together in large glass jars, from which they can be removed for study or demonstration.* Some of the dry preparations are also individually preserved under glass or in jars, for security when they are handled, and to make them more secure, also, than they can be when in the glazed cases alone; and, for the same reason, many, if not most, of the arterial preparations are mounted. Of the artistic specimens, there are two hundred and sixty-eight models by Thibert, and sixty-seven by Auzoux, of Paris. The casts in plaster amount to five hundred and seventy; but these include the phrenological collection, of which the number has been given above; twenty-one of the casts that were taken from recent specimens being colored somewhat after nature. There are also sixty photographs, and one hundred and three other specimens, including drawings, daguerreotypes, wax models, etc. As there are many dried specimens that are preserved, though essentially similar, so there are many others of great interest and of common occurrence, that are not generally preserved, except in regard to their external form, to the locality in which they are found, or their clinical history, — inasmuch as their appearances are entirely changed by any mode of preservation that is known.

A descriptive catalogue is essential in an anatomical museum; and one has been kept, in which the specimens that were given by Dr. Warren, and all that have since been added, have been entered as they were received. Many of them are simply enumerated; but the descriptions are often much detailed, though references are made, by volume and page, to the hospital records, and to the Medical Journal; it being understood that the Massachusetts General Hospital, and the Boston Medical and Surgical Journal are referred to, unless otherwise expressed. Lengthy as the descriptions sometimes are, however, they are almost always condensed from the original reports; and the liberty has always been taken of correcting errors, whenever such were known to exist. In the printed catalogue of Thibert's models many appearances are recorded that are not shown, and they are consequently not referred to. The donor's name, as a rule, is always given, whatever may be

* Designated by a mark (.) under the number.

INTRODUCTION. VII

his position, and if it is known, which is not always the case, though sometimes it is purposely withheld, and for various reasons; the donor being often the one who made the post-mortem examination, and not the one in whose practice the case occurred, and whose interest in it has not always disposed him to take any trouble in regard to the specimen. When the donor prepared the specimen, the fact has been or should be recorded. Many of the donors, and some of the best friends of the Museum, are now not living; but with a few exceptions, this does not appear. The specimens that are displayed in the cases are, of course, numbered to correspond with the descriptive catalogue; and a memorandum is kept of those that are preserved together, in spirit, and in the numbered jars. The specimens, also, as they have been entered in the catalogue, have been arranged according to a certain system, and briefly enumerated, with a repetition of the numbers and of the names of the donors.

The present volume has reached a most unexpected size, and would have been still larger if it had been as openly spaced throughout as it was at first. Figures, however, and other inelegant abbreviations are often• used, for the sake of brevity; and much is generally left to be inferred in regard to the specimens, — as the mode of preparation, the exhibition of certain parts, the fact that the history of a case was wholly or partially unknown, and generally the fact that a specimen was from the dissecting room. The date of the donation being given at the end of each case, the year is sometimes not referred to in the record, when the case was of short duration; and, if very short, the days of the week only are sometimes mentioned. In printed catalogues, generally, the different series or divisions are designated by letters, and separately numbered; but it seems to be more convenient for reference, to number the specimens regularly onward, and from first to last.

Besides the formal collection, there is another that consists mostly of indifferent specimens, and of what may be called duplicates; and they are very generally preserved in spirit. These amount altogether to two hundred and seventy-two; and fifty-eight of them belonged to Dr. Warren's original collection. They are all entered in a second and separate catalogue,

VIII   INTRODUCTION.

though very much less fully than in the other, but with references and a systematic index.

The Museum contains, for its size, many specimens of interest, and some that can hardly be surpassed. But there are a great many deficiencies; and it is to be hoped that many of them will be supplied by the zeal of the young men who are coming forward, and that the profession generally will continue to contribute, as they have heretofore, until there is no common form of injury or disease that will not be represented in the collection.

Since the above was in type, a manuscript " Catalogue of Preparations, belonging to the Anatomical Cabinet of the Massachusetts Medical College," has been received from Dr. J. Collins Warren, the son of Dr. J. Mason Warren, and grandson of the founder of the Museum. The date of this catalogue, of which I had never before heard, is not given; but it bears the marks of age, and, if it could have been consulted whilst the present volume was being prepared, it would have been of little use, as very few of the specimens can be identified; many are certainly not now in the collection, and it gives very generally little more than a mere enumeration of the specimens.

APRIL 29, 1870.

TABLE OF CONTENTS.

---◆◆---

9

anything like comminution, that at once suggests the idea of malformation. In the present case we must suppose, if the laminæ were broken upon the sides, that they were broken also, and most symmetrically, upon the posterior median line. 1862.   *Museum Fund.*

947. A deep incised wound in the body of the first dorsal vertebra.

From a young man who was stabbed in the middle of the right side of the neck, with a broad and sharp knife. The hemorrhage, which was very copious, was arrested; the common carotid being tied, though it was subsequently found uninjured. After this he rallied well; but on the second day phlegmonous inflammation came on about the wound, and he died seventy-eight hours after the injury. (Med. Jour. Vol. LXIX. p. 98.)   Vertebræ prepared by Dr. H., and dried. 1863.   *Dr. R. M. Hodges.*

948. The fifth and sixth cervical vertebræ, entirely separated, but not dislocated, and with only a trace of fracture.

From a man who was struck upon his breast, and thrown upon his back, when attempting to get upon the front platform of a horse-railroad car. Lived rather more than three days. Hospital, 97, 62. 1861.

Dr. George H. Gay.

949. Cranium of a man who lived twelve and one-half years after the passage of a large iron bar through his head.

The subject of this case was twenty-five years of age, of a strong constitution, and in vigorous health, and was engaged in blasting rocks, when the charge exploded. The bar, with which he was ramming or tamping it down, having been driven through his head, was thrown high into the air, fell at a distance of some rods, and was picked up smeared with blood and brain. The accident happened in the State of Vermont, Sept. 13th, 1848, and an account of the case was first published by Dr. Harlow, in the Boston Med. & Surg. Jour. in Dec. (Vol. XXXIX. p. 389).

In a few minutes he recovered his consciousness, was put into an ox-cart, and having been carried three-fourths of a

10

146   MORBID ANATOMY.

mile to his hotel, he got out with some assistance, and entered the house.   Two hours afterward, when he was seen by Dr. Harlow, he was quite conscious and collected in his mind, but exhausted by a profuse hemorrhage from the top of the head ; the scalp being everted, the bones very extensively fractured and upraised, and the brain protruding. In front of the angle of the lower jaw, upon the left side, was a linear wound through which the bar had entered, by the pointed end.   There was a protrusion of the left eye, equal to nearly one-half of its diameter ; and the left side of the face was more prominent than the right.   With a view to the presence, possibly, of any foreign bodies, Dr. H. passed one index finger down its whole length into the wound from above, and the other freely upward from below.   Frequent vomiting of blood from the stomach.   The pulse at this time was 60.

On the 15th the hemorrhage had ceased ; vision of the left eye was indistinct, and there was delirium.   On the 16th a fetid discharge, with particles of brain, from the head ; with a discharge also from the mouth.   23d : More rational, stronger, and asked for food.   Vision in left eye quite gone.   Pulse 60–84 since the accident.   On the 24th erysipelas appeared below the wound ; and for the next three days he was more comatose, with a large fungous growth from the upper wound, and a fungus from the inner canthus of the eye, that first appeared on the 19th.   27th : Discharge from the upper wound small, and exhalations from the mouth horribly fetid.   The large fungous growth was excised, and ℥ viii of pus were discharged by incision over the lower part of the frontal bone.   Eye very prominent.   The discharge after this was profuse and fetid. Oct. 6th he was better locally and generally, and sat up for a few minutes, but appeared demented.   Nov. 8th he was in every way doing well, and went abroad.   On the 14th he walked half a mile, exposed to dampness and cold, and there followed a febrile attack, with lancinating pain in the left side of the head and face.   For this he was bled and purged ; and on the 18th he was about the house again. On the twenty-fifth, about seven weeks and a half after the accident, he returned home, a distance of about thirty miles.

January 1st, 1849, the wound was quite closed. In April the left malar bone continued to be more prominent than the right. The eye, however, was less prominent than it had been; but the motions of the globe were limited, and there was ptosis of the lid, with a partial paralysis of the left side of the face. Upon the top of the head was a quadrangular prominence, and behind this a deep depression. No pain, but a queer feeling in the head. In regard to the state of his mind, he was very fitful and vacillating, though still very obstinate, as he always had been; and he was very profane, though never so before the accident.

After his recovery he travelled about with his bar, and exhibited himself in several of the large cities in this country; and in 1851 he got a situation, as a hostler, in a stable. In August, 1852, he went to S. America, and drove a six-horse stage-coach in Chili. . In 1859 and '60 his health began to fail, and early in 1860 he had a long sickness, but no particulars could be learned in regard to it. In June, 1860, he went to San Francisco, where his friends were residing; and as his health improved, he went to work upon a farm. In February, 1861, he had a fit, and soon two or three others. He had been ploughing on the day that he was attacked, and had had no premonitory symptoms. In a few days he was better, and did at different times various kinds of work. On the 20th of May he was attacked with severe convulsions, which recurred frequently; and on the following day he died.

In July, 1866, Dr. Harlow ascertained that his patient's mother was residing at San Francisco; and after a correspondence with her, and other members of the family who were with her, he not merely obtained the final history of the case, but in the most commendable spirit, and with a full appreciation of the scientific interest of the case, permission was given to have the cranium removed, and sent here for examination and preservation. In effecting this very desirable object, he was aided by D. D. Shattuck,

148   MORBID ANATOMY.

Esq., a brother-in-law of his patient, Dr. Coon, Mayor of the city, and Dr. J. D. B. Stillman, all of San F.

The cranium arrived in this city, with the bar, in 1868, and have been most generously presented, by Dr. Harlow, to the Medical College.

On examination of the cranium, it is generally, though not always, possible to distinguish between the bones that are gone, as the result of the injury, and those that have crumbled away and been lost since the man's death; the smoothness of the edges determining this point for the most part. The whole of the small wing of the sphenoid bone upon the left side is gone, with a large portion of the large wing, and a large portion of the orbital process of the frontal bone; leaving an opening in the base of the skull, 2 in. in length, 1 in. in width, posteriorly, and tapering gradually and irregularly to a point anteriorly. This opening extends from the sphenoidal fissure to the situation of the frontal sinus; and its centre is an inch from the median line. The optic foramen, and the foramen rotundum are intact. Below the base of the skull the whole posterior portion of the upper maxillary bone is gone. The malar bone is uninjured; but it has been very perceptibly forced outward, and the external surface inclines somewhat outward, from above downward. The lower jaw is also uninjured. The opening in the base above described is continuous with a line of old and united fracture that extends through the supra-orbitary ridge, in the situation of the foramen, inclines toward, and then from the median line, and terminates in an extensive fracture that was caused by the bar as it came out through the top of the head. This fracture is situated in the left half of the frontal bone, but, inferiorly, it extends somewhat over the median line. In form it is about quadrilateral; and it measures $2\frac{1}{2}$ x $1\frac{3}{4}$ in. Two large pieces of bone are seen to have been detached and upraised; the upper one having been separated at the coronal suture from the parietal bone, and being so closely united that the fracture does not show upon the outer surface. The lower piece shows the line of fracture all around. Owing to the loss of bone, two openings are left in the skull; one, that separates the two fragments, has nearly a triangular form, extends rather across the median line, and is 4 in. in circumference; the other, situated between the lower fragment, and the left half of the frontal bone, is long and irregularly narrow, and is 2⅜ in. in circumference. The edges of the fractured bones are smooth, and there is nowhere any new deposit. 1868.   *Dr. John M. Harlow, of Woburn.*

For the bar above referred to see No. 3106.

950. A cast of the head of the above individual. Soon after Dr. H. published the case, Dr. Bigelow wrote to him, and made arrangements, at a very considerable expense to himself, to have the man sent down to this city, and kept here for a full examination. After he had satisfied himself that the bar had actually passed through the man's head, and that he had essentially recovered from the accident, he was exhibited to the profession, the cast was taken, and a full account of the case, with illustrations, was published by Dr. B., in the American Jour. of Med. Sciences, July, 1850. 1856.   *Dr. H. J. Bigelow.*

The very small amount of attention that has been given to the above wonderful case, by the profession in this country, as well as in Europe, can only be explained by the fact that it far transcends any case of recovery from injury of the head that can be found in the records of surgery. It was too monstrous for belief, and yet Dr. Harlow has at last furnished evidence that leaves no question in regard to it.

951. A skull that was prepared by Dr. B., to show the course that the bar was supposed to have taken. 1856.
Dr. H. J. Bigelow.

952. Cast of the head of a man who was transfixed through the head by an iron gas-pipe, and who, to a very considerable extent, recovered from the accident.

The accident happened in the State of Ohio, May 14th, 1867, and the following is an abstract of the case, which was reported to Dr. Bigelow by the attending physicians, Drs. M. Jewett and F. W. Inman. The patient, a healthy and intelligent man, about twenty-seven years of age, was

150   MORBID ANATOMY.

blasting coal, when the charge exploded unexpectedly, and the pipe was driven through his head, entering at the junction of the middle and outer thirds of the right supra-orbitary ridge, and emerging near the junction of the left parietal, occipital, and temporal bones. One of his fellow-miners saw him upon his hands and knees, and struggling as if to rise; and, going to his assistance, he placed his knee upon his chest, supported his head with one hand, and with the other withdrew the pipe. This last projected about equally from the front and back of the head; and much force was required for its withdrawal. On being raised from the bottom of the shaft, which was about 100 ft. deep, he shivered as if he was very cold, groaned heavily, put both hands to his forehead, shook his head deprecatingly when spoken to, but moved his lips.

Three hours after the accident Dr. I was called, and found him comatose, and in a state of collapse; pulse 35, and weak; respirations nine per minute, and every breath seemed as if it would be the last. The right eye protruded half an inch, and blood, mixed with portions of brain, was oozing from the anterior wound, which was smooth, and about large enough to admit the index finger; the hemorrhage, however, being inconsiderable, though free at first. Posteriorly the opening was much larger, and the bones protruded; the extent of the fracture being about 3 in. The gas-pipe (No. 3107.) was shown, and about one-half of it was smeared with blood and brain; 4 ft. 2 in. in length, and $\frac{3}{8}$ in. in diameter. Some spiculæ of bone were removed from the back of the head; the free use of stimuli was ordered, with cold to the head, and warmth to the extremities. On the 16th his breathing was stertorous, with a pulse of 40; and calomel with podophyllin was given, with beef-tea. On the 17th there was some reaction; and as the medicine had had no effect, it was repeated, and, after an enema, free catharsis followed, with a tænia, 17 ft. long. On the 19th he was more restless, and, as it was difficult to keep him in bed, tart. antimony, with opium, was given.

In a very few days he began to swallow what was put into his mouth; about the twelfth day he began to take food freely, and in about three weeks from the time of the accident he ate voraciously. A pint of whiskey was given daily for the first five days, and on the 19th reaction commenced, with a pulse of 80. If he did not want food or whiskey, he would roll over and turn away. For six weeks the discharges from the bowels and bladder were involuntary. In seven weeks he sat up, and in one more he walked about a little. The right hand he used somewhat, but less well than the left. For about ten months after the accident his memory for some things was nearly lost, but during the next two months there was a considerable improvement.

When he was first seen, a probe, 4 in. in length, was passed into each of the wounds as far as it would reach, and without obstruction; and the chief point in the treatment consisted in the frequent passage of the probe, with a view to keeping the openings perfectly free. During the first ten days the probe was passed its whole length, and daily. If the orifices, and especially the posterior one, were at any time obstructed by a plug of brain, the coma would very much increase; and by shaving it off repeatedly, and passing the probe, the relief would often be very great. The discharge from the back wound was very considerable; and, as it became quite offensive, injections of chlorate of potash were frequently used. On the sixth day there was a slight ptyalism, and this Drs. J. and I. thought may have tended to prevent secondary inflammation.

Dr. Jewett visited Boston with the patient, at the invitation of Dr. Bigelow, and kindly presented to him the gas-pipe, and transferred to him the case, with liberty to make such use of it as he should see fit. Dr. B. exhibited the patient, with the gas-pipe, to the Mass. Medical Society, at their annual meeting in June, 1868, and then added the pipe to his collection in this museum; the cast being taken subsequently. The man appeared to be in a good state of general health; and, though his mental powers were considerably impaired, there was nothing unusual in his expression, nor would there be noticed, in a few minutes' conversation with him, any marked deficiency of intellect.

152 MORBID. ANATOMY.

He had done no work, however, since the time of the accident, and he had not fully recovered the use of his eye, nor of his right hand. Above the eye there was a small cicatrix, and a slight irregularity to the feel of the surface of the bone. Posteriorly there was a depression, quite defined, and nearly large enough to admit the top of the index finger, but without any elevation, or irregularity of the surrounding bone.

Drs. Jewett and Inman delivered to Dr. Bigelow, with their report, the statements of different physicians who saw the man with them, and no one of whom had the slightest doubt of the main fact in the case. Statements also were given by different non-professional persons. After Dr. J. returned to Ohio he sent to Dr. B. the hat that his patient wore at the time of the accident, and in it are holes corresponding to the openings in the skull. 1868. See **No. 3107.** *Dr. H. J. Bigelow.*

953. A skull, fractured so as to separate the whole anterior half from the posterior ; the bones being also separated to some extent at the coronal suture. 1847.
Dr. J. C. Warren.

954. A second specimen, in which the whole of the left side is beaten in. The patient fell from the top of a house. 1847. *Dr. J. C. Warren.*

955. Top of the skull, showing a fissure through the parietal bones ; and upon one side it may have extended to the base. Bones separated at the coronal suture, as in No. 953. Trephined. 1847. *Dr. J. C. Warren.*

956. Top of the skull, showing an extensive and comminuted fracture.

From a laborer, who was struck with the point of a pickaxe, in a fight, and lived about four days. Very drowsy. Quite conscious when first seen, without palsy, and with a pulse of 44 ; pupils acted. Several pieces of bone removed at the hospital (125, 164) by Dr. C. ; and these, having been with the other fragments dried

MORBID ANATOMY, 683

matter or concrete pus. The deposit consisted of minute globules or granular corpuscles, varying in size from those of tubercle to those of pus. The firm portion was fibrous. The right capsule was smaller than usual, though thicker at one part, and nowhere flat as usual; disease as in the left, but much less extensive. There was, also, some old disease of the brain, ecchymoses in the lungs, and a large quantity of blood in the heart, that was fluid, and continued so after removal from the body. 1857.

Dr. A. A. Gould.

3104. A third case. — The patient, a female, æt. thirty-one years, had been under the care of Dr. B., for about a year, with debility, a bronzed skin, and other anomalous symptoms ; the discoloration terminating near the margin of the hair, and leaving a narrow white line between the two. Occasionally there were attacks of indigestion ; and during her recovery from one of these, she indulged very grossly in indigestible food, and died in consequence. Both renal capsules were greatly enlarged ; texture firm ; and studded thickly with irregular, tubercular-looking deposits, from the size of a small shot to that of a chestnut. Other organs well. 1860.   *Dr. H. I. Bowditch.*

For other cases of Addison's disease, see p. 395.

3105. A thin cyst in the substance of the renal capsule. Collapsed ; but, if distended, would have been nearly as large as an English walnut. Traces of cretaceous matter in the parietes. — From a female dissecting-room subject, about twenty-five years of age, and almost anæmic in appearance. Lungs tubercular. 1857.   *Dr. R. M. Hodges.*

3106. An iron bar, that was driven through a man's head. He seemed to have entirely recovered from the accident, and lived twelve years and a half afterward, but died finally with cerebral symptoms. (See No. 949.)

The bar is 3 ft. 7 in. in length, and weighs $13\frac{1}{4}$ lbs. ; form cylindrical, and diameter $1\frac{1}{4}$ in. ; one end is square, as in a common crowbar, and the other tapers to a smoothly blunt point, — this last measuring $\frac{1}{4}$ in. 1868.

Dr. John M. Harlow, of Woburn.

684   MORBID ANATOMY.

3107. An iron gas-pipe, by which a man was transfixed through the head in May, 1867. (See No. 952.)

Dr. Bigelow mentions (April 1st, 1870) some important facts in regard to this case, and that were not referred to in the papers from which the history (p. 149) was drawn up. He says: " When addressed, his expression was intelligent and singularly pleasant. He evidently apprehended what was said to him, but rarely replied in words. His habitual reply on such occasions was ' mais, oui;' and this, with the word ' tabac,' of which article he was very fond, seemed to constitute his vocabulary. There could be no question that this was a case of what has been called aphasia. As far as could be judged, his intellectual functions were not disturbed. Being brought to a new city, he showed within a few days a singular faculty of finding his way home, through the streets, and from long distances, unaided." Dr. B. has also handed to me a letter from Dr. Jewett, that I had not before seen (dated April 29th, 1868), and in which he says: " To my request that he would go home with me, and work in my garden, he replied, ' No, sir-ee,' — the largest number of words I have heard him connect since the injury." — Dr. B. has heard nothing (1870) of the man since the middle of last summer, but he was then in fine health, and in regard to speech he had decidedly improved. There has never been, he says, any paralysis. 1868.   *Dr. H. J. Bigelow.*

3108. A wrought-iron spike, 3⅜ in. in length, that projected 2 in. from a barn floor, and upon which a man fell head foremost, 16½ ft. The case occurred (Dec. 1868) in the practice of Dr. C., who gave the following history of the case; and, at the request of Dr. J. B. Upham, presented the spike to the museum. (Med. Jour., March 24th, 1870.)

The patient was a laborer, twenty-eight years of age. The spike passed through the upper posterior part of the right parietal bone, and carried a portion of it, an inch square, into the substance of the brain, to the depth of about 2 in.; the fracture extending, also, downward nearly to the ear. The man was " firmly buttoned down to the floor" by the head of the spike, which measured 1½ in. across; and, in their attempts to extricate him, two strong

Appendix B

A Collation of Notes and Other Material on the Case

Introduction

This collation of the record of the case and the case notes themselves is a simple combination of Harlow 1848, Harlow 1868, and Bigelow 1850b. Although Bigelow's 1850 version of the case notes is a reproduction of what Harlow published in 1848, with only slight differences in punctuation and capitalization, in 1868 Harlow included some details omitted from the original. In their case note sections, neither Bigelow's 1850c nor Harlow's 1869 pamphlets differ from their respective originals, and therefore have not been referred to here.

Except for replacing the various symbols of the doses of the medications Harlow prescribed, I have attempted to reproduce these reports of Gage's accident as accurately as possible, and have not altered spelling, abbreviations, punctuation, or spacing. James Morse of the College of Pharmacy, University of Arizona, Tucson, first deciphered and discussed the various anti-phlogistic prescriptions and remedies with me. I later drew on Dr. David Koch of Marquette General Hospital and Prof. Barry Reed of the Victorian College of Pharmacy to check my translations of the quantities involved.

The Cause of the Accident (Medical Reports)

Harlow 1848

It appears from his own account, and that of the by-standers, that he was engaged in charging a hole, preparatory to blasting. He had turned in the powder, and was in the act of tamping it slightly before pouring on the sand. He had struck the powder, and while about to strike it again, turned his head to look after his men (who were working within a few feet of him), when the tamping iron came in contact with the rock, and powder exploded, driving the iron against the left side of the face.... The tamping iron is round, and rendered comparatively smooth by use. It is pointed at the end which entered first and is three feet, seven inches in length, one and one quarter inch in diameter, and weighs $13\frac{1}{4}$ pounds.

Bigelow 1850b

According to his own statement, he was charging with powder a hole drilled in a rock, for the purpose of blasting. It appears that it is customary in filling the hole to cover the powder with sand. In this case, the charge having been adjusted, Mr. Gage directed his assistant to pour in the sand; and at the interval of a few seconds, his head being averted, and supposing the sand to be have been properly placed, he dropped the head of the iron as usual upon the charge, to consolidate or "*tamp it in.*" The assistant had failed to obey the order, and the iron striking fire upon the rock, the uncovered powder was ignited and the explosion took place. Mr. Gage was at this time standing above the hole, leaning forward, with his face slightly averted; and the bar of iron was projected directly upwards in a line of its axis, passing completely through his head and high into the air.... The iron which thus traversed the skull weighs thirteen and a quarter pounds. It is three feet seven inches in length, and one and a quarter inches in diameter. The end which entered first is pointed; the taper being seven inches long, and the diameter of the point one quarter of an inch; circumstances to which the patient perhaps owes his life. The iron is unlike any other, and was made by a neighbouring blacksmith to please the fancy of the owner.

Harlow 1868

He was engaged in charging a hole drilled in the rock for the purpose of blasting, sitting at the time upon a shelf of rock above the hole. His men were engaged in the pit, a few feet behind him, loading rock upon a platform car, with a derrick. The powder and fuse had been adjusted in the hole, and he was in the act of "tamping it in," as it is called, previous to pouring in the sand. While doing this, his attention was attracted by his men in the pit behind him. Averting his head and looking over his right shoulder, at the same instant dropping the iron upon the charge, it struck fire upon the rock, and the explosion followed, which projected the iron obliquely upwards, in a line of its axis, passing completely through his head, and high into the air, falling to the ground several rods behind him, where it was afterwards picked up by his men, smeared with blood and brain.... The iron which thus traversed the head, is known with blasters as a "tamping iron," is round and rendered comparatively smooth by use, and is three feet seven inches in length, one and one-fourth inches in its largest diameter, and weighs thirteen and one-fourth pounds. The end which entered first is pointed, the taper being about twelve inches long, and the diameter of the point one-fourth of an inch.

The Passage of the Tamping Iron

Harlow 1848

[T]he powder exploded, driving the iron against the left side of the face, immediately anterior to the angle of the inferior maxillary bone. Taking a direction upward and backward toward the median line, it penetrated the integuments, the masseter and temporal muscles, passed under the zygomatic arch, and (probably) fracturing the temporal portion of the sphenoid bone, and the floor of the orbit of the left eye, entered the cranium ... and made its exit in the median line, at the junction of the coronal and sagittal sutures, lacerating the longitudinal sinus, fracturing the parietal and frontal bones extensively ... and protruding the globe of the left eye from its socket, by nearly one half its diameter.

Bigelow 1850b

The wound thus received ... was oblique, traversing the cranium in a straight line from the angle of the lower jaw on one side to the centre of the frontal bone above, near the sagittal suture, where the missile emerged; and the iron thus forcibly thrown into the air was picked up at a distance of some rods from the patient, smeared with brains and blood....

I procured a common skull, in which the zygomatic arches are barely visible from above; and having entered a drill near the left angle of the lower jaw, passed it obliquely upwards to the median line of the cranium just in front of the junction of the sagittal and coronal sutures. This aperture was then enlarged until it allowed the passage of the bar in question, and the loss of substance strikingly corresponds with the lesion said to have been received by the patient. From the coronoid process of the lower jaw is removed a fragment measuring about three-quarters of an inch in length. This fragment in the patient's case might have been fractured and subsequently reunited.

The hole now enters obliquely beneath the zygomatic arch, encroaching equally upon all its walls. In fact, it entirely occupies this cavity; the posterior wall of the antrum being partially excavated at the front of the hole, the whole orbitar portion of the sphenoid bone being removed behind, as also the anterior part of the squamous portion of the temporal bone, and the internal surface of the zygoma and malar bone laterally. In the orbit, the sphenoid bone, part of the superior maxillary below, and a large part of the frontal above, are cut away, and with these fragments much of the spheno-maxillary fissure; leaving, however, the optic foramen intact about a quarter of an inch to the inside track of the bar.

The base of the skull upon the inside of the cranium presents a cylindrical hole of an inch and a quarter diameter, and such as may be described by a pair of compasses, one leg of which is placed upon the lesser wing of the sphenoid bone at an eighth of an inch from its extremity, cutting the frontal, temporal and sphenoid bones; the other, half an inch outside the internal optic foramen.

The calvaria is traversed by a hole, two-thirds of which is upon the left, and one-third upon the right of the median line, its posterior border being quite near the coronal suture. The iron freely traverses the oblique hole thus described.

Harlow 1868

The missile entered by its pointed end, the left side of the face, immediately anterior to the angle of the lower jaw, and passing obliquely upwards, and obliquely backwards, emerged in the median line, at the back part of the frontal bone, near the coronal suture.

The missile entered, as previously stated, immediately anterior and external to the angle of the inferior maxillary bone, proceeding obliquely upwards in the line of its axis, passed under the junction of the superior maxillary and malar bones, comminuting the posterior wall of the antrum, entered the base of the skull, at a point the centre of which is one and one fourth inches to the left of the median line, in the junction of the lesser wing of the sphenoid with the orbitar process of the frontal bone—comminuting and removing the entire lesser wing, with one-half of the greater wing of the sphenoid bone—also fracturing and carrying away a large portion of the orbitar process of the frontal bone, leaving an opening in the base of the cranium, after the natural efforts at repair by the deposit of new bone, of one inch in its lateral, by two inches in its antero-posterior diameters, with a line of fracture or fissure leading anteriorly through the orbitar plate of the frontal bone, the anterior fossa, and deflecting laterally, towards the median line, divides the left frontal sinus, at the supra-orbitar notch, and ascends the forehead along the left margin of the ridge, for the attachment of the falx major. Inferiorly the line of separation begins at the infra-orbital foramen and the malar process of the supra-maxillary from the body of the bone, terminating at a point upon the superior maxillary opposite the last molar tooth. The bones implicated in its passage were the superior maxillary, malar, sphenoid, and frontal.... As the iron emerged from the head, it comminuted the central portion of the frontal bone, leaving an irregular oblong opening in the bone of three and one-half inches in its anterior-posterior, by two inches in its lateral diameter.

The Parts of the Brain That Were Injured

Harlow 1848
[The iron] entered the cranium, passing through the anterior left lobe of the cerebrum, and made its exit in the median line ... lacerating the longitudinal sinus, breaking up considerable portions of the brain.

Bigelow 1850b
It is obvious that a considerable portion of the brain must have been carried away; that while a portion of its lateral substance may have remained intact, the whole central part of the left anterior lobe, and the front of the sphenoidal or middle lobe must have been lacerated and destroyed. This loss of substance would also lay open the anterior extremity of the left lateral ventricle; and the iron, in emerging from above must have largely impinged upon the right cerebral lobe, lacerating the falx and the longitudinal sinus.

Harlow 1868
The iron, as you will perceive, entered the left cerebrum, at the fissure of Sylvius, possibly puncturing the cornu of the left lateral ventricle, and in its passage and exit must have produced serious lesion of the brain substance—the anterior and middle left lobes of the cerebrum—disintegrating and pulpifying it, drawing out a

considerable quantity of it at the opening in the top of the head, and lacerating unquestionably the upper aspect of the falx major and the superior longitudinal sinus.

Immediate Effects on Gage

Harlow 1848

I am informed that the patient was thrown upon his back, and gave a few convulsive motions of the extremities but spoke in a few minutes. His men (with whom he was a great favorite) took him in their arms and carried him to the road, only a few rods distant, and sat him into an ox cart, in which he rode, sitting erect, full three quarters of a mile, to the hotel of Mr Joseph Adams, in this village. He got out of the cart himself and with a little assistance walked up a long flight of stairs, into the hall, where he was dressed.

Bigelow 1850b

Dr. Harlow in the graphic account above alluded to, states that "immediately after the explosion the patient was thrown upon his back, and gave a few convulsive motions of the extremities but spoke in a few minutes. His men (with whom he was a great favourite) took him in their arms and carried him to the road, only a few rods distant, and sat him into an ox cart, in which he rode, sitting erect, full three quarters of a mile, to the hotel of Mr Joseph Adams, in this village. He got out of the cart himself and with a little assistance walked up a long flight of stairs, into the hall, where he was dressed."

Harlow 1868

The patient was thrown upon his back by the explosion, and gave a few convulsive motions of the extremities, but spoke in a few minutes. His men (with whom he was a great favorite) took him in their arms and carried him to the road, only a few rods distant, and put him into an ox cart, in which he rode, supported in a sitting posture, fully three-quarters of a mile to his hotel. He got out of the cart himself, with a little assistance from his men, and an hour afterwards (with what I could aid him by taking hold of his left arm) walked up a long flight of stairs, and got upon the bed in the room where he was dressed.

Initial Treatment

Williams 1848 in Bigelow 1850b

Dr. Harlow being absent at time of the accident, I was sent for, and was the first physician who saw Mr G., some twenty-five or thirty minutes after he received the injury; he at that time was sitting in a chair upon the piazza of Mr. Adam's hotel, in Cavendish. When I drove up, he said, "Doctor, here is business enough for you." I first noticed the wound upon the head before I alighted from my carriage, the pulsations of the brain being very distinct; there was also an appearance which, before I examined the head, I could not account for: the top of the head appeared somewhat like an inverted funnel; this was owing, I discovered, to the bone being fractured about the opening for a distance of about two inches in every direction. I ought to have mentioned above that the opening through the skull and integuments was not far from one and a half inch in diameter; the edges of this opening were everted, and the whole wound appeared as if some wedge-shaped body had passed from below upward. Mr. Gage, during the time I was examining this wound, was relating the manner in which he was injured to the bystanders; he talked so rationally and was so willing to answer questions, that I directed my inquiries to him in preference to the men who were with him at the time of the accident, and who were standing about at this time. Mr. G. then related to me some of the circumstances, as he has since done; and I can safely say that neither at that time nor on any subsequent occasion, save once, did I consider him to be other than perfectly rational. The one time to which I allude was about a fortnight after the accident, and then he persisted in calling me John Kirwin; yet he answered all my questions correctly.

I did not believe Mr. Gage's statement at that time, but thought he was deceived; I asked him where the bar entered, and he pointed to the wound on his cheek, which I had not before discovered; this was a slit running from the angle of the jaw forward about one and a half inch; it was very much stretched laterally, and was discoloured by powder and iron rust, or at least appeared so. Mr. Gage persisted in saying that the bar went through his head: an Irishman standing by said "Sure it was so, sir, for the bar is lying in the road below, all blood and brains." The man also said he would have brought it up with him, but he thought there would be an inquest, and it would not do.

About this time, Mr. G. got up and vomited a large quantity of blood, together with some of his food; the effort of vomiting pressed out about half a teacupful of the brain, which fell upon the floor, together with the blood, which was forced out at the same time. The left eye appeared more dull and glassy than the right. Mr. G. said he could merely distinguish light with it.

Soon after Dr. Harlow arrived, Mr. Gage walked upstairs, with little or no assistance, and laid down upon a bed, when Dr. H. made a thorough examination of the wounds, passing the whole length of his forefinger into the superior opening without difficulty; and my impression is that he did the same with the inferior one, but of that I am not absolutely certain; after this we proceeded to dress the wounds in the manner described by Dr. H. in the Journal. During the time occupied in dressing, Mr. G. vomited two or three times fully as freely as before. All of this time Mr. G. was perfectly conscious, answering all questions, and calling his friends by name as they came into the room.

Harlow 1848 (quoted in Bigelow 1850b, with only changes of abbreviations)

Being absent, I did not arrive at the scene of the accident until near 6 o'clock, P.M. You will excuse me for remarking here, that the picture presented was, to one unaccustomed to military surgery, truly terrific; but the patient bore his sufferings with the most heroic firmness. He recognised me at once, and said he hoped he was not much hurt. He seemed to be perfectly conscious, but was getting exhausted from the hemorrhage, which was very profuse both externally and internally, the blood finding its way into the stomach, which rejected it as often as every fifteen or twenty minutes. Pulse 60, and regular. His person, and the bed on which he was laid, were literally one gore of blood. Assisted by my friend, Dr Williams, of Proctorsville, who was first called to the patient, we proceeded to dress the wounds. From their appearance, the fragments of bone being up-lifted and the brain protruding, it was evident that the fracture was occasioned by some force acting from below upward. The scalp was shaven, the coagula removed, together with three small triangular pieces of the cranium, and in searching to ascertain if there were other foreign bodies there, I passed in the index finger its whole length, without the least resistance, in the direction of the wound in the cheek, which received the other finger in a like manner. A por-tion of the anterior superior angle of each parietal bone, and a semi-circular piece of the frontal bone, were fractured, leaving a circular opening of about $3\frac{1}{2}$ inches in diameter. This examination, and the appearance of the iron which was found some rods distant, smeared with brain, together with the testimony of the work-men, and of the patient himself, who was still sufficiently conscious to say that "the iron struck his head and passed through," was considered at the time suffi-ciently conclusive to show not only the nature of the accident, but the manner in which it occurred.

I have been asked why I did not pass a probe through the entire extent of the wound at the time. I think no surgeon of discretion would have upheld me in the trial of such a foolhardy experiment, in the risk of disturbing lacerated vessels, from which the hemorrhage was near being staunched, and thereby rupturing the attenuated thread, by which the sufferer still held to life. You will excuse me for being thus particular, inasmuch as I am aware that the nature of the injury has been seriously questioned by many medical men for whom I entertain a very high respect.

The spiculae of bone having been taken away, a portion of the brain, which hung by a pedicle, was removed, the larger pieces of bone replaced, the lacerated scalp was brought together as nearly as possible, and retained by adhesive straps, excepting at the posterior angle, and over this a simple dressing—compress, nightcap and roller. The wound in the face was left patulous, covered only by a simple dressing. The hands and fore arms were both deeply burned nearly to the elbows, which were dressed, and the patient was left with the head elevated, and the attendants requested to keep him in that position.

Harlow 1868

He seemed perfectly conscious, but was becoming exhausted from the haemor-rhage, which, by this time, was quite profuse, the blood pouring from the lacer-ated sinus at the top of his head, and also finding its way into the stomach, which ejected it as often as every fifteen or twenty minutes. He bore his sufferings with firmness, and directed my attention to the hole in his cheek, saying "the iron entered there and passed through my head." Pulse at this time 60, soft and regular. He recognised me at once, and said "he hoped he was not much hurt." His person, and the bed on which he lay, was one gore of blood. Assisted by my friend Dr Williams, who was first called to the patient in my absence, we proceeded to examine and dress his wounds. From the appearance of the wound in the top of the head, the fragments of bone being lifted up, the brain protruding from the opening and hanging in shreds upon the hair, it was evident that the opening in the skull was occasioned by some force acting from below, upward, having very much the shape of an inverted funnel, the edges of the scalp everted and the frontal bone extensively fractured, leaving an irregular oblong opening in the skull of two by three and one-half inches. The globe of the left eye was protruded from its orbit by half its diameter, and the left side of the face was more prominent than the right side. The pulsations of the brain were distinctly seen and felt.

The scalp was shaven, the coagula removed, with three small triangular pieces of the frontal bone, and in searching to ascertain if there were foreign bodies in the brain, I passed the index finger of the right hand into the opening its entire length, in the direction of the wound in the cheek, which received the left index finger in like manner, the introduction of the finger into the brain being scarcely felt. Aside from the triangular pieces already alluded to as removed, there were two other pieces detached from the frontal bone, the anterior being two and one-half by two inches, and the posterior one and one-half by two inches in size, leaving the antero-posterior diameter of the opening in the skull fully three and one-half inches.

This examination, and the appearance of the iron which was found some rods distant smeared with blood and brain, together with the testimony of the workmen and of the patient himself, who was sufficiently conscious to say that the iron "struck his head and passed through," was considered at the time as sufficiently conclusive, not only of the nature of the accident, but the manner in which it occurred. The small pieces of bone having been taken away, a portion of the brain, an ounce or more, which protruded, was removed, the larger pieces of bone replaced, the edges of the soft parts approximated as nearly as possible, and over all a wet compress, night cap and roller. The face, hands and arms were deeply burned. The wound in the cheek was left open, the hands and arms were dressed, and the patient was left with the head elevated, and the attendants directed to keep him in that position. This was at $7\frac{1}{2}$ o'clock, P.M.

Case Notes on Gage's Recovery

Note: In those of the following passages preceded by "Harlow 1848 and Bigelow 1850b," the only differences between Harlow and Bigelow are again in spelling or in the latter's expansion or contraction of abbreviations or terms used by Harlow.

13 September

Harlow 1848 and Bigelow 1850b

10, P.M., same evening.—The dressings are saturated with blood, but the hemorrhage appears to be abating. Has vomited twice only since being dressed. Sensorial powers remain as yet unimpaired. Says he does not wish to see his friends, as he shall be at work in a day or two. Tells where they live, their names &c. Pulse 65; constant agitation of the lower extremities.

Harlow 1868

At 10, P.M., same evening, the dressings are saturated with blood, but the haemorrhage is abating. Has vomited twice only, since being dressed. Mind clear. Says he "does not care to see his friends, as he shall be at work in a few days." Gives the names and residence of his relatives in Lebanon, N.H. Pulse 65. Constant agitation of his legs, being alternately retracted and extended like the shafts of a fulling mill.

14 September

Harlow 1848 and Bigelow 1850b

14th, 7, A.M.—Has slept some; appears to be in pain; speaks with difficulty, tumefaction of face considerable, and increasing; pulse 70; knows his friends, and is rational. Asks who is foreman in his pit. Hemorrhage internally continues slightly. Has not vomited since 12, M.

Harlow 1868

At 7, A.M., the 14th, has slept some during the night; appears to be in pain; speaks with difficulty; tumefaction of face considerable, and increasing. Recognises his mother and uncle. Bleeding into mouth continues. Asks who is foreman in his pit. Has not vomited since midnight.

15 September

Harlow 1848 and Bigelow 1850b

15th, 9, A.M.—Has slept well half the night. Sees objects indistinctly with left eye, when the lids are separated. Hemorrhage has ceased. Pulse 75.

8, P.M., same day—Restless and delirious; talks much, but disconnected and incoherent. Pulse 84, and full. Prescribed vin. colchicum, [0.5 dram or 1.85 ml] every six hours, until it purges him. Removed the night-cap.

Harlow 1868

On the following day, 15th, the haemorrhage entirely ceased. Slept well half of the night, and could see objects indistinctly with the left eye.

For a detailed and daily record of the progress of the case, I will refer you to the Boston Medical and Surgical Journal of Dec. 13, 1848. It is sufficient for my present purpose to call your attention to a brief abstract of some of the most important features of the case which followed. On the 15th Sept., two days after the accident, the patient lost control of his mind, and became decidedly delirious, with occasional lucid intervals. On that day a metallic probe was passed into the opening in the top of the head, and down until it reached the base of the skull, without resistance or pain, the brain not being sensitive.

16 September

Harlow 1848 and Bigelow 1850b

16th, 8, A.M.—Patient appears more quiet. Pulse 70. Dressed the wounds, which in the head have a foetid sero-purulent discharge, with particles of brain intermingled. No discharge from bowels. Ordered sulph. magnesia, [1 fluid ounce or 30 ml], repeated every four hours until it operates. Iced water to the head and eye. A fungus appears at the external canthus of the left eye. Says "the left side of his head is banked up."

Harlow 1868

16th, there began an abundant foetid, sanious discharge from the head with particles of brain intermingled, finding its way out from the opening in the top of the head, and also from the one in the base of the skull into the mouth.

17 September

Harlow 1848 and Bigelow 1850b

17th, 8, A.M.—Pulse 84. Purged freely. Rational, and knows his friends. Discharge from the brain profuse, very foetid and sanious. Wound in face healing.

18 September

Harlow 1848 and Bigelow 1850b

18th, 9, A.M.—Slept well all night and lies upon his right side. Pulse 72; tongue red and dry; breath foetid. Removed the dressings and passed a probe to the base of the cranium, without giving pain. Ordered a cathartic, which operated freely. Cold to the head. Patient says he shall recover. He is delirious, with lucid intervals.

Harlow 1868

On the 18th, he slept well nearly all night, but was as incoherent as ever in the morning.

19 September

Harlow 1848 and Bigelow 1850b

19th, 8, P.M.—Has been very restless during the day; skin hot and dry; tongue red; excessive thirst; delirious, talking incoherently with himself and directing his men.

20 and 21 September

Harlow 1848 and Bigelow 1850b

20th and 21st.—Has remained much the same.

22 September

Harlow 1848 and Bigelow 1850b

22d, 8, A.M.—Patient has had a very restless night. Throws his hands and feet about, and tries to get out of bed. Head hot. Says "he shall not live long so." Ordered a cathartic of calomel and rhubarb, to be followed by castor oil, if it does not operate in six hours.

4, P.M., same day—Purged freely twice, and inclines to sleep.

Harlow 1868

22d, at 8, A.M., I learn that he has had a very restless night. Throws his hands and feet about, tries to get out of bed. Head very hot. Says "he shall not live long so."

23 September

Harlow 1848 and Bigelow 1850b

23d.—Rested well most of the night, and appears stronger and more rational. Pulse 80. Shaved the scalp a second time, and brought the edges of the wound in position, the previous edges having sloughed away. Discharge less in quantity and less foetid. Loss of vision of left eye.

Harlow 1868

23d, I find he has rested and been quiet most of the night. Appears stronger and more rational. Pulse, which has varied from 60 to 84 since the injury, I find at 80. The scalp was reshaven and the edges of the wound brought into apposition as nearly as possible, the edges having sloughed away. The discharge is less in quantity and less foetid.

At this date, ten days after the injury, vision of the left eye, though quite indistinct before, was totally lost. Up to this time it had not occurred to me that it was *possible* for Gage to recover. The head had been dressed by myself three times every day; ice water kept on the head and face; the discharges carefully cleaned off, externally, while the attendants washed the mouth and fauces as often as necessary, with water and disinfecting solutions. The opening in the top of the head was always carefully covered in oiled silk underneath the wet compresses. Today he appears stronger and more rational than before; calls for food.

Period between 23 and 28 September

Harlow 1868

Sept. 24th, 9, A.M.. I find in my notes, taken at the time, that he has a pulse at 84; vision with right eye, and hearing with both ears, normal; bowels confined; can tell the day of the week and time of day; remembers persons who have visited him and incidents which have transpired since his injury. This improvement, however, was of short duration, though the discharge from the wounds had abated. I learned that in the night following he became stupid, did not speak unless aroused, and then only with difficulty; the integuments between the lower edge of the fracture in frontal bone and left nasal protuberance, swollen, hot and red, something like an erysipelatous blush. Pulse 96, soft. Failing strength. Is supported with food and stimulants. During the three succeeding days the coma deepened; the globe of the left eye became more protuberant, with fungus pushing out rapidly from the internal canthus. This fungus first made its appearance on the 19th, six days after the injury; also large fungi pushing up rapidly from the wounded brain, and coming out at the opening in the top of the head. On the 27th, the swelling upon the forehead horribly foetid. Pulse 84. Comatose, but will answer in monosyllables when aroused. Will not take nourishment unless strongly urged. Calls for nothing. Surface and extremities incline to be cool. Discharge from the wound scanty, its exit being interfered with by the fungi. The friends and attendants are in hourly expectancy of his death, and have his coffin and clothes in readiness to remove his remains immediately to his native place in New Hampshire. One of the attendants implored me not to do anything more for him, as it would only prolong his sufferings—that if I would only keep away and let him alone, he would die. She said he appeared like "water on the brain." I said it is not water, but matter that is killing the man—so with a pair of curved scissors I cut off the fungi which were sprouting out from the top of the brain and filling the opening, and made free application of caustic to them. With a scalpel I laid open the integuments, between the opening and the roots of the nose, and immediately there were discharged eight ounces [240 ml] of ill-conditioned pus, with blood, and excessively foetid. Tumefaction of left side of face increased. Globe of left eye very prominent.

Period from 23 September to 3 October

Harlow 1848 and Bigelow 1850b

From this time until the 3d. October, he lay in a semi-comatose state, seldom speaking unless spoken to, and then answering only in monosyllables. During this period, fungi started from the brain, and increasing rapidly from the orbit. To these was applied nitrate of silver cryst., and cold to the head generally. The dressings were renewed three times in every twenty-four hours; and in addition to this, laxatives, combined with an occasional dose of calomel, constituted the treatment. The pulse varied from 70 to 96—generally very soft. During this time an abscess formed under the frontalis muscle, which was opened on the 27th, and has been very difficult to heal. Discharged nearly [8 fluid ounces or 240 ml] at the time it was punctured.

Period between 27 September and 6 October

Harlow 1868

From this date, Sept. 28th, to Oct. 6th, the discharge from the openings was very profuse and foetid. Erysipelatous blush on the skin of the left side of face and head. Pulse ranging from 80 to 96. Speaks only when spoken to. Swallows well, and takes considerable nourishment, with brandy and milk; says he has no pain.

5 and 6 October

Harlow 1848 and Bigelow 1850b

Oct. 5th and 6th.—Patient improving. Discharge from the wound and sinus, laudable pus. Calls for his pants and wishes to get out of bed, though he is unable to raise his head from the pillow.

Harlow 1868

Oct. 6th—twenty-three days after the injury—I find entered in my note book as follows:—General appearance somewhat improved; pulse 90, and regular; more wakeful; swelling of left side of face abating; erysipelas gone; openings discharging laudable pus profusely; calls for his pants, and desires to be helped out of bed, though when lying upon his back cannot raise his head from the pillow. By turning to one side he succeeded in rising, and sat upon the edge of the bed for about four minutes. Says he feels comfortable. Appears demented, or in a state of mental hebetude.

7 October

Harlow 1848 and Bigelow 1850b

7th.—Has succeeded in raising himself up, and took one step to his chair, and sat about five minutes.

11 October

Harlow 1848 and Bigelow 1850b

11th.—Pulse 72. Intellectual faculties brightening. When I asked him how long since he was injured, he replied "four weeks this afternoon at $4\frac{1}{2}$ o'clock." Relates the manner in which it occurred, and how he came to the house. He keeps the day of the week and time of day, in his mind. Says he knows more than half of those who inquire after him. Does not estimate size or money accurately, though he has memory as perfect as ever. He would not take $1000 for a few pebbles which he took from an ancient river bed where he was at work. The fungus is giving way under the use of the crys. nitrate of silver. During all of this time there has been a discharge of pus into the fauces, a part of which passed into the stomach, the remainder being ejected from the mouth.

Harlow 1868

Oct. 11th—twenty-eighth day—Very clear in his mind; states how long he has been upon his bed, how he was injured, the particulars of the explosion, and the time in the day when it occurred.

15 October

Harlow 1868

Oct. 15th—thirty-second day.—Progressing favourably. Fungi disappearing; discharging laudable pus from openings. Takes more food, sleeps well and says he shall soon go home. Remembers passing and past events correctly, as well before as since the injury. Intellectual manifestations feeble, being exceedingly capricious and childish, but with a will indomitable as ever; is particularly obstinate; will not yield to restraint when it conflicts with his desires.

20 October

Harlow 1848 and Bigelow 1850b

20th.—Improving. Gets out and into bed with but little assistance. Sits up thirty minutes twice in twenty-four hours. Is very childish; wishes to go home to Lebanon, N. H. The wound in the scalp is healing rapidly.

Harlow 1868

Oct. 20th—thirty-seventh day—Improving; gets out and into bed with but little assistance; eats and sleeps well. Sensorial powers improving, and mind somewhat clearer, but very childish. The fungi have disappeared. The opening in the top of the head is closing up rapidly, with a firm membranous tissue.

8 November

Harlow 1848 and Bigelow 1850b

Nov. 8th.—Improving in every particular, and sits up most of the time during the day. Appetite good, though he is still kept upon a low diet. Pulse 65. Sleeps well, and says he has no pain in the head. Food digests easily, bowels regular, and nutrition is going on well. The sinus under the frontalis muscle has nearly healed. He walks up and down stairs, and about the house, into the piazza, and I am informed this evening that he has been in the street to-day.—I leave him for a week, with strict instructions to avoid excitement and exposure.

Harlow 1868

Nov. 8th—fifty-sixth day.—Improving in every respect. Sits up most of the time during the day. Appetite good, though he is not allowed on a full diet. Pulse 65. Sleeps well, and says he has not any pain in his head. He walks downstairs, about the house and into the piazza, and I am informed that he has been in the street to-day. I leave him today, with strict injunctions to avoid excitement and exposure.

15 November

Harlow 1848 and Bigelow 1850b

15th.—I learn on inquiry, that Gage has been in the street every day except Sunday, during my absence. His desire to be out and to go home to Lebanon has been uncontrollable by his friends, and he has been making arrangements to that effect. Yesterday he walked half a mile, and purchased some small articles at the store. The atmosphere was cold and damp, the ground wet, and he went without an overcoat, and with thin boots. He got wet feet and a chill. I find him in bed, depressed and very irritable. Hot and dry skin; thirst; tongue coated; pulse 110; lancinating pain in left side of head and face, rigors, and bowels constipated. Ordered cold to the head and face, and a black dose to be repeated in six hours, if it does not operate. He has had spiculae of bone pass into the fauces, which he expelled from the mouth within a few days.

Harlow 1868

Nov. 15th—sixty-fourth day—Returned last evening, and learn that Gage has been in the street every day during my absence, excepting Sunday. Is impatient of restraint and could not be controlled by his friends. Making arrangements to go home. Yesterday he walked half a mile, purchased some articles at the store, inquired the price, and paid the money with his habitual accuracy; did not appear to be particular as to the price, provided he had money to meet it. The atmosphere was cold and damp, the ground wet, and he went without an overcoat, and with thin boots; got wet feet and a chill. I find him in bed, depressed and very irritable; hot and dry skin; thirst; tongue coated; pulse 110; lancinating pain in left side of head and face; rigors, and bowels constipated. Ordered cold to the head and face and a cathartic, to be taken and repeated if it does not operate in six hours.

16 November

Harlow 1848 and Bigelow 1850b

16th, A.M.—No better. Cathartic has operated freely. Pulse 120; skin hot and dry; thirst and pain remain the same. Has been very restless during the night. Venesection [16 fluid ounces or 475 ml]. Ordered calomel, [10 grains or 650 mg] and ipecac. [2 grains or 130 mg] followed in four hours by castor oil.

8, P.M., same day.—Purged freely; pulse less frequent; pain in head moderated; skin moist. R. Antim. et potassa tart., [3 grains or 195 mg]; syr.simplex, [6 fluid ounces or 180 ml]. Dose a dessertspoonful every four hours.

Harlow 1868

Nov. 16th, A.M.—No better. Cathartic has operated freely. Pulse 120; has passed a sleepless night; skin hot and dry; pain and thirst unabated. Was bled from the arm [16 fluid ounces or 475 ml], and got: R. Hydrarg. chloridi, [10 grains or 650 mg], ipecac, [2 grains or 130 mg].

8, P.M., same day.—Pulse falling; heat and pain moderated. Took a solution of ant. pot. tart. during night, and slept well.

17 November

Harlow 1848 and Bigelow 1850b

17th.—Improving. Expresses himself as "feeling better in every respect;" has no pain in the head.

Harlow 1868

17th, A.M.—Much improved. Has purged freely during night, and says he feels better every way. Has no pain in head.

18 November

Harlow 1848 and Bigelow 1850b

18th.—Is walking about house again; says he feels no pain in the head, and appears to be in a way of recovering if he can be controlled. At this date I shall leave the case at present.

Final Clinical Status

Harlow 1848

The result, and a few remarks of a practical nature, together with the mental manifestations of the patient, I reserve for a future communication. I think the case presents one fact of great interest to the practical surgeon, and, taken as a whole, is exceedingly interesting to the enlightened physiologist and intellectual philosopher. In my effort to be brief, which I fear you will think an utter failure, I have omitted much in my notes, which might interest some readers. Allow me to say here, that I have seen a communication in "The Reflector and the Watchman," stating that "there is a piece of bone loose in the top of his head, as large as a dollar, which will have to be removed, should he live." The fractured portions of bone, excepting those which were removed at the first dressing, have united firmly, and the above remark was made unadvisedly. Should you think these notes of sufficient importance to deserve a place in your Journal, they are at your service.

Bigelow 1850b

Remarks—The leading feature of this case is its improbability. A physician who holds in his hand a crowbar, three feet and a half long, and more than thirteen pounds in weight, will not readily believe that it has been driven with a crash through the brain of a man who is still able to walk off, talking with composure and equanimity of the hole in his head. This is the sort of accident that happens in the pantomime at the theatre, but not elsewhere. Yet there is every reason for supposing it in this case literally true. Being at first wholly sceptical, I have been personally convinced; and this has been the experience of many medical gentlemen who, having first heard of the circumstances, have had a subsequent opportunity to examine the evidence.

18 November

Harlow 1868

18th.—Is walking about house again, free from pain in head, and appears to be in a way of recovering, if he can be controlled. Has recently had several pieces of bone pass into the fauces, which he expelled from the mouth. The discharge from the head very slight, and the opening steadily closing up.

25 November to April 1849

Harlow 1849 (note dated 3 January)
Gage at Lebanon is "walking about the house, and riding out, improving both mentally and physically."

Harlow 1868
On the 25th he was taken, in a close carriage, a distance of thirty miles, to Lebanon, N. H., his home, where I saw him in the succeeding week, and found him going on well. He continued to improve steadily, until on Jan. 1, 1849, the opening in the top of his head was entirely closed, and the brain shut out from view, though every pulsation could be distinctly seen and felt. Gage passed the succeeding winter months in his own house and vicinity, improving in flesh and strength, and in the following April returned to Cavendish, bringing his "iron" with him.

He visited me at that time, and presented something like the following appearances. General appearance good; stands quite erect, with his head inclined slightly towards the right side; his gait in walking is steady; his movements rapid and easily executed. The left side of the face is wider than the right side, the left malar bone being more prominent than its fellow. There is a linear cicatrix near the angle of the lower jaw, an inch in length. Ptosis of the left eyelid; the globe considerably more prominent than its fellow, but not as large as when I last saw him. Can adduct and depress the globe, but cannot move it in other directions; vision lost. A linear cicatrix, length two and one-half inches, from the nasal protuberance to the anterior edge of the raised fragment of the frontal bone, is quite unsightly. Upon the top of the head, and covered with hair, is a large unequal depression and elevation—a quadrangular fragment of bone, which was entirely detached from the frontal and extending low down upon the forehead, being still raised and quite prominent. Behind this is a deep depression, two inches by one and one-half inches wide, beneath which the pulsations of the brain can be perceived. Partial paralysis of left side of face. His physical health is good, and I am inclined to say that he has recovered. Has no pain in the head, but says it has a queer feeling which he is not able to describe.

Appendix C

The Statement of Walton A. Green

Introduction

The original of Walton A. Green's statement is held by the Norman Williams Public Library in Woodstock, Vermont, where it is catalogued as part of "WP 080 Williams, Edward Higginson 1824." The statement is on pages 7 and 8 of the typescript of what purports to be an article from an undated issue of the *Vermont Tribune*. The article, entitled "Recovery from the Passage of an Iron Bar through the Head," is clearly based on a copy of Harlow's 1868 report on Gage. According to its opening sentence, it was sent to the *Tribune* by Judge Charles H. Scott, of Tyson.

The first three words with which Green's statement is introduced ("The following was"), the whole of the last sentence ("The above is a true statement … Adams and myself"), a flourish rather like the finish to a statutory declaration, and the signature are handwritten, presumably by Green.

Nancy Bacon, then librarian of the Norman Williams Public Library in Woodstock, Vermont, who sent me this copy of Green's statement in January 1990, had no idea of its source. Sandra Stearns of the Cavendish Historical Society later gave me another, slightly different, copy with the words "Published V Tribune 7-12-1929" written by hand on it, with the date August 11, 1943, typed under Green's name, and omitting the handwritten introduction and declaratory flourish. In this reproduction, I have retained the typing errors, spelling, punctuation, and capitalization of the original. I am grateful to the Norman Williams Public Library for permission to reproduce Green's statement.

Walton Green's Statement

The following was

Written February 26, 1938, by Walton A. Green, Proctorsville, Vt.

This certifies that I served with Christopher W Goodrich (aged 82) and Joseph H. Adams (aged about 75) popularly known as "Deaf Joe" as one of the Listers or Tax Assessors, in 1906. While we were appraising real estate in the vicinity of the accident to Phineas Gage, Mr. Goodrich showed us the exact spot where the accident occured, and then explained how he took him in his ox cart to his boarding place in Cavendish village. Gage boarded at the tavern, or hotel, which then stood directly across the road from where the solier's monumentiis (where the Aura Austin house now stands).

Let it be remembered that in those days ox teams were the usual mode of heavy hauling as horses were mostly too light for such work. Mr. Goodrich, who at that time was about 24, was known to have kept one of the best ox teams in town and made a business of working out with his teams all his life. He owned a fine pair when he was 82.

The accident took place at the second cut south of Cavendish where many potholes in the rock give indisputable evidence that black river once went this way near where Roswell Downer built his lime kiln later.

Thomas Winslow, who had a cabinet shop below where Floyd Gay's garage is now situated, was called in to measure Gage (as was the custom in those days) and he made a coffin for him in readiness to use.

Dr. Harlow, at that time lived where Will Butler now lives. He sold out to Dr. Hazelton, who in turn sold to Dr. Spafford, and Mrs. Butler is Dr. Spafford's daughter.

Dr. Williams, who Dr. Harlow speaks of, lived and practiced medicine in Proctorsville village at the time.

The above is a true statement of facts made by
Christopher W Goodrich in the presence
of Joseph H Adams and myself.   *Walton A. Green*

Appendix D

Ferrier's Letters to Bowditch about Gage

The set of letters transcribed here from David Ferrier to Henry Pickering Bowditch are held as autographs by the Countway Library of Harvard University where they are catalogued as "H MS, c 5.2. Ferrier, Sir David, 1843–1929. 4 A.L.s. to Henry Pickering Bowditch; London, 1877–1879."

Each letter is written on two sheets of paper in the form seen here. After folding the sheets of paper in two, Ferrier began each letter on the right hand side of sheet one, then continued on sheet two, first on the left hand and then the right hand side, before finishing on the left-hand side of sheet one. Keeping to Ferrier's format makes the task of comparing the transcriptions with the originals easier. I have transcribed the letters as accurately as possible, but Ferrier's writing is so difficult to read that it would not surprise me if they contained errors. The whole set of the letters is reproduced; each letter is also complete, and all retain Ferrier's punctuation, spelling, abbreviations, and capitalization.

The paper on which the third letter of February 10, 1878 is written is edged in black.

I am pleased to be able to thank Richard Wolfe of the Countway for permission to reproduce the letters, and a typescript of the set has now been deposited there. Unfortunately, the whereabouts of Bowditch's replies to Ferrier are not known.

16, Upper Berkeley Street,
Portman Square. W.
October 12, 1877

My Dear Bowditch,

I am writing to ask you to do me a little favour.

It is in reference to a rather celebrated specimen which I believe exists in the museum of your University—the skull of the man who had a tamping-iron projected through his head.

From the account given by Dr. Bigelow in the American Journal of the Medical Sciences, July 1850 and the drawing which he there gives of his experiments on a skull with the object of determining the exact seat of the lesion I came to the conclusion that the injury was confined to the region in advance of the coronal suture. Dr. Dupuy has lately been writing in the Medical Times & Gazette that he can prove conclusively that it destroyed the Island of Reil and what not.

Now I should be very much obliged to you if you would examine the skull carefully & tell me exactly the line [lines?] of entrance & exit of the iron bar & the appearance presented. Better still it would be if you could furnish me with a sketch of the preparation In investigating the reports on diseases and injuries of the brain I am constantly being amazed at the inexactitude and distortion to which they are subjected by men who have some pet theory to support. The facts suffer so frightfully that I feel obliged always to go to the fountain head—dirty and muddy though this frequently turns out

Trusting to hear from you soon. With kind regards to yourself & to Putnam.

Yours very sincerely

David Ferrier.

16 , Upper Berkeley Street,
Portman Square. W.
December 28, 1877

My Dear Bowditch,

I can't say how much I feel indebted to you and Putnam for the magnificent photographs of the "Crowbar Case" which I received yesterday. They practically bring the skull itself before me and I look forward with intense satisfaction to presenting them before the London Physicians in my lectures in March next. Now I am going to ask you still another favour. Of course you will write a paper on the subject and reproduce the photographs. If it is not too much to ask I should like to be the publisher myself in my lectures, at least in the first instance, as in this way a charm of novelty will be given to my remarks on this case in my lectures. So that if you are not in a great hurry perhaps you can wait till then before bringing out your paper in extenso.

I should have been glad to have had in your own words, a brief statement of the locality of the lesion, for though the photographs are so good that I can make one for myself, still a few lines from you might have been an apt paragraph for quotation in my lectures

I should like if you would compare the diagram given by Bigelow in the Amer. Jour. Med. Sc. July 1850 & tell me if you agree with me in thinking that Bigelow has represented the track of the bar a little too much towards the middle line & beyond it & also somewhat nearer the coronal suture than was actually the case. It seems to me from the opening at the left-side of the middle line that the bar did not cross the middle line at all, & that it emerged more in front raising the flap of bone hanging on the line of fracture on the right side of the frontal. In which case the left anterior lobe was alone injured.

Bigelow also represents the hole in the base of the skull a little further outwards from the middle line than the photograph warrants. As it is however I think I shall have a triumphant case against Dupuy and others.

Is there any further account of the case, with post-mortem etc. beyond that given by Bigelow? I have an idea there is, but I cannot find any reference to it.

I am very anxious to have this case definitely settled as it is one of more than usual interest and importance in a localisation point of view.

With kind regards & many thanks to yourself & Putnam.

Yours very sincerely
David Ferrier

16 Upper Berkeley Street
London W
February 10, 1878

My Dear Bowditch,

I hope that long ere this time you have got the telegram I sent off the other day and which I hope was sufficiently clear as to its meaning. I found in looking at Dr. Harlow's account of the Crowbar case that the woodcuts he gives would be a very desirable accompaniment to my lectures which I am to give early in March & which I shall publish in the Med. Journals & perhaps separately.

To avoid delay & ensure my getting the woodcuts in time, always supposing the possibility of getting them at all, I thought it desirable to employ a swifter form of message than by letter. I do hope you will be able to get at least clichés of the woodcuts from Dr Harlow or the publisher (Clapp & Son Boston) and I shall be everlastingly grateful. I did not know of their existence till you sent me Harlow's paper which has been of the greatest value to me.

I think your proposal to simulate the lesion with the brain in situ would be a most desirable experiment. I am sure I cannot suggest anything to you in the way of carrying it out as the indications furnished by Turner, Broca, Féré &cc will guide you sufficiently.

Bucknell, Crichton-Browne, Hughlings-Jackson and I are about to bring out a new Journal of Neurology entitled "Brain". We propose to get the first no out in April, and every quarter after. I have been asked by my brother editors to solicit contributions from you and from Putnam. Kindly ask Putnam for me, until I get time to write to him directly at more length. I hope your answer will be in the affirmative. Contributions, anatomical, physiological, pathological & therapeutical in the nervous system of any kind will form the subject of our Journal.

The paper on which I write is the sign of a grievous bereavement I have recently sustained—my only child, a daughter of 2½ years. I have been quite [unfitted?] for all work of late. Kindest regards to Putnam & yourself.

Yours very sincerely
David Ferrier

16, Upper Berkeley Street,
Portman Square. W.
January 15, 1879

My Dear Bowditch,

I have given orders to my publishers Smith Elder & Co to transmit to you the woodcuts of the crowbar case for which I was so very much indebted to you. I think you will find them unworn [illegible word], as my illustrations were all taken from clichés of the blocks.

The case has excited very considerable interest here, & your photographs created quite a sensation at the College of Physicians—as they brought the facts home in such a telling manner.

I hope—Bigelow notwithstanding—that Putnam & you will really carry out your proposed investigation. I can do no experimental work now—I am quite relegated to clinical medicine & therapeutics.

I used in former days to be able to retire in the evening & do a lot of work quietly in my private laboratory. All this is done away with as I cannot work under the accursed antivivisection laws which hamper private research so much.

I suppose there is no use in asking you to give us a paper for "Brain", but still if you should relent we should be delighted to have a contribution from you.

Please give my kindest regards to Putnam & believe me

Yours very sincerely
David Ferrier

Appendix E

The CT Scans of Phineas Gage's Skull

The CT images of Phineas Gage's skull reproduced here were made for Dr. H. Richard Tyler and Dr. Kenneth L. Tyler. When the CT scan first became available, Drs. Ken and Rick Tyler, with the cooperation of Mr. D. Gunner, Curator of the Warren Museum, and Dr. Rumbaugh, Head of the Neuroradiology Section of the Brigham and Womens Hospital, utilized the instrument to demonstrate the actual defects of Phineas Gage's skull caused by the passage of the crowbar. The images were used in the presentation by the Drs. Tyler to the 1982 meeting of the Academy of Neurology, but have not otherwise been published. I am greatly indebted to the Drs. Tyler for making them available for inclusion in *An Odd Kind of Fame*, and especially to Dr. H. Richard Tyler for his comments about them.

The most immediately relevant images are reproduced in chapter 5, but a fuller set is reproduced here. The images are of two kinds: lateral and frontal. The lateral scans contain information about the healing of the larger pieces of frontal bone that were wholly or partly detached at the time of the accident. From them, some judgment of how vertical was the trajectory of the tamping iron can be made. They also indicate how close the area in which the tamping iron emerged was to the junction of the coronal and sagittal sutures. The frontal images also gradually move from the front of the skull toward the back. They contain most of the information about the relation of the area of emergence to the midline. Taken together, they suggest that the larger part of the area in which the tamping iron emerged lay in front of the junction of the coronal and sagittal sutures and to the left of the midline.

The Drs. Tyler make the point that they used the skull landmarks to hypothesize the *minimal* lesion the crowbar would have caused in the brain. They point out that secondary bone fragments and the subsequent infection made a larger lesion than the minimal one almost a certainty.

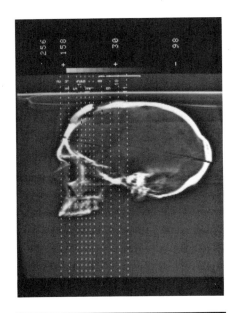

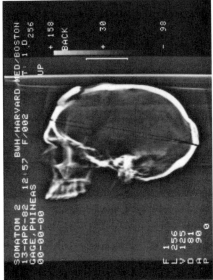

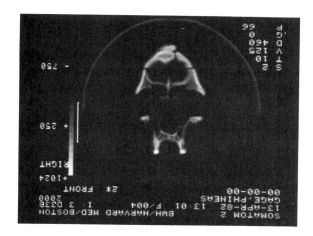

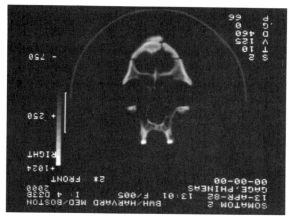

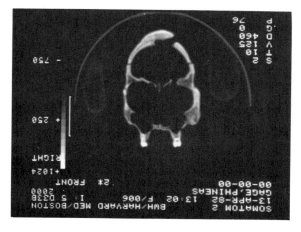

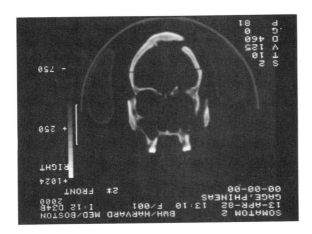

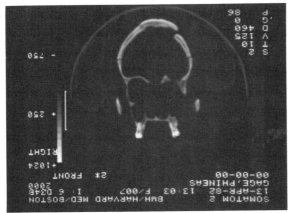

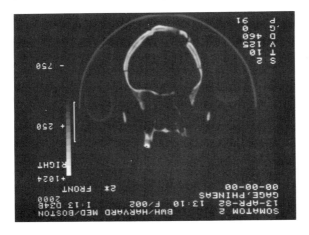

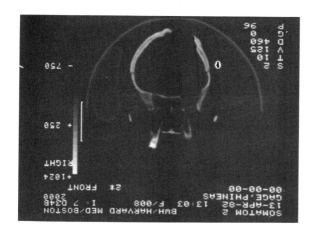

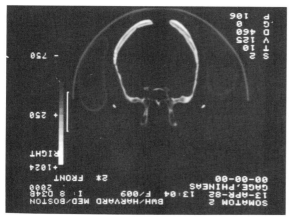

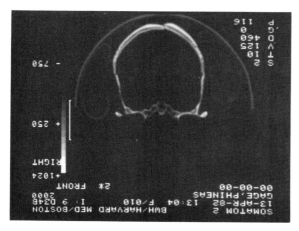

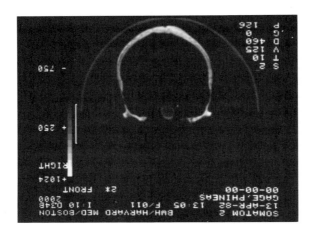

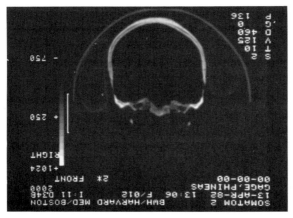

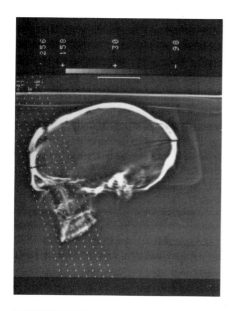

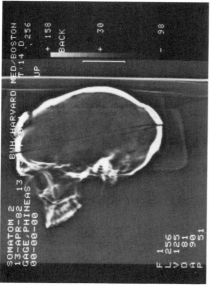

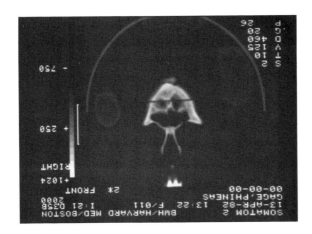

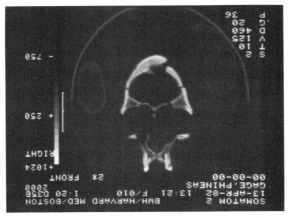

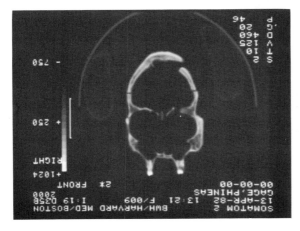

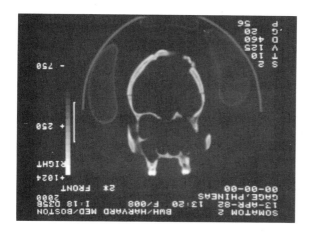

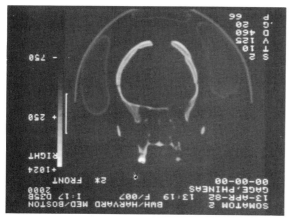

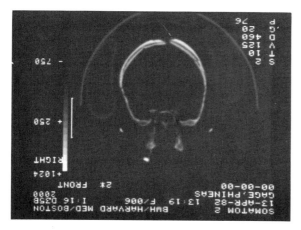

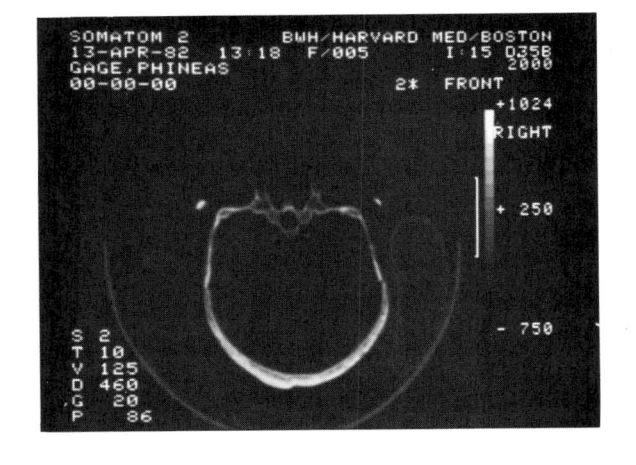

Appendix F

Harlow's Presentations to the Middlesex East District Medical Society

Introduction

The material reproduced in Appendix F comes from the collection of papers of the Middlesex East District Medical Society held by the Woburn Public Library, Woburn, Massachusetts. I am very appreciative of the effort made by the Librarian, Kathleen O'Doherty, to find them and to Tom Smith for having copies made for me of the photographs of Gage's skull that were originally made for Harlow. I am also extremely grateful to the Trustees of the Library for permission to reproduce them.

Here I have included in narrative form the short entries about Harlow's donating photographs of Gage's skull to the society. The other material reproduces in whole or in part the papers Harlow gave to the society or the versions of them recorded in the minutes. It is the four cases and the expert appreciation of them that are the most valuable and important. However, I could not resist extracting that part of the discussion at another of the meetings provoked by the tapeworm Harlow presented.

Harlow's Presentation of the Photographs of Gage's Skull

The minutes of the December 1868 meeting of the Middlesex East District Medical Society note that "Dr. Harlow exhibited some plates [i.e., photographic prints] [*of* crossed out] taken from the Skull and Crowbar, from the case published in the proceedings of the State Society" (Middlesex East District Medical Society, Record Book, vol. 1, p. 147). At the next meeting of the Society, on 27 January, the proceedings opened with, "Donations being called for, Dr. Harlow gave to the Society a set of Plates illustrating the case of Injury to the Head, alluded to at the last meeting. A vote of thanks was given him for this gift" (p. 47). The photographs were then fixed into the Record book between pages 148 and 150 and bibliographic details of Harlow's and Bigelow's papers written on the pages.

The photographs Harlow exhibited and donated are those of Gage's skull and the tamping iron taken for him by S. Webster Wyman, photographer of Woburn. Mentioned in chapter 5, they seem to be the basis for the blocks used in Harlow's

1868 paper and also used by J. B. S. Jackson as the frontispiece to the Warren Museum *Catalogue* (1870). They may also be the photographs Bowditch sent to Ferrier and which seem to have been obtained from Harlow. The original glass plate negatives no longer seem to exist. Possibly they were lost in the massive fire of 1873 that destroyed four acres of Woburn's business district, including Wyman's studio in Kelly's block. But they may still exist in that same limbo where Harlow's case notes and other material now apparently missing from the Warren are stored.

Harlow's Tapeworm

Record Book of the Middlesex East District Medical Society, Volume III. July 13, 1881–Aug 22, 1888.
Extract from minutes of meeting of 4th. November, 1884:

Woburn, November 4th, 1884

The society held its 259th monthly meeting at the Central House, Woburn, being entertained by Dr. Bartlett. The following members were present: Drs. Down, Cowdery, Bartlett, Harlow, Sheldon, Nickerson, Hodgdon, Winsor, Putney, March, Odlin, F. F. Brown, W. S. Brown, also Drs. C. D. Homans and Hon. Ingalls of Boston.

Dr. Harlow, apologizing that he had no rarer specimen to offer, presented a tape worm 8 feet in length which he had obtained from a patient (a Harvard college student) whose symptoms at first seemed to indicate that he had typhoid fever but who recovered after the passage of the worm. His method of obtaining the tape worm he had mentioned to the society on previous occasions and was sufficiently common and simple. On being urged he gave it once more. He directs an emulsion of the common pumpkin seed, *circurbita pepo*. Take [4 ounces or 125 gm] fresh seeds and boil in [6 fluid ounces or 180 ml] milk. Divide into three parts. After a preliminary fast of six hours give one portion of the emulsion every three hours until all has been taken. After the last dose give an ounce of castor oil with two drams of turpentine. The worm follows. He never succeeded without the aid of turpentine.

Dr Holmes remarked that in thirty years of all the specimens of tænia presented to this society he believed that the head had never once been shown. In a recent case he had used an infusion of the Bermuda pumpkin seed, four ounces in coffee, which he administered in three doses at intervals of two hours, following the last dose with first 10 grs [10 grains or 648 mgm] calomel and 5 grs [5 grains or 324 mgm] jalap, then [fluid ounce 15 ml] castor oil. He feels confident that the whole worm was expelled but he cannot find the head. A patient to whom he gave the castor oil and turpentine combined complained that the remedy was worse than the disease and asserted that he should prefer the disease to the remedy.

Harlow's cases

The following reports of Harlow's cases are the only four located in the Woburn collection of papers. Cases 2 and 4 are separate, fully written-out manuscripts, the former appearing to me to be in Harlow's own hand, and those of Cases 1 and 3 are included in the minutes of meetings.

Ian Cope, MD, [Fellow of the Royal College of Surgeons, Fellow of the Royal Australasian College of Surgeons, Fellow of the Royal College of Obstetricians and Gynaecologists and Fellow of the Royal Australian College of Obstetricians and Gynaecologists], examined the manuscripts for me with a view to evaluating Harlow's medical knowledge and skill against the standards of the time. Dr. Cope is Chairman of the Archives, Library and College Collection of the Royal Australian College of Obstetricians and Gynaecologists. He has a considerable knowledge of the history of nineteenth-century medicine, especially of obstetrics and gynaecology. His opinions and comments are as follows:

The management of the cases of placenta praevia (1878 and 1891) was appropriate and indicate expertise for the times. The principles of management had not changed significantly since Denman's Textbook of 1802 (Thomas Denman [1802]. *An Introduction to the Practice of Midwifery*. New York: James Oram for William Falconer and Evert Duyckinck) but as Braxton Hicks (1889) indicates, the maternal mortality rate had been reduced from 30% to somewhere near 5% over the previous 30 years (presumably because of increased expertise demonstrated by the doctors). It was not until the late 1920's that caesarean section came to be used.

The case of imperforate hymen and his report of true knot in the umbilical cord are not exceptional. The management was appropriate.

The discussion 1884 of the case of abdominal pain may have been one of intussusception but more likely appendicitis—"typhlitis." Howard Kelly and E. Burdon 1905 in their volume of the Vermiform Appendix and its Diseases discuss the early reports of appendicitis, 1759 to 1886, and "typhlitis." They describe (p. 28) how Reginald Fitz, of Boston in 1886 cleared up the entire subject leading to the understanding of the morbid conditions affecting the vermiform appendix. The discussion of 1884 is in keeping with the understanding of the time and is interesting as it details the situation shortly before Fitz's paper was presented.

In summary, Harlow's medical knowledge for the times was good and his level of skill appears to be above average.

Case 1:   Placenta Praevia

(From minutes)
Record Book of the Middlesex East District Medical Society, Volume II. Beginning March 1870, pp. 166–169. [The period covered in Volume II is actually 30 March 1870 to 13 July 1881.]
Full record of meeting of 13th, November 1878

Woburn Mass
November 13th. 1878.

The Society held this evening its one hundred and ninety fifth meeting as the guests of Dr. Kelly at the Central House.
Present Drs. Abbott, W. S. Brown, F. F. Brown, Bartlett, Baiss [?], Chase, Cutter, Graves, Harlow, Hodgdon, Holmes, Kelley, Weight & Winsor.

The president in the chair.
The records of previous meeting not being present were dispensed with.
Dr. Abbott appointed secretary position.
Voted on motion of Dr. Winsor that the Secretary be authorized to prepare & keep on hand an index of all papers read before the Soc. & specimens exhibited for future reference.
Dr. Kelley reports a case of typhoid fever, a boy 10 years old, after convalescence began an ulcer appeared near each angle of the mouth, which increased until there was a slough in each cheek about 2 inches in diameter. Boy is now recovering with considerable loss of substance.

The Society adjourned to supper, after which the records of previous meeting were read & [*approved* crossed out] amended.

Dr. Harlow read the notes of the following case of Placenta Prævia, Twins, mother & children saved.
Mrs. ———. aet. 42, had a miscarriage 14 months ago at 4th month: about the 4th month of present pregnancy she was threatened with miscarriage [*which* crossed out].
On the morning of Nov. 2nd pt awoke to find herself flowing, no pain. Dr. H——— made an examination oss not dilated, but felt over it a pulpy mass which he judged to be placenta. ordered rest, she remained in bed a week, & on the 10th awoke flowing severely. Dr. H——— was called, found oss about the size of half dollar, felt the placenta but no head, at this time there was not much bleeding; four hours later the oss had dilated to the size of a dollar & the head was pressing down, ruptured membranes, bleeding slight & for $\frac{1}{2}$ an hour no pains, then they came frequently & regularly, at 9AM delivered a boy weighing $6\frac{1}{2}$ lbs. [*illegible word*] seemed very short. on examining for placenta found something in vagina which he supposed was it, but which proved not to be placenta of child delivered, it was soon followed, however, by the other placenta, he then discovered the breech of a second child presenting, which he delivered, it being a female child weighing 5 lbs, alive though delivered about 10 minutes after its placenta. Dr. Harlow thought about a quarter of the placenta had been detached for a week previous. In the conduct of this case, as the hemorrhage was not great, Dr. H. had left the case to nature.

Dr. W. S. Brown thought that if the diagnosis of placenta prævia was made, he might be inclined to induce premature labor. In answer to Dr. Cutter's question "What he would do if placenta was central," Dr. Harlow said if oss was dilated or dilatable would separate it & bring down the feet & deliver, if it was not would plug: thought the practice of going through the placenta was wrong.

Dr. Cutter thought the fact of Dr. Harlow's child being delivered alive 10 minutes after the placenta, would be in favor of separating the placenta & delivering.

Dr. Harlow's experience was that children born at 7th mon. were more likely to live than those at 8th mo. why it was so he was unable to say.

Dr. Abbott said that the popular idea about seven months children being more viable was a very old one, even mentioned by Hypocrates; but the medico-legal authority he had recently consulted, considered it absurd.

Dr. Hodgdon thought it difficult to establish any specific rule for such cases, it seemed to him that in many cases of p.p. the uterus did not seem to act as well as in ordinary cases, he had had two cases of central implantation; both cases did well, in the second he thought he went through the placenta, of this however he was not positive: he would not induce labor unless symptoms were urgent as he considered child's chances less & there was more difficulty in dilating he could not appreciate the great objection to penetrating placenta.

Dr. Winsor had had one case of partial prævia, but it attended to its self agreed with Dr. Hodgdon to treat each case according to circumstances should be inclined to tell the parents previous to delivery that the child would probably die, would like to know rate of mortality in the practices of the members. Dr. Cutter's one case central p.p. died. Dr. W. S. Brown about $\frac{1}{2}$ dozen cases partial p.p. about $\frac{1}{2}$ saved.

Dr. Dow 2 cases partial recovered; one complete both mother & child died.

Dr. Harlow reported a case of brain disease & showed the specimen of the brain, containing a small tumor of the left hemisphere of the cerebellum, which pressing on a large vein had deprived the surrounding parts of part of its nutrition & caused quite a large cyst.

Dr. Harlow showed the specimen of a portion of duodenum from the late Dr. Bickford. there was quite a deep ulcer, the remarkable feature in the case was that the pancreas had become firmly attached to the intestine just behind the [*illegible word* crossed out] ulcer, thus forming a floor for it & preventing perforation.

adjourned

I. Richmond Bass
Secretary

Case 2: Imperforate Hymen

(Separate paper)
Envelope 7 in the papers of the Middlesex East District Medical Society

A Case of Imperforate Hymen.
Read Oct 17, 1883
by
Dr. Harlow.
A Case of Imperforate Hymen Reported Oct 17. 1883

B. E. M. a well developed & robust looking girl of 14 years has had uniform health from infancy. Fell from a hammock on the [*three largely illegible words* crossed out] 10th of Aug. 1883, striking upon the left hip & back. Complained of pain & tenderness in the hip & pain in the back, but in a few days was better & went to her school. The case was managed by her mother without the advice of a physician. About the 1st of September the pain in the hip & back increased, [*illegible word* crossed out] a limp in the walk was [*more* crossed out] noticeable & patient left school & took her bed. The writer requested to see her on the 7th [*two illegible words*, first crossed out] when the aforegoing history was attained with the added particulars as to these then present conditions. A remarkably healthy & robust girl with temperature & pulse was before me with pain in the left hip & back extending down the leg in knee & the heel—so great was the pain that patient made the loudest outcries from her sufferings—diligent inquiry elicited the fact that the pain was somewhat paroxysmal, patient often having intervals of several hours rest. When first seen she was in bed, decubitus dorsal, turned to the right side, with the left leg partly flexed. No marks of injury were seen upon the painful hip, but there was tenderness over and around the great trochanter. Leg & foot normal as to appearance & sensation. The mother stated that patient had pain in the back passage & had internal piles for nearly a year, that there were no external tumors. Patient had never menstruated nor shown any indication of doing so—Rest [*with* crossed out] dry cups to the hip with a suppository of opium and belladonna were advised—the cups were applied by the mother several times and in two weeks the patient was walking about the house feeling well & free from pain in the hip & leg without [*illegible word*].

On the 1st Oct inst. the mother called upon the writer for a suppository as she said her daughter was troubled with the "piles" again—nothing further was heard from the patient until the 11th inst. in the evening when the writer was requested to see patient immediately as she was in great pain. Arriving at the house I learned that patient had been about the house & out of doors thinking about going back to her school. In the afternoon she was entertaining a company of her mates & after the tea was over & the company about to retire patient was suddenly seized with "the old pain in the back passage" as the mother phrased it & " it seemed as if the child would die."

Regarding the fact that so well developed and robust a girl did not assume "the custom of women" the writer insisted upon making an examination to ascertain the extent of the "internal piles." The index finger well in the rectum found that cavity in a perfectly normal condition but pressed upon by a fluctuating mass in front. An attempt to enter the vagina in the same manner was not as successful as that passage was closed by a firm inelastic membrane just within the labia—with a finger in the rectum & pressure upon this membrane unmistakable fluctuation was found. An enema containing $\frac{1}{4}$ gr morph was given and retained & patient was soon at rest and passed the night and next forenoon [*free* written over illegible word] from pain.

Next day the 12th in the afternoon patient was etherized & placed upon the [*lithotomy* written over illegible word] position & examination revealed a tense & and highly vascular membrane stretched across & completely closing the vaginal outlet with evident fluctuation above.

This membrane was punctured in its centre with a larger trocar & thirty fluid ounces of dark <u>treacle</u> like fluid withdrawn. The opening was extended [*through to the* crossed out] with the fingers & [*illegible word*] where the uterus would be felt in is place & normal as to size. There was no external tenderness in either illeac fossæ.

The nervous shock from the withdrawal of the fluid was considerable, the pulse becoming very frequent & feeble & the face pallid. The vagina was washed daily first with a weak sol. of Carbol. acid and later with permanganate of potash. Patient has progressed thus far without a symptom & today was in her chair making patchwork. The noteworthy features of this case appear to be that so large a quantity of the menstrual could be retained in the vagina for so long a time as this probably had been without constitutional disturbance—there having been neither rigors or [*illegible word*]—& that the fluid was absolutely without [*illegible word*].

Case 3: Pain and Inflammation in the Ilio-Caecal Region

(From minutes)
Record Book of the Middlesex East District Medical Society, Volume III. July 13, 1881–Aug 22, 1888, pp. 145–149.
Full record of meeting of August 6th., 1888

Woburn. August 6th. 1884.

This eve the Society held its 256th regular monthly meeting at the Central House, the guests of Dr. Abbott.
Dr. Dow the president in the chair.
Present, Drs. Hodgdon, Holmes, Abbott, Putney, Graves, Odlin, Clark, Cowdrey, March, Winsor, Dow, Harlow, F. F. Brown, Heath, Jordan, Nickerson and [?] Stevens.
The records of the last meeting were read and approved.

In lieu of a paper, Dr. Harlow gave the following points in a case that he first saw on the 5th day of illness.
A healthy Irishman aged 35 was suddenly attacked with [*typhlitis* crossed out] pain in the ilio-caecal region followed by inflammation that soon extended over the whole abdomen. The pulse was not remarkable.
Dr. Harlow immediately gave a hypodermic injection of morphia with good effect and ordered a pill to contain 1 grain each of opium and calomel with one sixth of a grain of ipecac, to be given every 4 hours for 24 hours.
Within 24 hours the bowels moved freely after having been confined eight days. In the feces was found what was supposed to be a small fragment of the intestine: made up of mucous and muscular tissues. [The specimen was here shown to the Society.] No serous coat could be found. The patient rapidly recovered. At the onset of the attack the patient was thoroughly tho unsuccessfully plied with cathartics. Dr. Harlow said he located the problem at the ilio-caecal valve.
There was considerable enteritis—but the peritoneum was not much affected.

Dr. Holmes queried whether an invagination could free [?] itself. He said he once met a man who claimed that he had repeatedly suffered from symptoms of invagination.

Dr. Harlow spoke of a boy who had had symptoms of invagination, and subsequently passed a portion of the descending colon—three inches long. The boy recovered and is now a robust young man.

Dr. Putney cited a similar case.

Dr. Cowdrey reported that he had under his case care [?] a boy, with what he had diagnosticated a scrofulous ankle. The patient looked healthy but was lame. The ankle was swollen and tender. Tr Iodine followed by a months rest in a plaster splint had effected no change. Over the metatarsal bones there was what looked like an enlarged bursa about the size of a pig nut.

In answer to Dr. Hodgdon, Dr. Cowdrey answered, "The patient can bend the ankle and can bear his weight on it."

Dr. Winsor suggested aspirating with a subcutaneous syringe.

Dr. Cowdrey had thought of that.

Dr. Abbott said he treated [*bursa* crossed out] ganglions by compression.

Dr. Odlin asked whether typhlitis ever became chronic—or [*if* crossed out] recurred.

Dr. Harlow said he could count 4 females and one male with chronic typhlitis. One lady had had frequent attacks: the last one was superinduced by a carriage ride and a severe cold. Previous to leaving home she was well. She now has tenderness and inflammation over the ileo-caecal region.

He thought it took years to recover from typhlitis, even under the best treatment. Eight years ago the high school teacher of Woburn had a very severe attack of typhlitis. The man fully recovered and had had no recurrence of the disease. For a considerable time he had a tender spot about 4 inches across in the ilio-caecal region. Another case that occurred 10 or 12 years ago. The patient had all the attendant symptoms of typhlitis, and recovered in 2 or 3 years, and has remained well.

Dr. Odlin said that 4 years ago he had typhlitis and was 6 weeks in bed. Within 2 years he had had 3 severe attacks of the disease.

Dr. F. I. Knight to whom he [*had* crossed out] related the history of his first attack told him that he knew of 2 similar cases that were caused by riding in a two wheeled chaise.

Several months later Dr. Odlin used a two wheeled chaise a few days and [*suffered from* crossed out] had his second attack.

He had recently had another seizure which came on immediately after running a lawn mower.

He felt satisfied that long rides over rough roads caused his [*illness while* crossed out] earlier attacks of typhlitis, while his recent experience with a lawn mower had convinced him that he ought not—only to a slight extent—indulge in manual labor.

In reply to Dr. Cowdrey, Dr. Odlin said he had a tender bunch [?] over the ilio-caecal region.

Dr. Harlow said he attached much importance to Dr. Odlin's remarks, as he had heard of numerous similar cases.

Dr. Winsor said he had recently disch'd a gentleman aged 50 years—with the following history. He took a horse-back ride—the next day he felt lame and stiff, and supposed he had taken cold—[*took a bath and* crossed out] On the 2nd day pain settled in his abdomen and a tumor about 3 inches in diameter developed in the ilio-caecal region.

He vomited once.

The tumor and attendant symptoms gradually disappeared.

Dr. Odlin said he took a calomel purge when he felt his last attack developing.

Dr. Abbott said he had seen good results follow the use of large doses of calomel. He mentioned a case of intestinal obstruction. A maid 19 or 20 years old died with symptoms of peritonitis. The autopsy showed a diverticulum that formed a loop in which was a strangulated knuckle of intestine.

Dr. Winsor asked if any member present had noticed illness follow the use of impure milk. He said that there had been over 200 cases of mouth and throat disease reported from Dover Eng. These cases were all supplied with milk from one dairy where several cows were found with foot and mouth disease.

He thought similar cases might develop [*here* crossed out] among us.

Dr. Abbott said that many of the diseases that arise in England following milk routes are carefully investigated.

Dr. F. F. Brown read a short thesis from the Medical Brief in which the author maintained that oxyuris vemicularis was propagated from animated cats hairs.

Dr. Harlow showed a specimen of a reef knot in an umbilical cord.

Dr. Putney showed a simple knot in a cord, an enlarged prostate, a portion of invaginated intestine, and a portion of a heart and aorta showing extensive calsification of the aortic valve and ascending arch.

Adjourned

G. E. Putney, Secy

Case 4:   Placenta Lateralis

(Separate paper)

Envelope 7 in the papers of the Middlesex East District Medical Society

[Although the peculiarity of the concluding "signature" may suggest that J. M. Harlow was not the author, he is listed in the Index of papers as such.]

Read at Woburn

Oct 14, 1891.

Case of Placenta Lateralis.

On night of Sept. 29th, '91 was called to attend Mrs. W. in confinement. On the way to the house her husband informed me that the waters had broken & labor well under way. Found Mrs. W in bed. On questioning her said that the pains had ceased, that she was only seven or eight months along. I made a digital examination, had difficulty in reaching the os but found it undilated. Found that the waters that came away was a gush of blood. After remaining about one hour and finding that the hemorrhage had ceased prescribed $\frac{1}{8}$ gr. morphia and perfect rest in bed. Called the next forenoon. Patient in bed, pulse 76, having a pain occasionally, commencing in the center over the pubes & radiating in all directions as she said. Gave $\frac{1}{8}$ gr. morphia as before, hoping she might go to term. About 9 o'clock P.M. Mr. W called me, saying that Mrs. W was having pains regular & fast. Found patient pale, rapid and feeble pulse, with history of flowing for nearly four hours with an occasional pain. On examination found os well down in pelvis, soft, flabby, and dilated so as to admit the fingers easily. Found on entering the fingers into the os a soft boggy mass which I could not make out to be any part of the child. Called it the placenta and told Mr. W to go after Dr. Morse or anyone he could get. Dr. Morse came and I stated to him what I thought the case was and asked him to examine. He found and detached on examination about $2\frac{1}{2}$ in. [*square* crossed out] of the placenta which covered the os completely. The os readily admitting of dilatation Dr. Morse decided to use the forceps. Administered ether and delivered by forceps a dead child. Recovered well from ether but was very low from loss of blood. I gave brandy in teaspoonfull doses all night. She had no nurse or any woman in the house to bathe or clean up the bed and she laid in the same bed for three or four days. When some of the neighbors came in and cleaned out the room, bathed her & changed the bed. She had no rise in temperature. Pulse remained about 80 and she made a good recovery, within two weeks was up and dressed.

CW Harlow M.D.

Appendix G

Lineages of Phineas Gage and John Martyn Harlow

The Phineas Gage Line

What I have been able to establish about the lineage of Phineas Gage relies heavily on documents and information kindly made available to me by L. Winston Ham, a Gage relative and genealogical researcher of Hollis, New Hampshire; Robert Leavitt, City Historian, Lebanon, New Hampshire; Carol Rifelj of Middlebury College, Vermont; Kenneth Cramer and Anne Ostendarp, archivists of the library of Dartmouth College, New Hampshire; and Virginia Dennerley of Concord, New Hampshire, also a Gage relative. The more specific references are to W. M. Gage 1922; C. V. Gage 1964?, pp. 3, 35; Roberts 1957; and Stearns, Whitcher, and Parker 1908, p. 1651. The copy of C. V. Gage's otherwise undated work in the New England Historic and Genealogical Society has the date "1964" stamped on it.

For the archival dating of the marriage of Jesse and Hannah Gage, I am indebted to Robert Drake of Hanover, New Hampshire. Except for the dates of the birth and marriage of Sarah Foster Little to Roswell Rockwell Gage, which come from the Little (1882) genealogy, and the dates of the marriage and death of Phebe Jane, which come from the Shattuck genealogy, the date of birth, marriage, and deaths of their children are from Roberts and C. V. Gage. The Shattuck genealogy is partly in Shattuck 1855 and Larson 1977 but is much more complete on the World Family Tree collection of family files on Compact disc (WFT CDs, vol. 6, file 3455), and I am most grateful to Mr. Robert Askew of Cherokee Village, Arkansas, for finding this for me. My web searches, responses to the Phineas Gage site, and Pamela Storm Wolfskill's skillful management of her genealogy page have brought me information from Gage and Harlow descendents or others having information about members of the Harlow, Gage, and Shattuck families. They include Marion Calvert of Houston, Texas; Charles Gage of Dallas, Texas; Joanne Harriman of Gorham, New Hampshire; Paul Hershey of Redondo Beach, California; Jill Kane of Oakland, California; Barbara Trussell of Danville, New Hampshire, and Jahan Byrne, Kathi Gori, and "Colleen," all net-dwellers. I am similarly grateful to the descendents of Edward Higginson Williams: David Butler, Susan Cazja, and especially the Rev. Edward Williams, IV.

Where the sources differ over dates and places (and I have indicated only a small number of such discrepancies) I have chosen from the sources that seemed the most reliable. In the absence of an archival or similar documented date, broadly speaking, I preferred C. V. Gage and Roberts.

Variant Names

Hannah Trussell Swetland: Her names are given variously as "Hanna," "Trusel" or "Trussel," and "Sweetland" or "Sweatland." I have chosen the spellings given in the Swetland (1907) genealogy.

Phineas P. Gage: There seems to be no record of Phineas's second name. Most often it is stated to begin with "P" but occasionally with "B." In the former case, traditional New England naming practice might suggest it was also Phineas, but I am told that it would be very unlikely for the one first name to be used twice. Because there are no predecessors whose first names begin with "P," the second name may come from the Swetland side of the family. I know almost nothing about that family, but one should note that the second name of brother Dexter was "Pritchard."

Lura G.: Her name is sometimes given as "Laura," and I have not found her second name.

Roswell Rockwell: His second name comes from the Little (1882) genealogy.

Phebe Jane: Her rarely given second name comes from the notice of her husband's death in the *San Francisco Examiner*, 21 March 1904, p. 6. In some later records it is given as "Phoebe."

The Lineage of Phineas Gage

1. *John* Gage
born 1604 in England
died 1673 at Ipswich, Massachusetts
married (1) date unknown
Amy (Amee) Wilford, died in June 1658 at Ipswich, Massachusetts
married (2) on 7 November 1658
Sarah Keyes, died on 7 July 1681, widow of Robert Keyes
2. *Benjamin* Gage
born 1643
died 10 October 1672 at Andover, Haverhill County, Massachusetts
married (1) on 16 February 1663 at Salem, Massachusetts
Mary Keyes, born 16 June 1645, died 20 December 1668, daughter of Robert and Sarah Keyes
married (2) on 11 October 1671
Prudence Leaver, born 11 June 1644, died 26 October 1716
3. *John* Gage
born 15 July 1672
died 10 October or December 1751 at Bradford, Massachusetts
married on 13 June 1694
Sarah Hazleton, born 11 March 1673, died 27 May 1753

4. *John* Gage
born 13 September 1708
died at Chester, Concord County, New Hampshire
married on 25 May 1738
Elizabeth Haynes, born 4 February 1717
5. *Solomon* Gage
born 8 February 1739 [1738?]
died Concord, Enfield, New Hampshire
married (1) [1767?]
married (2) on 7 June 1782
Sarah Stevens
6. *Phineas* Gage
born in 1772 at Concord, New Hampshire
died on 17 September 1849 at Enfield, New Hampshire, and buried in Lot 232, Enfield Town Cemetery
married on 19 February 1797 at Enfield, New Hampshire
Phebe Eaton, born 4 July 1776, Chester, New Hampshire (Candia, New Hampshire), died 8 March 1860 at Enfield, New Hampshire, and buried in Enfield Town Cemetery
7. *Jesse Eaton* Gage
born 1 April 1798 at Enfield, New Hampshire
died date and place unknown
married on 27 April 1823 in Lebanon, New Hampshire
Hannah Trussell Swetland, born 27 December 1797 in East Lebanon, New Hampshire, died 9 March 1887 in San Francisco, and buried in Vault 962, Pioneer Mound, Cypress Lawn Cemetery, Colma, California
8.1 *Phineas P.* Gage
born 9 July 1823, at Lebanon, New Hampshire
died 21 May 1860 in San Francisco, and buried in Vault 962, Pioneer Mound, Cypress Lawn Cemetery, Colma, California
8.2 *Lura G.* Gage
born 2 [3] December 1826 at Enfield, New Hampshire
died 25 February 1902 at Caanan, New Hampshire
married 9 December 1850
John Trissel Milton, born 2 December 1823 [1826?] at Caanan, New Hampshire, died 4 January 1886 in Caanan, New Hampshire
8.3 *Roswell Rockwell* Gage
born 28 March [April] 1829 at Grafton, New Hampshire
died 12 July 1915 at Enfield, New Hampshire
married (1) on 7 [13] May 1850 in Springfield, New Hampshire
Sarah Foster Little, born 24 February 1832, died 2 December 1892 at Grafton, New Hampshire
married (2) on 6 March 1894 in Wilmot, New Hampshire
Addie Josephine Cole, born 12 October 1850

8.4 *Dexter Prichard* Gage
born 17 April 1831 [1833] at Enfield, New Hampshire
died 19 April 1869 at Enfield, New Hampshire, and buried in Lot 265 in Village Cemetery, Lebanon, New Hampshire
married on 9 June 1853
Mary Baker Eastman
8.5 *Phebe Jane* Gage
born 20 November 1832 at New Ipswich, New Hampshire
died August 1914 at San Rafael, Marin County, California
married 10 November 1853 in San Francisco
David Dustin Shattuck, born 28 May 1830 at Bradford, New Hampshire, died 20 March 1904, San Francisco

The John Martyn Harlow Line

I am grateful to Mr. Stan Shaw, historian of the Harlow Family Association, for his letter to me of 18 August 1998, in which he provided most of the details of the line. The few dates and names I have added come either from town records (*Vital Records of Acton* 1923 for Charlotte Davis) or from wills and Woburn, Massachusetts, newspapers (for Frances Kimball Harlow).

The Lineage of John Martyn Harlow

1. *Sgt. William* Harlow
born between 25 August 1624 and 25 August 1625, probably in England
died 25 August 1691 at Plymouth, Massachusetts
married (1) on 20 December 1649, at Plymouth, Massachusetts
Rebecca Bartlett, daughter of Robert Bartlett and Mary Warren
married (2) on 25 January 1665/1666 at Plymouth, Massachusetts
Mary Shelley
2. *William* Harlow
born 2 June 1657 at Plymouth, Massachusetts
died 28 January 1711/1712 at Plymouth, Massachusetts, aged 54 years
married circa January 1683 at Plymouth, Massachusetts
Lydia Cushman
3. *William* Harlow
baptized in 1689 at Plymouth, Massachusetts
died 18 February 1750 at Bridgewater, Plymouth, Massachusetts
married 18 June 1713 at Plymouth, Massachusetts
Joanna Jackson
4. *Isaac* Harlow
born 21 April 1726 at Plymouth, Massachusetts
died 1817
married circa 1750
Mary Byram, widow of Aaron Thompson

5. *Isaac* Harlow
born 26 July 1757 at Sussex, New Jersey
died January 1829 at Whitehall, Washington County, New York, aged 71, and buried at Whitehall
married circa 1777 at Whitehall, Washington County, New York
Mehitable Lothrop
6. *Ransom* Harlow
born 22 December 1780 at Whitehall, Washington County, New York
died 24 February 1855, aged 74
married 15 May 1803 at Whitehall, Washington County, New York
Annis Martyn
7. *John Martyn* Harlow
born 25 November 1819 at Whitehall, Washington County, New York
died Woburn, Massachusetts, 13 May 1907, aged 87
married (1) on 5 January 1843 at Acton, Massachusetts
Charlotte Davis of Acton, Massachusetts, died 5 July 1886 at Woburn, Massachusetts
married (2) on 2 August 1888 at Woburn, Massachusetts
Frances Kimball Ames of Woburn, Massachusetts, died on 2 May 1914 at Woburn, Massachusetts

Appendix H
The Sources Searched

Seven kinds of material were searched for information about Gage:

1. Manuscripts such as letters and diaries held by historical society and university libraries, some of which occasionally also existed in printed form
2. Material relating to Barnum
3. Collections of posters, broadsheets, and illustrations
4. Folklore collections
5. Holdings of newspapers
6. Holdings of nonmedical magazines
7. Medical, psychological, and psychiatric serial publications

The search was usually of the whole material, but where the material or its contents was indexed, the indexes were searched under the following headings: accidents, American crowbar case, bar, Bigelow, brain, brain injury, cases, Cavendish, cranium, crowbar, Duttonsville, Gage, Harlow, iron rod, Massachusetts, medical, railroad, railroad accidents, rod, skull, skull injury, tamping iron, Vermont, Yankee.

Each source is listed here in some detail, primarily to serve as a guide to later searchers, although it cannot be assumed that because we found nothing, there was nothing to be found. Why we searched where we did, and why we concentrated on particular time periods, follows directly from Harlow's account of Gage's case. A short introduction has been given to some sections of this Appendix to clarify these points where that may not be reasonably evident.

Manuscripts

California

California Historical Society: newspapers included in later general list for relevant items on Gage and Shattuck in relation to travels, death, exhumation.

California State Library, Sacramento: death and exhumation records for Phineas in the California Information File: 1846–1985.

California State Library, Sutro: ship passenger records.

Green Library, Stanford University: newspapers included in later general list for relevant items on Gage and Shattuck in relation to travels, death, exhumation.

San Francisco Public Library San Francisco History Center: Biography Index and related files for David Dustin Shattuck, Henry Perrin Coon, and Jacob Davies Stillman; San Francisco Municipal Reports; Shuck's Official Roll of San Francisco; newpapers included in the later general list for relevant items on Gage and Shattuck in relation to travels, death, and exhumation; and printed historical works by Hubert Howe Bancroft, Stuart Dagett, Julian Dana, Clifford Merrill Drury, John Shertzer Hittell, Bailey Millard, Oscar Tully Shuck. Unsuccessful search for exhumation records.

San Francisco Genealogical Society: San Francisco Census Records, family records of Gage and Shattuck.

University of California, Berkeley: Papers of Henry Perrin Coon and Jacob Davies Stillman

Connecticut

Bridgeport Public Library: An unrewarding search for relevant local holdings was made while searching the Barnum material.

Connecticut Historical Society, Hartford: Papers of Nathan Adams, Wm. Bridgeman, Clifford Chaffee, Jefferson Church, James Gray, Samuel Graves, John Hooker, Chas. Kibbee, Alfred Lambert, Hugh K. Prentice, George F. Ramsdell, James M. Smith, G. W. Swazey, William Tulley, and Henry R. Vaille, most of whom were physicians; notebook of Seth Chase Gordon, a medical student at Dartmouth Medical College; Records of the Worcester Society for Medical Improvement; diaries of David and Jocelyn Frances Peck; diary of James Hosner; diary of John Flavell Judd; journal of Marie Howard; the Gage and Woodward family papers; and the indexed manuscript material of Benjamin Franklin Heywood. After 2 April 1846, the Worcester Society for Medical Improvement did not meet again until 26 October 1857.

Yale University, New Haven: Papers of Edward Elisha Phelps, and Cushing's collection of material on Henry Jacob Bigelow.

Massachusetts

Acton: Acton Memorial Library and Acton Historical Society: searches of Town records, local newspapers, and the records of the Acton Evangelical Society for Harlow at the Ashby Academy and in the Acton schools, for Harlow's marriage to Charlotte Davis, and for Charlotte in relation to the Acton Evangelical Society and Harlow's bequest to it.

American Antiquarian Society, Worcester: Manuscripts cited are those of Caroline Bennett White Papers, 1844–1915; the Salisbury Family Papers, #65, Diaries 1848–1850 (cf. #33, School Diaries 1850–1852); Benjamin Eddy Cotting papers; and the Cushing papers and printed genealogy (Cushing 1905). Other manuscripts searched included those of the Adams family, Peter Child Bacon, Enoch Bartlett, Frances Bennett, Andrew Bigelow, James Bernard Blake, David Hewes, the Foster family, Elizabeth Peabody, the Paine family, Theodore Parker, Franklin Benjamin Sanborn, the Shaw-Webb family, Edward Ashwell Teulon, the Ward family, John White Webster, the Winchester family, and the papers relating to the Boston Police. The printed version of Benjamin Browne Foster's *Down East Diary*, edited by Charles H. Foster, Orono, Maine: University of Maine; printed diaries from the *California Historic Society Quarterly*, particularly those of Thomas Kerr and Marco Thorne; and the printed and manuscript versions of Florence M. Christman's *One Man's Gold*, McGraw-Hill, 1976.

Boston Athenaeum: Searches were made of *Old Crichton's Faces*, Cornelius Weeks Walter's Extract Book (a scrapbook kept by the editor of the *Boston Evening Traveller*), and the diaries and letters for the relevant periods of Samuel Eliot in his personal and family papers.

Countway Library, Harvard University, Boston: Casebooks, diaries, lecture notes, letters under the names of those members of the Boston Society for Medical Improvement present at the 10 November meeting or who usually attended (Boston Society for Medical Improvement, 1849), and for each of the students in the 1850 *Catalogue* of Harvard Medical School (Harvard University, 1850), respectively. Holdings of casebooks for the relevant periods are small, and J. B. S. Jackson's was the only one belonging to a member of any of the groups. Neither the correspondence of these individuals nor the Bowditch and Putnam papers at the Countway yielded any mention of Gage.

Fitchburg: Fitchburg Memorial Library and Fitchburg Historical Society: searches of Town records and Fitchburg *Sentinel* for Harlow's marriage to Charlotte Davis and for Harlow at the Ashby Academy.

Massachusetts Historical Society, Boston: Manuscripts of Walter Channing II and John Collins Warren, and letters of Henry Jacob Bigelow.

New Hampshire

Andover Historical Society: Papers of Charles Edward Abbot and Nathan Foster Abbott; papers of Mary Byers Smith, chiefly for those of John and Peter Smith; the Taft collection; the Bell papers, especially those of Charles Upham Bell, James Bell, Judith Almira Upham Bell, Luther V. Bell, and Mary Anne Bell White.

Dartmouth College Libraries: Manuscripts of Edward Elisha Phelps at Dartmouth (and Yale). The Dartmouth academic staff and medical students for 1848–1852 considered were Josiah Whitney Barstow, Mills Olcott Heydock, Henry Laurens Rodimon, James Austin Smith, and the Johnson journals and diaries in Dartmouth College and Dana Libraries. Other Dartmouth College papers searched, mainly of those holding academic appointments, were those of Charles Frederick Boyden, Benjamin Hatch Bridgeman, Phineas Sanborn Conner, Dixi Crosby, Theodore French, Carleton Pennington Frost, Reuben Dimond Massey, and Albert Smith.

New Hampshire Historical Society, Concord: Papers of Silas Cummings; David Parker Stowell, including his diary of a voyage around the Horn to Valparaiso and his notes of a lecture by Edward Elisha Phelps; records of the New Hampshire Medical Society.

The *Enfield Historical Society, Lebanon Historical Society*, and *Manchester Historical Society.*

Vermont

University of Vermont Library and Archives, Burlington: Searches were made of the diaries of Batchelder, Rosewell Farnham, William Henry Hoyt, Royal Whitman Peake, Willis R. Peake, Franklin Olmsted, Willard Stevens, Lucius Swett, George Augustus Weeks, and the Rev. John Wheeler.
Vermont State Historical Society, Montpelier: Fairbank letters and Hagerman papers.
Sheldon Museum, Middlebury: Index to the Henry Sheldon Collection of his diaries, scrapbook, and papers on the R&BRR.
The *Cavendish Historical Society, Norman Williams Library* in Woodstock, *Middlebury College Library, Rutland Historical Society*, and the *Woodstock Historical Society*.

Barnum

Material about Gage in relation to Barnum was searched at the Barnum Archive at the Barnum Museum, Bridgeport, Connecticut; in the historical collections of the Bridgeport Public Library; in Barnum's correspondence with Moses Kimball, his Boston agent, held by the Boston Athenæum Library; at the Barnum Collection of the New York Historical Society; a systematic sampling of Barnum's advertisements for his Museum attractions in the *New York Times* for 1850; the entries for Barnum's Museum in George C. D. Odell's *Annals of the New York Stage* (Volumes 5 and 6, covering the years 1843–1853), posters and similar material in the Crawford Theater collection held in the Sterling Library, Yale University; and the broadsheet collections of the American Antiquarian Society, Worcester, Massachusetts, and the Vermont Historical Society, Montpelier. Early and late editions of Barnum's published autobiography were also searched.

None of the following authorities on Barnum, his museum, and his circus, or on the exhibitions of what were then called "freaks," or on the American circus in general had ever heard of Gage in connection with Barnum, or otherwise: Fred Dahlinger, Director, Parkinson Library and Research Center, Circus World, Baraboo, Wisconsin; A. H. Saxon, editor of Barnum's correspondence and author of *P. T. Barnum: The Legend and the Man*; circus historians Stuart Thayer, author of *Annals of the American Circus*, and Thomas Ogden, author of *Two Hundred Years of the American Circus*; and Donald Wilmeth, Department of Theatre Arts, Brown University, author of *Variety, Entertainments and Amusements: A Reference Guide*.

Posters, Broadsheets, and Illustrations

Poster, broadsheet, illustration, portrait, and photograph collections were searched at the American Antiquarian Society, Boston Athenaeum, and Vermont State Historical Society, and, as mentioned above, in the Crawford Theater

Collection at Yale University (searched partly by Christine Weideman), at the Barnum Archives, and at the New York Historical Society.

Folklore

The index to the ballad collection of Henry Sheldon at the Sheldon Museum, Vermont, was searched. Authorities consulted were Richard Baumann, Editor, *Journal of American Folklore* and Director, Center for Intercultural Studies in Folklore and Ethnomusicology, University of Texas at Austin; Roger deV. Renwick, Department of English, University of Texas at Austin; Edward D. Ives, Director, Northeast Archives of Folklore and Oral History, Department of Anthropology, University of Maine at Orono; and W. Edson Richmond, Chairman, Folklore Institute, Indiana University. Richmond did find Gage's name "not entirely unfamiliar," and Ives recalled seeing the Ripley cartoon in the 1930s.

Newspapers

The periods covered in searches of newspapers are coded (a) for the period of Gage's accident, that is, from September 1848 to January 1849, (t) for the period of supposed travel in New England, that is, November 1849 to January 1851, (h) for his subsequent history, and (f) for the time of Harlow's report on Gage's final status. There is much variation from this ideal pattern, usually because holdings of the papers were incomplete. A number of Lebanon and Hanover newspapers was searched by Kenneth Cramer, Dartmouth College Library Archives, as well as by Robert Leavitt, Lebanon historian.

f *Alta California*
a, t *Bellows Falls Gazette*
a, t *Bennington State Banner*
a, t *Boston Daily Advertiser*
a *Boston Daily Courier*
a, t, f *Boston Daily Evening Transcript*
a *Boston Daily Journal*
a *Boston Evening Journal*
a *Boston Weekly Transcript*
f *The Bulletin* (San Francisco)
a, t *Burlington Sentinel*
a *Christian Reflector and Christian Watchman* (Boston)
f *Daily Herald and Mirror* (San Francisco)
a *Daily Free Press* (Burlington, Vermont)
a, t, f *Globe and Mail* (Toronto)
a *Granite State Whig* (Lebanon, New Hampshire) (later *Granite State Free Press*)
a *Green Mountain Freeman* (Montpelier, Vermont)
f *The Leader* (Toronto)
a, t *The Liberator* (Boston)

f *The Londoner* (Toronto)
a, t *National Eagle* (Claremont, New Hampshire)
f *New York Times:*   Annual index under the headings mentioned earlier and the
regularly featured California or San Francisco letters.
t, f *Public Ledger and Daily Transcript* (Philadelphia)
a, t *Rutland County Herald* (Rutland, Vermont)
a, f *Traveller* (Boston) in all four varieties: *Morning Traveller* or *Daily Traveller*,
Evening Traveller or *Daily Evening Traveller*, *Semi-Weekly*, and *Weekly* (sometimes this last was *American Traveller*)
a, t *Vermont Daily Free Press*
a *Vermont Mercury* (Woodstock, Vermont) (later the *Woodstock Mercury*)
a *Vermont Patriot*

Magazines

Magazines were usually searched for the period covering Gage's accident and
recovery and for the six-month period following Harlow's 1868 paper. The Table
of Contents of most magazines was examined first, then the volumes themselves
were leafed through. For those magazines that were indexed, the search was
based on the headings mentioned earlier.

American Phrenological Journal and Miscellany (and its variously titled con-
tinuations):   Vol. 1, 1848, to Vol. 48, 1868.
American Register and Magazine (Boston) (later the *Atlantic Monthly*):   The
Register contained an occasional (and hard to locate) "Miscellany" section that,
like the *Monthly*, often reported on scientific and medical matters.
Brownson's Quarterly Review (Boston and New York):   A Roman Catholic
journal with idiosyncratic notices of matters of literary and scientific interest.
Some of the 1870 numbers were missing.
Every Saturday (Boston):   A popular monthly reproducing articles from mainly
English sources but with occasional local gossip. Began in 1866.
Harper's (New York):   Had a very detailed and cross-referenced index with
regular sections "Historical record," "Scientific record," and the like, and in
1865, sections devoted to Barnum's Museum. Editor's essay commented on
matters of special interest.
Living Age (also *Little's Living Age*) (Boston):   Considerable coverage of medical and scientific matters (e.g., Helmholtz's measurement of the velocity of the
nerve impulse).
Massachusetts Quarterly Review (Boston):   Only three volumes, 1848–1850.
Poole's Index to Periodical Literature (New York):   Searched for 1848–1881
using those of the list of subject headings mentioned earlier that appeared in its
index.
Putnam's Magazine (New York):   Began in 1868 and number 2 for that
year missing. Had wide coverage, especially of minor medical and scientific
matters.

Medical Serials

Medical serials were also searched during the period of Gage's accident and recovery, for the period following Harlow's 1868 paper, and for 1878 for the time after Ferrier's *Gulstonian Lectures*. Except for "Ferrier" being added to the index terms, the search was made in the same way as that for the magazines. The *Index-Catalogue of the U.S. Surgeon-General's Library* was searched under the medical terms or their equivalents from the magazine indexes, with "aphasia" and related terms added.

Medical, Psychological, and Psychiatric Serials

American Journal for the Advancement of Science
American Journal of Insanity
American Journal of Phrenological Science (and variant titles)
American Journal of Psychology
American Journal of the Medical Sciences
American Medical Recorder
Annals of Medical History
Annual of the Universal Medical Sciences
Association for Research in Nervous and Mental Disease (Monographs)
Australian Medical Journal
Brain
British and Foreign Medical Review
British and Foreign Medico-Chirurgical Review
British Medical Journal
Boston Medical and Surgical Journal
Buffalo Medical Journal
Bulletin of the History of Medicine
Bulletin of the Medical Library Association
Clinical Neurosurgery
Dublin Medical Press
Edinburgh Medical and Surgical Journal
Edinburgh Medical Journal
Half Yearly Abstract of the Medical Sciences
Journal of Anatomy and Physiology
Journal of Psychological Medicine
Lancet
London Journal of Medicine
London Medical Gazette (later the *Medical Times and Surgical Gazette*)
London Medical Record
Medical and Surgical Reporter
Medico-Chirurgical Transactions
Medical Journal and Monthly Record

Medical News and Library
Medical Press and Circular
The Medical Record (New York)
Medical Reporter (Periscope)
Medical Times (London) (became *Medical Times and Gazette*)
Neurology
New York Journal of Medicine
North Western Medicine and Surgical Journal
Pacific Medicine and Surgical Journal
The Practitioner (London)
Psychological Monographs
Psychological Record
The Retrospect of Practical Medicine and Surgery (Braithwaite)
Surgery
Western Journal of Medicine

References

Ackerknecht, I. (1982). *A Short History of Medicine*. Baltimore: Johns Hopkins University Press.

Ackerly, S. S. (1935). Instinctive, emotional and mental changes following prefrontal lobe extirpation. *American Journal of Psychiatry* 92: 717–729.

Ackerly, S. S. (1964). A case of paranatal bilateral frontal lobe defect observed for thirty years. In J. M. Warren and K. Akert., eds., *The Frontal Granular Cortex and Behavior* (pp. 192–218). New York: McGraw-Hill.

Ackerly, S. S., and Benton, A. L. (1948). Report of a case of bilateral frontal lobe defect. *Research Publications of the Association for Research in Nervous and Mental Disease* 27: 479–504.

Adey, W. R. (1974). Information processing in sensory and motor systems. In W. R. Adey, L. C. Birch, D. B. Lindsley, J. Maddox, R. M. May, J. Olds, and W. M. O'Neil., eds., *Brain Mechanisms and the Control of Behaviour* (pp. 326–342). London: Heinemann.

Aitchison, J. (1989). *The Articulate Mammal: An Introduction to Psycholinguistics* (3d ed.). London: Unwin Hyman.

Aldrich, L. C., and Holmes, F. R. (1891). *History of Windsor County, Vermont*. Syracuse, NY: Mason.

Alford, H. J. (1869). Fracture of base of skull: Recovery. *British Medical Journal* ii: 347–348.

Alford, L. B. (1948). Cerebral localization; outline of a revision. *Nervous and Mental Disease Monograph Series*, Whole Number 77.

Althaus, J. (1873). *A Treatise on Medical Electricity* (3d ed.). London: Longman's Green.

Altrocchi, J. (1980). *Abnormal Behavior*. New York: Harcourt, Brace, Jovanovich.

Anderson, W. (1888). A case of compound fracture of the cranium, with depression and escape of cerebral matter; operation; recovery; remarks. *Lancet* ii: 265–266.

Angell, J. R. (1904). *Psychology*. New York: Holt.

Annandale, T. (1877). Case in which a knitting needle penetrated the brain through the orbit. Recovery, with loss of sight in one eye. *Edinburgh Medical Journal* 104: 891–894.

Anstie, F. E. (1864a). *Stimulants and Narcotics, Their Mutual Relations*. London: Macmillan.

Anstie, F. E. (1864b). On the action of opium as an "astringent" in diabetes. *Lancet*, *ii*, 602–603.

Anstie, F. E. (1865). On the physiological and therapeutical action of alcohol. *Lancet*, *ii*, 343–345.

Aristotle. (1911). *The Parts of Animals* (A. L. Peck, trans.). London: Heinemann.

Armour, J. (1831). Case of severe injury of the head, fungus, and removal of a large portion of the brain, with remarks. *Glasgow Medical Journal* 4: 341–349.

Arndt, R. (1892a). Electricity, use of, in the treatment of the insane—Historical sketch. In D. H. Tuke, ed., *A Dictionary of Psychological Medicine* (pp. 426–431). London: Churchill.

Arndt, R. (1892b). Neurasthenia. In D. H. Tuke, ed., *A Dictionary of Psychological Medicine* (pp. 840–850). London: Churchill.

Ashby Academy. (1840). *Catalogue of the Officers and Students of Ashby Academy for the Year Ending November, 1840*. Fitchburg, MA: [Ashby Academy?].

Ashhurst, J. (1865). On the treatment of gunshot injuries of the head. *American Journal of the Medical Sciences* 50: 383–390.

Ashworth, B. (1986). *The Bramwells of Edinburgh: A Medical Dynasty*. Edinburgh: Royal College of Physicians.

Association for Research on Nervous and Mental Disease. (1934). Localization of Function in the Cerebral Cortex: An Investigation of the Most Recent Advances. *Proceedings of the Association, December 1932 Meeting* (Vol. 13). Baltimore: Williams and Wilkins.

Association for Research on Nervous and Mental Disease. (1948). The Frontal Lobes. *Proceedings of the Association, December 1947 Meeting* (Vol. 27). Baltimore: Williams and Wilkins.

Atkinson, W. B. (1880). *A Biographical Dictionary of Contemporary Physicians and Surgeons* (2d ed.). Philadelphia: Brinton.

Atrens, D. M., and Curthoys, I. S. (1982). *The Neurosciences and Behaviour: An Introduction* (2d ed.). Sydney, Australia: Academic Press.

Austin, K. A. (1977). *A Pictorial History of Cobb and Co.: The Coaching Age in Australia, 1854–1924*. Adelaide, Australia: Rigby.

Babbit, W. M. (1867–1868). Pistol-shot wound of the forehead. *Boston Medical and Surgical Journal* 77: 346–347.

Bacq, Z. M. (1975). *Chemical Transmission of Nerve Impulses: A Historical Sketch*. Oxford: Pergamon. (Original work published 1974)

Bain, A. (1855). *The Senses and the Intellect*. London: Parker.

Bain, A. (1859). *The Emotions and the Will*. London: Parker.

Bain, A. (1873). *Mind and Body*. New York: Appleton-Century.

Bain, A. (1882a). *James Mill: A Biography*. London: Longmans, Green.

Bain, A. (1882b). *John Stuart Mill: A Criticism with Personal Recollections*. London: Longmans, Green.

Bain, A. (1904). *Autobiography*. London: Longmans, Green.

Baine, D. (1742). A fracture of the skull, with loss of part of the substance of the brain. In *Medical Essays and Observations* (pp. 401–403). Edinburgh: [A Medical Society].

Bakan, D. (1975). The authenticity of the Freud memorial collection. *Journal of the History of the Behavioral Sciences* 11: 365–367.

Baker, F. (1909). The two Sylviuses: An historical study. *Bulletin of the Johns Hopkins Hospital* 20: 329–339.

Baker, G. P. (1937). *The Formation of the New England Railroad Systems*. New York: Greenwood Press.

Baker, W. M. (1880). *Kirkes' Hand-Book of Physiology* (10th ed.). London: John Murray.

Ballance, C. A. (1922). *A Glimpse into the History of the Surgery of the Brain*. London: Macmillan.

Ballantyne, J. W., ed. (1915). *Encyclopaedia Medica* (2d ed.). Edinburgh: Green.

Barfoot, M. (1995). *"To Ask the Suffrages of the Patrons": Thomas Laycock and the Edinburgh Chair of Medicine, 1855* (Medical History, Supplement No. 15). London: Wellcome Institute for the History of Medicine.

Barker, II, F. G. (1993). Treatment of open brain wounds in America, 1810–1880: A survey. *Journal of Neurosurgery* 78: 364A.

Barker, II, F. G. (1995). Phineas among the phrenologists: The American Crowbar Case and nineteenth century theories of cerebral localization. *Journal of Neurosurgery* 82: 672–682.

Barlow, E. (1802). History of a considerable wound of the brain, attended with singular circumstances. *Annals of Medicine* (Edinburgh) 7(ii): 382–389.

Bartholinus, T. (1641). *Institutiones Anatomicæ*. Leiden, Netherlands: Hack.

Bartholow, R. (1874a). Experimental investigations into the functions of the human brain. *American Journal of the Medical Sciences* 67: 305–313.

Bartholow, R. (1874b). Correspondence: Experiments on the function of the human brain. *British Medical Journal* i: 727.

Bartholow, R. (1877). General correspondence: Letter from Dr. Roberts Bartholow. *Medical Times and Gazette* ii: 371–372.

Bartlett, J. R. (1859). *A Dictionary of Americanisms (2d ed.)*. Boston: Little Brown (Johnson reprint New York, 1968).

Barton, J. K. (1881). Penetrating gunshot wound of the skull; lodgement of bullet in interior of cranium; recovery. *Lancet* i: 248.

Bassett, T. D. S. (1992). *The Growing Edge: Vermont Villages, 1840–1880.* Montpelier: Vermont Historical Society.

Bateman, F. (1865). Aphasia, or loss of the power of speech, with remarks on our present knowledge of its pathology. *Lancet* i: 532–533.

Bayliss, L. E. (1915). *Principles of General Physiology.* London: Longmans.

Beaumont, J. G. (1983). *Introduction to Neuropsychology.* Oxford: Blackwell.

Beekman, F. (1945). A celebrated case of cerebral injury. *Bulletin of the History of Medicine* 17: 521–526.

Beers, F. W. (1869). *Atlas of Windsor Co., Vermont From Actual Surveys by and Under the Direction of F. W. Beers.* New York: Beers, Ellis, and Soule.

Bell, C. (1823). On the motions of the eye in illustration of the muscles and nerves of the orbit. *Philosophical Transactions of the Royal Society* 113: 166–186, 289–307.

Bennett, A. H., and Godlee, R. J. (1882–1885). Case of cerebral tumour. *Proceedings of the Royal Medical and Chirurgical Society* i: 438–444.

Bennett, A. H., and Godlee, R. J. (1884). Excision of a tumour from the brain. *Lancet* ii: 1090–1091.

Bennett, A. H., and Godlee, R. J. (1885a). Sequel to the case of excision of a tumour from the brain. *Lancet* i: 13.

Bennett, A. H., and Godlee, R. J. (1885b). Case of cerebral tumour. *Transactions of the Royal Medical and Chirurgical Society of London* 58: 243–275.

Bennett, A. H., and Gould, A. P. (1887). Case of epilepsy of six years' duration. Complete recovery after surgical operation on the skull and brain. *British Medical Journal* i: 12–13.

Berker, E. A., Berker, A. H., and Smith, A. (1986). Translation of Broca's 1865 report. Localization of speech in the third left frontal convolution. *Archives of Neurology* 43: 1065–1072.

Berman, A. (1978). The heroic approach in 19th century therapeutics. In J. W. Leavitt and R. L. Numbers, eds., *Sickness and Health in America* (pp. 77–86). Madison: University of Wisconsin Press.

Best, C. H., and Taylor, N. B. (1937). *The Physiological Basis of Medical Practice.* Baltimore: Wood.

Bianchi, L. (1922). *The Mechanism of the Brain and the Function of the Frontal Lobes* (J. H. McDonald, trans.). New York: William Wood. (Original work published 1921)

Bibliographical notices. *Recovery From the Passage of an Iron Bar Through the Head.* By John M. Harlow of Woburn. Boston, David Clapp. (1869). *Boston Medical and Surgical Journal* 80: 116–117.

Bibliographic and literary notes. Art. 1. *A Descriptive Catalogue of the Warren Anatomical Museum, Harvard University.* (1870). *New York Medical Journal* 12: 552–554.

Bigelow, H. J. (1850a). *An Introductory Lecture Delivered at the Massachusetts Medical College, November 6th, 1849.* Boston: n.p.

Bigelow, H. J. (1850b). Dr. Harlow's case of recovery from the passage of an iron bar through the head. *American Journal of the Medical Sciences* 20: 13–22.

Bigelow, H. J. (1850c). *Dr. Harlow's Case of Recovery from the Passage of an Iron Bar through the Head.* Philadelphia: Collins.

Bird, B. L. (1865). Compound comminuted fracture of the left temporal region of the skull, with loss of bone, and about six drachms of brain, resulting from the kick of a horse, followed by complete recovery. *American Journal of the Medical Sciences* 49: 552–553.

Bixby, M. (1927). *The Diary of Marcellus Bixby from 1852 to 1856.* Los Angeles: The Historical Society of Southern California.

Blackington, A. (1956). The man with a hole in his head. In *More Yankee Yarns* (pp. 73–80). New York: Dodd, Mead.

Blakemore, C. (1977). *Mechanics of the Mind.* Cambridge: Cambridge University Press.

Blakeslee, S. (1994). Old accident points to brain's moral center. *New York Times*, May 24, Science Section, pp. B5, B8.

Bloom, F. E., and Lazerson, A. (1988). *Brain, Mind, and Behavior* (2d ed.). New York: Freeman.

Bloom, F. E., Lazerson, A., and Hofstadter, L. (1985). *Brain, Mind, and Behavior.* New York: Freeman.

Blumer, D., and Benson, D. F. (1975). Personality changes with frontal and temporal lobe lesions. In D. F. Benson and D. Blumer, eds., *Psychiatric Aspects of Neurologic Disease* (pp. 151–170). New York: Grune and Stratton.

Boardman, A. (1851). *A Defence of Phrenology.* New York: Fowler and Wells.

Bodkin, T. (1830). Case of recovery from extensive injury of the left hemisphere. *Edinburgh Medical and Surgical Journal* 34: 319–323.

Bolton, A. (1878–1879). Compound comminuted fracture of the skull, extensive laceration, and loss of brain substance. Operation-Recovery-Paralysis. *Brain* 1: 566–569.

Bonin, G. von (1960). *Some Papers on the Cerebral Cortex.* Springfield, IL: Thomas.

Boon, A. (1881). Case of compound fracture of the skull; trephining; recovery. *Lancet* ii: 788–789.

Bootzin, R. R., and Acocella, J. R. (1984). *Abnormal Psychology: Current Perspectives* (4th ed.). New York: Random House.

Bootzin, R. R., Acocella, J. R., and Alloy, L. B. (1993). *Abnormal Psychology: Current Perspectives* (6th ed.). New York: McGraw-Hill.

Boring, E. G. (1950). *A History of Experimental Psychology* (2d ed.). New York: Appleton-Century-Crofts.

Boston Society for Medical Improvement. (1849). *Records of Meetings* (Vol. 6). Countway Library, Harvard University, Boston. Manuscript B. Ms b 92.2.

Botkin, B. A. (1944). *A Treasury of American Folklore*. New York: Crown.

Botkin, B. A., and Harlow, A. F. (1953). *A Treasury of Railroad Folklore*. New York: Crown.

Bowditch, H. P. (1874). Report on physiology. *Boston Medical and Surgical Journal* 89: 79–84.

Bramwell, J. M. (1903). *Hypnotism: Its History, Practice, and Theory*. London: Richards. (New York: Julian Press reprint, 1956.)

Brazier, M. A. B. (1959). The historical development of neurophysiology. In J. Field, H. W. Magoun, and V. E. Hall, eds., *Handbook of Neurophysiology* (Vol. 1, pp. 1–58). Baltimore: Waverly Press.

Breese, B. B. (1899). On inhibition. *Psychological Review, Monograph Supplements* 3(1): 1–65.

Brickner, R. M. (1934). An interpretation of frontal lobe function based upon the study of a case of partial bilateral frontal lobectomy. *Research Publications of the Association for Research in Nervous and Mental Disease* 13: 259–351.

Brickner, R. M. (1936). *The Intellectual Functions of the Frontal Lobes*. New York: Macmillan.

Bridgman, A. M., ed. (1895). *A Souvenir of Massachusetts Legislators, 1895* (Vol. 4). Stoughton, MA: Bridgman.

Bridgman, A. M., ed. (1896). *A Souvenir of Massachusetts Legislators, 1896* (Vol. 5). Stoughton, MA: Bridgman.

British Medical Journal. (1874a). Editorial: Experiments on the human subject. *British Medical Journal* i: 687.

British Medical Journal. (1874b). Editorial note. *British Medical Journal* i: 723.

Broadbent, W. H. (1878–1879). A case of peculiar affection of speech, with commentary. *Brain* 1: 484–503.

Broca, P. (1861a). Loss of speech, chronic softening and partial destruction of the left anterior lobe of the brain. In R. H. Wilkins, ed., *Neurological Classics* (pp. 63–64). New York: Johnson Reprint. (Original work published 1861 as Perte de la parole, ramoillissement chronique et destruction partielle du lobe antériur gauche du cerveau, *Bulletins de la Société d'Anthropologie de Paris* 2: 235–238)

Broca, P. (1861b). Remarks on the seat of the faculty of articulate language, followed by an observation of aphemia. In G. von Bonin, ed. and trans., *Some Papers on the Cerebral Cortex* (pp. 49–72). Springfield, IL: Thomas. (Original work published 1861 as Remarques sur la siège de la faculté du langage articulé, suivies d'une observation d'aphémie (perte de la parole), *Bulletin et Mémoires de la Société Anatomique de Paris* 36: 330–357)

Broca, P. (1861c). New observation of aphemia produced by a lesion of the posterior half of the second and third frontal convolutions. In R. H. Wilkins, ed., *Neurological Classics* (pp. 64–68). New York: Johnson Reprint. (Original work published 1861 as Nouvelle observation d'aphémie produite par une lésion de la moitié postérieure des deuxième et triosième circonvolutions frontales, *Bulletin et Mémoires de la Société Anatomique de Paris* 36: 398–407)

Broca, P. (1986). On the site of the faculty of articulated speech. In E. A. Berker, A. H. Berker, and A. Smith, Translation of Broca's 1865 report. Localization of speech in the third left frontal convolution. *Archives of Neurology* 43: 1065–1072. (Original work published 1865 as Sur la siège de la faculté du langage articulé, *Bulletins de la Société d'Anthropologie Paris* 6: 377–393)

Broca, P. (1991). The diagnosis and subsequent drainage of a brain abscess situated at the level and region of language. In J. L. Stone, Paul Broca and the first craniotomy based on cerebral localisation. *Journal of Neurosurgery* 75: 154–159. (Original work published 1876 as Diagnostic d'un abcès situé au niveau de la région du langage; trépanation de cet abcès, *Revue d'Anthropologie* 5: 244–248.)

Brooke, [?]. (1861). Compound fracture of the skull, with protrusion of the substance of the brain; Recovery. *Lancet* ii: 373.

Brooks, N. (1869). The man with the hole in his head. *The Overland Monthly* 3: 30–37.

Browder, J. (1941). Advances in neurological surgery during the past fifty years. *American Journal of Surgery* 51: 164–187.

Brown, B. (1860). Case of extensive compound fracture of the cranium. Severe laceration and destruction of a portion of the brain, followed by fungus cerebri, and terminating in recovery. *American Journal of the Medical Sciences* 40: 399–403.

Brown, H. (1976). *Brain and Behavior: A Textbook of Physiological Psychology.* New York: Oxford University Press.

Brown, J. W. (1991, January). *Phrenological studies of aphasia before Broca.* Paper presented at the History of Brain Functions Conference, Ft. Myers, Florida.

Browne, W. A. F. (1833). Derangements of the faculty of language from injury to the anterior lobe of the cerebrum. *Lancet* ii: 330–333.

Brunton, T. L. (1874). Inhibition, peripheral and central. *West Riding Lunatic Asylum Reports* 4: 179–222.

Brunton, T. L. (1883). On the nature of inhibition, and the action of drugs upon it. *Nature* 27: 419–422, 436–439, 467–468, 485–487.

Buell, P. L., and Sizer, N. (1842). *A Guide to Phrenology.* Woodstock, VT: Mercury Press.

Bull, J. W. D. (1982). The history of neuroradiology. In F. C. Rose and W. F. Bynum, eds., *Historical Aspects of the Neurosciences* (pp. 255–264). New York: Raven Press.

Burckhardt, G. (1891). Ueber rinderexcisionen, als heitrag zur operativen therapie der psychosen. *Allgemeine Zeitschrift fur Psychiatrie* 47: 463–548.

Burrage, W. L. (1923). *A History of the Massachusetts Medical Society 1781–1922*. Norwood, MA: Plimpton Press.

Cabot, S. (1856–1857). Severe injury to the head, followed by hernia cerebri; death; autopsy. *Boston Medical and Surgical Journal* 55: 227–232.

Cabot, S. (1860). Fracture of the skull; hernia cerebri. *Boston Medical and Surgical Journal* 61: 180–183.

Caldwell, C. (1839). Thoughts on the most effective condition of brain as the organ of mind, etc. *American Phrenological Journal* 1: 393–430.

Calkins, M. W. (1901). *An Introduction to Psychology*. New York: Macmillan.

Campbell, A. W. (1905). *Histological Studies on the Localization of Cerebral Function*. Cambridge: The University Press.

Capen, N. (1881). *Reminiscences of Dr. Spurzheim and George Combe*. New York: Fowler and Wells.

Capon, H. J. (1879). Two cases of fracture of the skull with depression (one with loss of brain substance), in which recovery took place without complication. *Medical Times and Gazette* i: 563–564.

Cardno, J. (1955). Bain and physiological psychology. *Australian Journal of Psychology* 7: 108–120.

Carola, R., Harley, J. P., and Noback, C. R. (1992). *Human Anatomy and Physiology* (2d ed.). New York: McGraw-Hill.

Carlson, N. R. (1994). *Physiology of Behavior* (5th ed.). Boston: Allyn and Bacon.

Carlson, N. R. (1995). *Foundations of Physiological Psychology* (3d ed.). Boston: Allyn and Bacon.

Carmichael, [?]. (1841). Untitled discussion. *Dublin Medical Press* 5: 179–181.

Carpenter, W. B. (1851). *The Principles of Physiology, General and Comparative* (3d ed.). London: Churchill.

Carpenter, W. B. (1874). *Principles of Mental Physiology*. London: King.

Carter, K. C. (1982). On the decline of bloodletting in nineteenth century medicine. *Journal of Psychoanalytic Anthropology* 5: 219–234.

Castaigne, P., Lhermitte, F., Signoret, J. L., and Abelanet, R. (1980). Description et étude scannographique du cerveau de Leborgne: Le découverte de Broca. *Revue Neurologique* 136: 563–583.

Castiglioni, A. (1958). *A History of Medicine*. New York: Knopf.

Castleton Medical College. (1842). *Catalogue of the Students and Graduates of the Fall Term, 1842*. Albany, NY: [Castleton Medical College?].

Chance, E. J. (1858). On a case of complicated injury to the brain and skull, with remarkable persistence of consciousness. With post mortem examination, and clinical remarks. *Lancet* i: 82–84, 134–136.

Chandler, A. D. (1977). *The Visible Hand: The Managerial Revolution in American Business*. Cambridge: Harvard University Press.

Changeux, J.-P. (1985). *Neuronal Man: The Biology of Mind* (L. Garey, trans.). New York: Pantheon. (Original work published 1983)

Changeux, J.-P. and Connes, A. (1995). *Conversations on Mind, Matter, and Mathematics* (M. B. DeBevoise, ed. and trans.). Princeton, NJ: Princeton University Press. (Original work published 1989)

Charcot, J.-M. (1876). *Leçons sur les localisations dans les maladies du Cerveau*. Paris: Bureaux du Progrès Médical.

Charcot, J.-M. (1878). *Lectures on Localization in Diseases of the Brain* (E. P. Fowler, trans.). New York: Wood. (Original work published 1876)

Charcot, J.-M. (1883). *Lectures on the Localization of Cerebral and Spinal Diseases* (W. B. Haden, trans.). London: New Sydenham Society. (Original work published 1876–1880)

Charcot, J.-M., and Pitres, A. (1883). Étude critique et clinique de la doctrine des localisations motrices dans l'écorce des hémisphère cérébraux de l'homme. *Revue de Médicine* 31: 329–354, 426–468, 641–661, 844–875.

Cheney, B. H. (1867). Gunshot wound of the skull. Recovery. *American Journal of the Medical Sciences* 53: 146–148.

Child, H. (1886). *Gazetteer of Grafton County, N.H., 1709–1886*. Syracuse, NY: Syracuse Journal Co.

Childs, F., ed. (1961). *Hanover, New Hampshire: A Bicentenial Book*. Hanover, NH: Hanover Bicentennial Committee.

Chowdhury, R. R. (1941). *Handbook of Mica*. New York: Chemical Publishing Company.

Christison, J. S. (1900). *Brain in Relation to Mind*. Chicago: Meng.

Christman, E. (1931). *One Man's Gold: The Letters and Journal of a Forty-Niner*. London: Whittelsey House.

Clarke, E. S. (1968). Brain anatomy before Steno. In G. Scherz, ed., *Steno and Brain Research in the Seventeenth Century*. *Annalecta Medico-Historica* (Vol. 3, pp. 27–34). Oxford: Pergamon.

Clarke, E. S., and Dewhurst, J. (1972). *An Illustrated History of Brain Function*. Oxford: Sandford Publications.

Clarke, E. S., and Jacyna, L. S. (1987). *Nineteenth-Century Origins of Neuroscientific Concepts*. Berkeley and Los Angeles: University of California Press.

Clarke, E. S., and O'Malley, C. D. (1968). *The Human Brain and Spinal Cord: An Historical Study Illustrated by Writings from Antiquity to the Twentieth Century*. Berkeley and Los Angeles: University of California Press.

Clawson, D. (1980). *Bureaucracy and the Labor Process: The Transformation of U.S. Industry, 1860–1920*. New York: Monthly Review Press.

Cobb, S. (1940). Review of neuropsychiatry for 1940. *Archives of Internal Medicine* 66: 1341–1354.

Cobb, S. (1943). *Borderlands of Psychiatry*. Cambridge: Harvard University Press.

Coleman, J. C., Butcher, J. N., and Carson, R. C. (1984). *Abnormal Psychology and Modern Life* (7th ed.). Glenview, IL: Scott, Foresman.

Coleman, T. (1965). *The Railway Navvies: A History of the Men Who Made the Railways*. London: Hutchinson.

Collins, H. L. (1941). *Philadelphia: A Story of Progress*. Philadelphia: Lewis Historical Publishing.

Columbia-Greystone Associates. (1949). *Selective Partial Ablation of the Frontal Cortex*. New York: Hoeber.

Combe, A. (1823). On the effects of injuries of the brain on the manifestations of the mind. *Transactions of the Phrenological Society* (Edinburgh) 1: 183–208. (Reprinted in G. Combe, 1825, pp. 522–546)

[Combe, A.?] (1827). [Review of] *Physiologie des Tempéramens ou Constitutions, &c. Phrenological Journal* (Edinburgh) 4: 438–454, 604–608. (Attributed to Combe by Cooter, 1989)

Combe, G. (1825). *A System of Phrenology* (2d ed.). Edinburgh: Anderson.

Combe, G. (1830). *A System of Phrenology* (3d ed.). Edinburgh: Anderson.

Constantian, H. M. (1972). The country doctor and his illustrious patient. *Worcester Medical News* 36: 12–15.

Coon, D. (1986). *Introduction to Psychology: Exploration and Adaptation* (5th ed.). Minneapolis-St. Paul, MN: West.

Cooter, R. (1989). *Phrenology in the British Isles: An Annotated, Historical Biobibliography and Index*. London: Scarecrow Press.

Corban, F. (1825). Case of fracture and depression of a part of the frontal bone, with an escape of a considerable portion of the brain; and from which the patient recovered. *London Medical and Physical Journal* 53: 182–185.

Craigie, W. A., and Hulbert, J. R. (1938). *A Dictionary of American English on Historical Principles*. Chicago: University of Chicago Press.

Cranefield, P. F. (1974). *The Way In and the Way Out*. Mt. Kisco, NY: Futura.

Crawford, C. K. (1816). Case of fracture of the skull, in which a quantity of brain was lost and a real hernia cerebri successfully treated by pressure; etc. *Edinburgh Medical and Surgical Journal* 12: 22–25.

Crawford, M. P., Fulton, J. F., Jacobsen, C. F., and Wolfe, J. B. (1948). Frontal lobe ablation in chimpanzee: A résumé of "Becky" and "Lucy." *Research Publications of the Association for Research in Nervous and Mental Disease* 27: 3–58.

Creager, J. (1992). *Human Anatomy and Physiology* (2d ed.). Dubuque, IA: Brown.

Crider, A. B., Goethals, G. R., Kavanagh, R. D., and Solomon, P. R. (1983). *Psychology* (2d ed.). Glenview, IL: Scott, Foresman.

Critchley, M. (1979). God and the brain: Medicine's debt to phrenology. In *The Divine Banquet of the Brain and Other Essays* (pp. 235–253). New York: Raven.

Critchley, M., and Critchley, E. (1998). *John Hughlings Jackson: Father of English Neurology*. New York: Oxford University Press.

Croker, G. (1867). Compound fracture of the skull, with loss of a portion of the substance of the brain. *Medical Press and Circular* (Dublin) 4: 567–568.

Crosier, B. (1975, October 4). Memories Prevail of a Man with a Hole in His Head. *Rutland Daily Herald*, Vermont. p. W-15.

Crowfoot, W. H. (1825). A case of wounded brain. *Edinburgh Medical and Surgical Journal* 24: 260–261.

Cullin, [?]. (1893). Gunshot wound of the head with laceration of the brain; hernia cerebri; Recovery. *Lancet* i: 1517.

Cummings, J. L. (1991). Frontal sub-cortical circuits and human behavior. *Archives of Neurology* 50: 873–880.

Currier, P. J. (1984). *Currier Family Records of USA and Canada* (Vol. 1). Henniker, NH: Author.

Cushing, J. S. (1905). *The Genealogy of the Cushing Family*. Montreal: Perrault.

Cushing, K. R. (1992). *Isinglass, Timber and Wool: A History of the Town of Grafton, New Hampshire*. Grafton: Author.

Dalton, J. G. (1859). *A Treatise on Human Physiology*. Philadelphia: Blanchard and Lea.

Dalton, J. G. (1875). *A Treatise on Human Physiology* (6th ed.). Philadelphia: Blanchard and Lea.

Damasio, A. R. (1985). The frontal lobes. In K. H. Heilman and E. Valenstein, eds., *Clinical Neuropsychology* (2d ed., pp. 339–375). New York: Oxford University Press.

Damasio, A. R. (1993, April). *Memory and language systems in humans*. Paper presented to the 1993 Decade of the Brain Plenary Session, 45th Annual Meeting, American Academy of Neurology, New York. (Available as Audiotape no. 11-47-93 from National Audio Video Inc., Denver, Co)

Damasio, A. R. (1994). *Descartes' Error. Emotion, Reason, and the Human Brain*. New York: Grosset/Putnam.

Damasio, A. R., and Van Hoesen, G. W. (1983). Emotional disturbances associated with focal lesions of the limbic frontal lobe. In K. H. Heilman and P. Satz, eds., *Neuropsychology of Human Emotion* (pp. 85–110). New York: Guilford.

Damasio, H., Grabowski, T., Frank, R., Galaburda, A. M., and Damasio, A. R. (1994). The return of Phineas Gage: Clues about the brain from the skull of a famous patient. *Science* 264: 1102–1105.

Dandy, W. E. (1922). Treatment of non-encapsulated brain tumors by extensive resection of contiguous brain tissue. *Bulletin of the Johns Hopkins Hospital* 33: 188.

Dandy, W. E. (1928). Removal of right cerebral hemisphere for certain tumors with hemiplegia. Preliminary report. *Journal of the American Medical Association* 90: 823–825.

Dandy, W. E. (1933). Physiological studies following extirpation of the right cerebral hemisphere in man. *Bulletin of the Johns Hopkins Hospital* 53: 31–51.

Dandy, W. E. (1966). *The Brain*. Hagertown, MD: Prior.

Danziger, K. (1982). Mid-nineteenth-century British psycho-physiology: A neglected chapter in the history of psychology. In W. R. Woodward and M. G. Ash, eds, *The Problematic Science: A Neglected Chapter in the History of Psychology* (pp. 119–146). New York: Praeger.

D'Auvergne Collings, C. (1893). Case of compound depressed fracture of the skull with loss of brain substance. *Lancet*, i: 926–927.

Davidson, W. (1838). Report of surgical cases treated in the Glasgow Royal Infirmary during the years 1836–1837. *Edinburgh Medical and Surgical Journal* 49: 41–47.

Davidson, W. L. (1904). Supplementary chapter. In A. Bain, *Autobiography* (pp. 400–424). London: Longmans, Green.

Davies, J. D. (1955). *Phrenology: Fad and Science*. New Haven, CT: Yale University Press. (Facsimile reprint 1971, Archon Books)

Davison, G. C., and Neale, J. M. (1974). *Abnormal Psychology: An Experimental Clinical Approach*. New York: Wiley.

Dax, M. (1865). Lesions de la moitié gauche de l'encéphale coïncidant avec l'oubli des signes de las pensée. *Gazette Hebdomadaire de Médicine et de Chirurgie* (Paris) 2: 259–262.

Deaver, J. B. (1901). *Surgical Anatomy: A Treatise on Human Anatomy in Its Application to the Practice of Medicine and Surgery* (Vols. 1–3). Philadelphia: Blakiston.

Denny-Brown, D. (1951). The frontal lobes and their functions. In A. Feiling, ed., *Modern Trends in Neurology* (pp. 13–89). London: Butterworth.

Diamond, S., Balvin, R. S., and Diamond, F. R. (1963). *Inhibition and Choice: A Neurobiological Approach to Problems of Plasticity in Behavior*. New York: Harper and Row.

Dimond, S. J. (1980). *Neuropsychology: A Textbook of Systems and Psychological Functions of the Human Brain*. London: Butterworths.

Dodds, W. J. (1877–1878). On the localisation of functions of the brain. *Journal of Anatomy and Physiology* 12: 340–363, 454–494, 636–660.

Dodge, R. (1926a). The problem of inhibition. *Psychological Review* 33: 1–12.

Dodge, R. (1926b). Theories of inhibition: Parts I and II. *Psychological Review* 33: 106–122, 167–177.

Donaldson, H. H. (1896). Central nervous system. In W. H. Howell, ed., *An American Textbook of Physiology* (pp. 605–743). Philadelphia: Saunders.

Doton, H. (1855). *Map of Windsor County, Vermont.* Pomfret, VT: n.p.

Downs, R. N. (1871). Punctured fracture of the skull, penetrating the brain; apparent recovery; death from cerebral suppuration four months subsequently. *American Journal of the Medical Sciences* 62: 429–433.

Draper, J. W. (1856). *Human Physiology: Statical and Dynamical.* New York: Harper.

Drayton, H. S., and McNeill, J. (1892). *Brain and Mind* (6th ed.). New York: Fowler and Wells.

Dunkel, H. B. (1970). *Herbart and Herbartianism: An Educational Ghost Story.* Chicago: University of Chicago Press.

Dunlap, K. (1912). *A System of Psychology.* New York: Scribner's.

Dunn, R. (1845). Case of suspension of the mental faculties, of the powers of speech, and special senses. *Lancet* ii: 536–538, 588–590.

Dunn, R. (1850). On a case of hemiplegia, with cerebral softening, and in which loss of speech was a prominent symptom. *Lancet* ii: 473–475, 499–500.

Du Pont. (1969). *The Blaster's Handbook.* Wilmington, DE: Du Pont.

Dupuis, T. R. (1872). Compound fracture of the skull-loss of bone and brain-recovery. *Canadian Lancet* 4: 354–358.

Dupuy, E. (1873). *Examen de quelques points de la physiologie du Cerveau.* Paris: Delahaye.

Dupuy, E. (1877a). A critical review of the prevailing theories concerning the physiology and the pathology of the brain. *Medical Times and Gazette* ii: 11–13, 32–34, 84–87, 356–358, 474–475, 488–490.

Dupuy, E. (1877b). Physiology of the brain: An attempt to explain the mode of production of movements following electrical irritation of the cortex cerebri. *New York Medical Journal* 25: 478–490.

Dupuy, E. (1892). The Rolandic area cortex. *Brain* 15: 190–214.

Dworetzky, J. P. (1988). *Psychology* (3d ed.). Minneapolis-St. Paul, MN: West Publishing Co.

Eckstein, G. (1970). *The Body Has a Head.* New York: Harper and Row.

Edes, R. T. (1868). *Dissertations on the Part Performed by Nature and Time in the Cure of Diseases; For Which Prizes Were Awarded by the Massachusetts Medical Society to Robert T. Edes, M.D., James F. Hibberd, M.D., and John Spare, M.D. 1868.* Boston: Clapp & Son.

Edmonson, J. (1823). Case of fracture of the os frontis, with a loss of considerable portion of brain. *Edinburgh Medical and Surgical Journal* 19: 199–202.

Eissler, K. R. (1979). Bericht über die sich in den Vereinigten Staaten befindenden Bücher aus S. Freud's Bibliothek. *Jahrbuch der Psychoanalyse* 11: 10–50.

Elcan, A. L. (1880). Case of extensive traumatic injury of the skull, abscess of the brain, right hemiplegia, aphasia, recovery. *American Journal of the Medical Sciences* 79: 426–429.

Elder, W., and Miles, A. (1902). A case of tumour of the left pre-frontal lobe removed by operation. *Lancet* i: 363–366.

Eriksson, R., ed. (1959). *Andreas Vesalius' First Public Anatomy at Bologna 1540: An Eyewitness Report*. Uppsala, Sweden: Almqvist and Wiksells.

Evans, T. M. (1865). Compound fracture of the skull, followed by extensive cerebral protrusion; recovery. *British Medical Journal* ii: 521.

Fenner, R. (1899). Recovery after bullet wound of the head and destruction of brain tissue. *Lancet* i: 367.

Ferrier, D. (1873). Experimental researches in cerebral physiology and pathology. *West Riding Lunatic Asylum Medical Reports* 3: 30–96.

Ferrier, D. (1876). *The Functions of the Brain*. London: Smith, Elder.

Ferrier, D. (1877–1879). *Correspondence with Henry Pickering Bowditch. Countway Library, Harvard University, Boston*. Manuscript H MS c 5.2.

Ferrier, D. (1878a). The Goulstonian lectures of the localisation of cerebral disease. *British Medical Journal* i: 397–402, 443–447.

Ferrier, D. (1878b). *The Localisation of Cerebral Disease: Being the Gulstonian Lectures of the Royal College of Physicians for 1878*. London: Smith, Elder.

Ferrier, D. (1878c). *Les Fonctions du Cerveau* (H. C. de Varigny trans.). Paris: Germer Baillère. (Original published 1876.)

Ferrier, D. (1879). *Die Functionen der Gehirnes*. (Deutsche ausgabe übers von Heinrich Obersteiner). Braunschweig, Germany: Vieweg.

Ferrier, D. (1880). *Die Localisation der Hirnerkrankungen*. (Deutsche ausgabe übers von R. H. Pierson). Braunschweig, Germany: Vieweg.

Ferrier, D. (1886). *The Functions of the Brain* (2d ed.). London: Smith, Elder.

Ferrier, D. (1889–1890). Cerebral localisation in its practical relations. *Brain* 12: 36–58.

Ferrier, D. (1890a). The Croonian lectures on cerebral localisation (I), (II), (III), (IV). *Lancet* i: 1225–1231, 1287–1293, 1343–1349, 1409–1416.

Ferrier, D. (1890b). Abstract of the Croonian lectures on cerebral localisation (V), (VI). *Lancet* ii: 8–11, 64–66.

Ferrier, D. (1890c). *The Croonian Lectures on Cerebral Localisation*. London: Smith, Elder.

Finger, S. (1994). *Origins of Neuroscience: A History of Exploration into Brain Function*. New York: Oxford University Press.

Finger, S., and Buckingham, H. W. (1994). Alexander Crichton (1763–1856). Disorders of fluent speech and associationist theory. *Archives of Neurology* 51: 498–503.

Finger, S., and Roe, D. (1996). Gustave Dax and the early history of cerebral dominance. *Archives of Neurology* 53: 806–813.

Fisher, R. G. (1951). Psychosurgery. In A. E. Walker, ed., *A History of Neurological Surgery* (pp. 272–284). Baltimore: Williams and Wilkins.

Fitch, J. C. (1852). Case of fracture of the skull, with loss of a portion of the substance of the brain; recovery. *Canada Medical Journal and Monthly Record of Medical and Surgical Science* 1: 96–101.

Fitzpatrick, J. (1840). Case of depressed fracture of the cranium, with paralysis of the left arm. *Dublin Medical Press* 4: 54–55.

Flint, A. (1866). Cases of loss of speech, or aphasia, as connected with hemiplegia, with remarks. *Medical Record* (New York), i: 4–6.

Flint, A. (1901). *A Text-Book of Human Physiology* (4th ed.). New York: Appleton.

Flourens, P. (1846). *Phrenology Examined*. (C. D. Meigs, trans.) Philadelphia: Hogan and Thompson. (Original work published 1842)

Folsom, A. C. (1868–1869). Extraordinary recovery from extensive saw-wound of the skull. *Pacific Medical and Surgical Journal* 2: 550–555.

Forbes, J. G. (1849). Cases of fracture of the skull. *Lancet* i: 579–581.

Foster, B. B. (1975). *Down East Diary* (C. H. Foster, ed.). Orono: University of Maine.

Foster, M. (1897). *A Text Book of Physiology* (7th ed.). London: Macmillan.

Foulis, D. (1879). A case in which the third left frontal convolution was absent, without aphasia. *British Medical Journal* i: 383–384.

[O. S. Fowler?]. (1839). The temperaments. *American Phrenological Journal* 1: 361–369.

Fowler, O. S. (1873). *Human Science: Or, Phrenology*. Philadelphia: National.

Fowler, O. S. (1877). *Works on Phrenology, Physiology, and Kindred Subjects*. Manchester, England: Heywood.

Fox, G. (1849). Compound comminuted fracture of skull removal of a large portion of right parietal bone recovery. *American Journal of the Medical Sciences* 17: 43–44.

Franz, S. I. (1906). On the functions of the cerebrum. The frontal lobes. *Archives of Psychology* 2: 5–64.

Freeman, W. (n.d.). *Adventures in Lobotomy*. Unpublished manuscript. Himmelfarb Health Sciences Library, George Washington University Medical Center, Washington, D.C.

Freeman, W., and Watts, J. W. (1942). *Psychosurgery: Intelligence, Emotion, and Social Behavior Following Prefrontal Lobotomy for Mental Disorders.* Springfield, IL: Thomas.

Freeman, W., and Watts, J. W. (1950). *Psychosurgery in the Treatment of Mental Disorders and Intractable Pain* (2d ed.). Springfield, IL: Thomas.

French, W. (1792). A case of a fractured cranium, attended with a loss of a small portion of the brain. *Medical Society of London Memoirs* 3: 604–605.

Freud, S. (1953a). *On Aphasia: A Critical Study* (E. Stengel, trans.). New York: International Universities Press. (Original work published 1891)

Freud, S. (1953b). *The Interpretation of Dreams.* In *The Standard Edition of the Complete Psychological Works of Sigmund Freud* (Vols. 4–5, pp. 1–621). (Original work published 1900)

Freud, S. (1961a). *The Ego and the Id.* In *The Standard Edition of the Complete Psychological Works of Sigmund Freud* (Vol. 19, pp. 12–59). (Original work published 1923)

Freud, S. (1961b). A note on the "Mystic writing pad." In *The Standard Edition of the Complete Psychological Works of Sigmund Freud* (Vol. 19, pp. 227–232). (Original work published 1925)

Freud, S. (1964). *An Outline of Psycho-Analysis.* In *The Standard Edition of the Complete Psychological Works of Sigmund Freud* (Vol. 23, pp. 144–207). (Original work published 1940)

Freud, S. (1966). *Project for a Scientific Psychology.* In *The Standard Edition of the Complete Psychological Works of Sigmund Freud* (Vol. 1, pp. 295–387). (Unpublished manuscript written 1895)

Fritsch, G., and Hitzig, E. (1960). On the electrical excitability of the cerebrum. In G. von Bonin, ed. and trans., *Some Papers on the Cerebral Cortex* (pp. 73–96). Springfield, IL: Thomas. (Original work published 1870 as Über die electrische Erregbarkeit des Grosshirns, *Archiv für Anatomie, Physiologie, und Wissenschaftliche Medizin* 37: 300–332)

Fritsch, G., and Hitzig, E. (1963). The electrical excitability of the cerebrum. In R. H. Wilkins, trans., *Journal of Neurosurgery* 20: 904–916. (Original work published 1870 as Über die electrische Erregbarkeit des Grosshirns, *Archiv für Anatomie, Physiologie, und Wissenschaftliche Medizin* 37: 300–332)

Fromkin, V., and Rodman, R. (1983). *An Introduction to Language* (3d ed.). New York: Holt, Rinehart and Winston.

Fromkin, V., Rodman, R., Collins, P., and Blair, D. (1990). *An Introduction to Language* (2d Australian ed.). Sydney, Australia: Holt, Rinehart and Winston.

Fulham, V. S. (1910). *The Fulham Genealogy.* Burlington, VT: Free Press Printing.

Fulton, J. F. (1949a). *Functional Localization in the Frontal Lobes and Cerebellum.* Oxford: Oxford University Press.

Fulton, J. F. (1949b). *Physiology of the Nervous System* (3d ed.). New York: Oxford University Press.

Fulton, J. F. (1951). *Frontal Lobotomy and Affective Behavior: A Neurophysiological Analysis.* New York: Norton.

Fulton, J. F., ed. (1966). *Readings in the History of Physiology* (2d ed.) Springfield, IL: Thomas.

Fuster, J. M. (1980). *The Prefrontal Cortex: Anatomy, Physiology, and Neurophysiology of the Frontal Lobe.* New York: Raven.

Gaffney, C. (1860). Case of compound comminuted fracture of skull with loss of brain-substance, treated successfully. *Medical Times and Gazette* ii: 156.

Gage, C. V. ([1964?]). *John Gage of Ipswich, Mass., and his Descendants.* Worcester, NY: Author.

Gage, W. M. (1922). *Gage Families.* Chico, CA: No publisher.

Gainotti, G. (1996). Personality disorders. In J. G. Beaumont, P. M. Kennedy, and M. J. C. Rogers, eds., *The Blackwell Dictionary of Neuropsychology* (pp. 565–569). Oxford: Blackwell.

Gall, F. J. (1835). *On the Functions of the Brain and Each of Its Parts: With Observations on the Possibility of Determining the Instincts, Propensities, and Talents, or the Moral and Intellectual Dispositions of Men and Animals, by the Configuration of the Brain and Head* vols. 1–6 (W. Lewis, trans.). Boston: Marsh, Capen, and Lyon. (Original work published 1822–1825)

Gall, F. J. (1838). Petitions and remonstrances by Dr. Gall against an order by Francis the First, Emperor of Germany. In F. J. Gall, J. Vimont, and F. J. V. Broussais, *On the Functions of the Cerebellum by Drs. Gall, Vimont, and Broussais* (G. Combe, trans. pp. 309–335). Edinburgh: McLachlan and Stewart. (Original work published 1804)

Gall, F. J. (1994). Letter from Dr. F. J. Gall to Mr. Josef F. von Retzer on the prodromus he has completed on the functions of the human and animal brain. In R. Eling, ed., *Reader in the History of Aphasia: From Franz Gall to Norman Geschwind* (pp. 17–27). Amsterdam: John Benjamins. (Original work published 1798)

Gall, F. J., and Spurzheim, J. G. (1810–1819). *Anatomie et Physiologie du Système Nerveux en Général, et du Cerveaux en Particulier, avec des Observations sur la Possibilité de Reconnoitre Plusiers Dispositions Intellectuuells et Morales de L'homme et des Animaux, par la Configuration de leurs Têtes* (Vols. 1–5). Paris: Schoell.

Gardner, M. (1981). *Science: Good, Bad and Bogus.* Buffalo, NY: Prometheus.

Garrison, F. H. (1913). *An Introduction to the History of Medicine.* Philadelphia: Saunders.

Geison, G. L. (1972). Social and institutional factors in the stagnancy of English physiology, 1840–1870. *Bulletin of the History of Medicine* 46: 30–58.

Georget, A. (1998). *Sur les Traces de Phineas Gage*. Paris: Interscoop/Arté.

German, W. J., and Fox, J. C. (1934). Observations following unilateral lobectomies. *Research Publications of the Association for Research in Nervous and Mental Disease* 13: 378–430.

Goonetilleke, J. K. D. A. (1979). Long term survival following firearm injury to the head. *Medicine, Science, and the Law* 19: 205–207.

Gould, G. M., and Pyle, W. L. (1896). *Anomalies and Curiosities of Medicine*. Philadelphia: Saunders.

Government of the Commonwealth of Massachusetts. (1885). *A Souvenir. Historical, Descriptive and Biographical Sketches*. Boston: Tichner.

Gowers, W. R. (1879). Cases of cerebral tumour illustrating diagnosis and localisation. *Lancet* i: 327–329, 363–365.

Gowers, W. R. (1885). *Diagnosis of Diseases of the Brain and of the Spinal Cord*. New York: Wood.

Gray, F. J. (1868). Gunshot wound in the head. Injury to brain without severe symptoms; recovery. *Lancet* i: 374.

Greenblatt, M., Arnot, R., and Solomon, H. C. (1950). *Studies in Lobotomy*. New York: Grune and Stratton.

Greenblatt, S. H. (1965). The major influences on the early life and work of John Hughlings Jackson. *Bulletin of the History of Medicine* 39: 346–376.

Greenblatt, S. H. (1977). The development of Hughlings Jackson's approach to diseases of the nervous system 1863–1866: Unilateral seizures, hemiplegia, and aphasia. *Bulletin of the History of Medicine* 51: 412–430.

Griesinger, W. (1867). *Mental Pathology and Therapeutics* (2nd German ed., C. Lockhart and J. Rutherford, trans). London: New Sydenham Society. (Original work published 1861)

Groves, P. M., and Schlesinger, K. (1982). *Introduction to Biological Psychology* (2d ed.). Dubuque, IA: Brown.

Guthrie, G. J. (1842). *On Injuries of the Head Affecting the Brain*. London: Churchill and Renshaw.

Guyton, A. C., and Hall, J. E. (1996). *Textbook of Medical Physiology* (9th ed.). Philadelphia: Saunders.

Hall, M. (1832). On a particular function of the nervous system. *Proceedings of the Committee of Science and Correspondence of the Zoological Society of London*, Part 2, vol. 25: 190–192.

Hall, M. (1837a). On the reflex function of the medulla oblongata and medulla spinalis. In *Memoirs of the Nervous System* (Part 1, pp. 1–31). London: Gilbert, Sherwood, and Piper. (Original work published 1833)

Hall, M. (1837b). *On the True Spinal Marrow and on the Excito-Motory System of the Nerves*. London: Sherwood, Gilbert and Piper.

Hall, M. (1839). Memoirs on some principles of pathology in the nervous system. *Medico-Chirurgical Transactions* 22: 191–217.

Hall, M. (1843). *New Memoirs on the Nervous System*. London: Baillère.

Halliburton, W. D. (1896). *Kirkes' Hand-Book of Physiology* (14th ed.). London: John Murray.

Halliburton, W. D. (1909). *Handbook of Physiology* (9th ed.; 22d ed. of Kirkes' *Physiology*). London: John Murray.

Halliburton, W. D., and McDowall, R. J. S. (1937). *Handbook of Physiology and Biochemistry* (35th ed.). London: John Murray.

Hamby, W. B. (1967). *Ambroise Paré: Surgeon of the Renaissance*. St. Louis, MO: Green.

Hamilton, F. H. (1864). Lectures on gunshot injuries of the head. *American Medical Times* 8: 61–62, 73–74, 85–86, 97–99.

Hammond, W. A. (1871). *A Treatise on the Diseases of the Nervous System*. New York: Appleton.

"Hard to Believe but Absolutely True" (1930, August 30) *New York Sun*, p. 20.

Hargrave, [?]. (1861). Compound and depressed fracture, with loss of cerebral substance; recovery. *Dublin Medical Press* 46: 387.

Harlow, J. M. (1848). Passage of an iron rod through the head. *Boston Medical and Surgical Journal* 39: 389–393.

Harlow, J. M. (1849). Letter in "Medical miscellany." *Boston Medical and Surgical Journal* 39: 506–507.

Harlow, J. M. (1868). Recovery from the passage of an iron bar through the head. *Publications of the Massachusetts Medical Society* 2: 327–347.

Harlow, J. M. (1869). *Recovery from the Passage of an Iron Bar through the Head*. Boston: Clapp.

Harmatz, M. G. (1978). *Abnormal Psychology*. Englewood Cliffs, NJ: Prentice-Hall.

Harris, J. (1993). "The Sage of Manchester Square": A glance at Hughlings Jackson and his ideas on brain function. *Perception* 22: 1383–1388.

Harris, R. P. (1847). Case of compound fracture of the skull, with escape of cerebral substance, ending in recovery. *American Journal of the Medical Sciences* 13: 67–70.

Harrup, R. (1814). Singular case of recovery, after the loss of a considerable portion of the brain. *London Medical and Physical Journal* 32: 184–187.

Hart, L. A. (1975). *How the Brain Works: A New Understanding of Human Learning, Emotion, and Thinking*. New York: Basic Books.

Harvard University. (1850). *Catalogue of Students Attending Medical Lectures in Boston 1849–1850*. Boston: Author.

Harvey, G. (1846). Instance of fracture of the cranium, with depression, and subsequent hernia cerebri. *Lancet* ii: 503–506.

Hayes, L. S. (1907). *History of the Town of Rockingham, Vermont Including the Villages of Bellows Falls*. Rockingham, VT: Town of Rockingham.

Hayes, L. S. (1929). *The Connecticut River Valley in Southern Vermont and New Hampshire: Historical Sketches*. Rutland, VT: Tuttle.

Head, H. (1926). *Aphasia and Kindred Disorders of Speech* (Vol. 1). Cambridge: Cambridge University Press.

Heard, L. (1863). Punctured wound of the brain. *Boston Medical and Surgical Journal* 68: 380–382.

Hearnshaw, L. S. (1964). *A Short History of British Psychology 1840–1940*. London: Methuen.

Hebb, D. O., and Penfield, W. (1940). Human behavior after extensive bilateral removal from the frontal lobes. *Archives of Neurology and Psychiatry* 44: 421–438.

Henderson, D. K., and Gillesipie, R. D. (1944). *A Text-book of Psychiatry* (6th ed.). London: Oxford University Press.

Herbart, J. F. (1891). *A Textbook in Psychology: An Attempt to Found the Science of Psychology on Experience, Metaphysics, and Mathematics* (2d ed., M. K. Smith, trans.). New York: Appleton. (Original work published 1834)

Heustis, J. W. (1829). Inquiry into the causes, nature, and treatment of hernia cerebri. *American Journal of the Medical Sciences* 4: 315–330.

Hildebrandt, H. (1991, September). *Der psychologische Versuch in der Psychiatrie: Was wurde aus Kraepelins (1895) Programm?* Paper presented to 3. Fachtagung der Fachgruppe "Geschichte der Psychologie," Passau.

Hilgard, E. R. (1987). *Psychology in America: A Historical Survey*. San Diego, CA: Harcourt, Brace, Jovanovich.

Hippocrates. (1849). On the sacred disease. In F. Adams, ed. and trans., *The Genuine Works of Hippocrates* (pp. 347–360). London: New Sydenham Society.

Hippocrates. (1923–1931). The sacred disease. In *Selected Works* (Vol. 2, W. H. S. Jones, ed. and trans., pp. 139–183). London: Heinemann.

Hitzig, E. (1870). Über die electrische Erregbarkeit des Grosshirns. *Berliner Klinische Wochenschrift* 19: 227–228.

Hockenbury, D. H., and Hockenbury, S. E. (1997). *Psychology*. New York: Worth.

Hoff, T. (1991, January). *Gall's concept of internal function; in reply to Dallenbach (1915) and Young (1970)*. Paper presented at the History of Brain Functions Conference, Ft. Myers, FL.

Hollander, B. (1901). *The Mental Functions of the Brain*. London: Grant Richards.

Hollander, B. (1931). *Brain, Mind, and the External Signs of Intelligence*. London: George Allen and Unwin.

Holmes, O. W. (1891). *Memoir of Henry Jacob Bigelow*. Cambridge: Wilson.

Home, E. (1814). Observations on the functions of the brain. *Philosophical Transactions of the Royal Society, London* 104: 469–486.

Hooper, E. S. (1920). Alexander Bain. In S. Lee, ed., *Dictionary of National Biography. Twentieth Century, Supplement 1901–1911* (pp. 79–81). Oxford: Oxford University Press.

Horlbeck, E. (1848). Case of compound fracture of the cranium with loss of cerebral substance. *American Journal of the Medical Sciences* 17: 239–240.

Horsley, V. (1884–1885). Case of occipital encephalocele in which a correct diagnosis was obtained by means of the induced current. *Brain* 7: 228–243.

Horsley, V. (1886). Brain-surgery. *British Medical Journal* ii: 670–675.

Horsley, V. (1887a). Note on the means of topographical diagnosis of focal disease affecting the so-called motor regions of the cerebral cortex. *American Journal of the Medical Sciences* 95: 342–369.

Horsley, V. (1887b). Remarks on ten consecutive cases of operations upon the brain and cranial cavity to illustrate the details and safety of the method employed. *British Medical Journal* i: 863–866.

Howard, B. (1871). A case of trephining and removal of a minié bullet which had passed into the brain through a trap-door fracture of the os frontis, followed by recovery. *American Journal of the Medical Sciences* 52: 385–389.

Howell, W. H. (1937). *A Text-Book of Physiology for Medical Students and Physicians*. Philadelphia: Saunders.

Hugan, G. H. (1956). The Rutland Railway: The little train that could. *Vermont Life* 11(1): 2–7.

Hughes, C. D. (1897). Neurological progress in America. *Journal of the American Medical Association* 29: 315–323.

Hughes, C. H. (1875). On the vicarious function of the cerebral hemispheres and convolutions, considered in relation to unilateral wounds of the head and insanity. *American Journal of Insanity* 32: 184–197.

Humphreys, C. E. (1885). Compound depressed fracture of the skull; loss of cerebral substance; non interference; recovery. *Lancet* ii: 243.

Hunter, W. B. (1881). Fracture of the base of the skull; recovery. *Lancet* ii: 788.

Hurd, D. H., ed. (1890). *History of Middlesex County, Massachusetts* (Vol. 1). Philadelphia: J. W. Lewis.

Hutter, O. F. (1961). Ion movements during vagus inhibition of the heart. In E. Florey, ed. *Nervous Inhibition* (pp. 114–123). Oxford: Pergamon.

Huxley, T. (1923). *Lessons in Elementary Physiology* (J. Barcroft, ed.). New York: Macmillan.

Jackson, J. B. S. (1849). *Medical Cases* (Vol. 4, Cases no. 1358–1929, pp. 720, 610). *Countway Library Harvard University, Boston.* Manuscript H MS b 72.4.

Jackson, J. B. S. (1870). *A Descriptive Catalogue of the Warren Anatomical Museum.* Boston: Williams.

Jackson, J. H. (1861). Syphilitic affections of the nervous system. *Medical Times and Gazette* i: 642–652, ii: 59–60, 83–85, 133–135.

Jackson, J. H. (1863). *Suggestions for Studying the Diseases of the Nervous System on Professor Owen's Vertebral Theory.* London: np.

Jackson, J. H. (1864). Clinical remarks on cases of defects of expression (by words, writing, signs, etc) in diseases of the nervous system. *Lancet* ii: 604–605.

Jackson, J. H. (1869). A study of convulsions. *St. Andrews' Medical Graduates Association: Transactions* 3: 162–204.

Jackson, J. H. (1873). On the anatomical and physiological localisation of movements in the brain. *Lancet* i: 84–85, 162–164, 232–234.

Jackson, J. H. (1874a). Observations on the localisation of movements in the cerebral hemispheres as revealed by cases of convulsion, chorea, and "aphasia." *West Riding Lunatic Asylum Medical Reports* 3: 175–195.

Jackson, J. H. (1874b). On the scientific and empirical investigations of epilepsies. *Medical Press and Circular* 69: 325–327, 347–352, 389–393, 409–412, 475–478, 497–499, 519–521.

Jackson, J. H. (1875). Temporary mental disorders after epileptic paroxysms. *West Riding Lunatic Asylum Reports* 5: 105–129.

Jackson, J. H. (1884). Croonian Lectures on evolution and dissolution of the nervous system. *Lancet* i: 555–558, 649–652, 739–744.

Jackson, J. H. (1887). An address on the psychology of joking. *Lancet* ii: 800–801.

Jackson, J. H. (1888–1889). Discussion of Dr. Mercier's "Inhibition." *Brain* 11: 386–393.

Jacobs, L. M., Berrizbeitia, L. D., and Ordia, J. (1985). Crowbar impalement of the brain. *Journal of Trauma* 25: 359–361.

Jacobsen, C. F. with Elder, J. H., and Haselrud, G. M. (1936). Studies of cerebral functions in primates: I. The functions of the frontal association areas in monkeys. *Comparative Psychology Monographs* 13(3): 3–60.

Jacobsen, C. F., Wolfe, J. B., and Jackson, T. A. (1935). An experimental analysis of the functions of the frontal association areas in primates. *Journal of Nervous and Mental Disease* 82: 1–29.

James, A. (1881). The reflex inhibitory centre theory. *Brain* 4: 287–302.

James, W. (1890). *The Principles of Psychology* (Vols. 1 and 2). New York: Holt.

Janson, H. (1840). Case of gun-shot wound of the head and brain recovery. *American Journal of the Medical Sciences* 26: 248–249.

Jasper, H. H. (1995). A historical perspective: The rise and fall of prefrontal lobotomy. In H. H. Jasper, S. Riggio, and P. S. Goldman-Rakic, eds., *Epilepsy and the Functional Anatomy of the Frontal Lobe* (pp. 97–114). New York: Raven.

Jefferson Medical College. (1843). *Annual Announcement of Jefferson Medical College of Philadelphia: Session 1843–1844* Philadelphia: [Jefferson Medical College?].

Jefferson Medical College. (1844). *Catalogue of the Students and Faculty of Jefferson Medical College of Philadelphia for the Session 1843–1844*. Philadelphia: [Jefferson Medical College?].

Jefferson Medical College. (1845). *Catalogue of the Students and Faculty of Jefferson Medical College of Philadelphia for the Session 1844–1845*. Philadelphia: [Jefferson Medical College?].

Jewett, M. (1868). Extraordinary case of recovery after severe injury to the head. *Western Journal of Medicine* 3: 151–152.

Joanette, Y. (1990, July). *The early diagram makers: The point of view of a contemporary*. Paper presented at the World Federation of Neurology—Research Group on Aphasia, Toulouse, France.

Johnson, A. B. (1928). *Two Sons of Vermont*. Woodstock, VT: Elm Tree Press.

Johnson, T. H., and Ward, T., eds. (1965). *The Letters of Emily Dickinson* (Vols. 1 and 2). Cambridge: Harvard University Press.

Jones, A. (1826). Case of fractured skull, with loss of portion of the brain. *Philadelphia Journal of Medical and Physical Sciences* 4: 158–160.

Joynt, R. J., and Benton, A. L. (1964). The memoir of Marc Dax on aphasia. *Neurology* 14: 851–854.

Judd, C. H. (1907). *Psychology. General Introduction*. New York: Scribner's.

Kalat, J. W. (1981). *Biological Psychology*. Belmont, CA: Wadsworth.

Kalat, J. W. (1996). *Introduction to Psychology* (4th ed.). Pacific Grove, CA: Brooks/Cole.

Kantor, J. R. (1924). *Principles of Psychology*. New York: Knopf.

Kebbell, A. (1876). Case of compound comminuted fracture of skull; laceration and escape of brain matter; partial paralysis of right arm; removal of thirteen fragments of bone; recovery. *Lancet* i: 11–12.

Keen, W. W. (1888). Three successful cases of cerebral surgery. *American Journal of the Medical Sciences* 96: 329–357, 453–465.

Keith, A. (1911). An address on the position of Sir Charles Bell among anatomists. *Lancet* i: 290–293.

Kelly, H. A. (1912). *A Cyclopedia of American Medical Biography* (Vol. 1). Philadelphia: Saunders.

Kemper, G. W. H. (1885). A case of lodgement of a breech-pin in the brain; removal on the second day; recovery. *American Journal of the Medical Sciences* 89: 128–130.

[Kennedy, J.?] (1829). Remarks on Mr. Stone's "Evidences against the System of Phrenology," No. VII, including a Comprehensive View of the New Theory of Temperament. By Dr. Thomas des Trosievères. *London Medical and Surgical Journal* 2: 507–530. (Attributed to Kennedy by Cooter, 1989)

Kimble, D. P. (1963). *Physiological Psychology: A Unit for Introductory Psychology*. Reading, MA: Addison–Wesley.

Kirkes, W. S. (1848). *Hand-Book of Physiology*. London: John Murray.

Kirkland, E. C. (1948). *Men Cities and Transportation: A Study in New England History 1820–1900*. Cambridge: Harvard University Press.

Knapp, P. C. (1891). *The Pathology, Diagnosis, and Treatment of Intra-Cranial Growths*. Boston: Rockwell and Churchill.

Kolb, B., and Whishaw, I. Q. (1985). *Fundamentals of Human Neuropsychology* (2d ed.). New York: Freeman.

Krech, D. (1963). Cortical localization of function. In L. Postman, ed., *Psychology in the Making: Histories of Selected Research Problems* (pp. 31–72). New York: Knopf.

Kulpe, O. (1909). *Outlines of Psychology* (E. B. Titchener, trans.). New York: Macmillan. (Original work published 1901)

Kuntz, A. (1970). Eduard Hitzig. In W. Haymaker and F. Schiller, eds., *The Founders of Neurology* (2d ed., pp. 229–233). Springfield, IL: Thomas.

Lacy, B. (1984, December 10). He survived this injury. *Valley News* (White River Junction, Vermont), p. 17.

Ladd, G. T. (1894). *Psychology. Descriptive and Explanatory*. New York: Scribner's.

Ladd, G. T. (1898). *Outlines of Descriptive Psychology*. New York: Scribner's.

Lahey, B. B. (1992). *Psychology: An Introduction* (4th ed.). Dubuque, IA: Brown.

Lamere, B. (1964–1965). Phineas Gage had a headache. *The Rural Vermonter* 3: 28–29.

Landois, L. (1887). *A Text-Book of Human Physiology* (2d American ed., W. Stirling, trans.). Philadelphia: Blakiston.

Lanphear, E. (1895). Lectures on intracranial surgery. XI—The surgical treatment of insanity. *Journal of the American Medical Association* 24: 883–886.

Larson, B. M. (1977). *Memorials No. 2 of the Descendents of William Shattuck*. Wisconsin, Rickland Center: Rickland County Publishers.

Laycock, T. (1841). *A Treatise on the Nervous Diseases of Women; Comprising an Inquiry into the Nature, Causes, and Treatment of Spinal and Hysterical Disorders*. London: Longmans.

Laycock, T. (1845). On the reflex function of the brain. *British and Foreign Medical Review* 19: 298–311.

Laycock, T. (1854). The correlation of psychology and physiology. *Journal of Psychological Medicine* 7: 511–519.

Laycock, T. (1855). Further researches into the function of the brain. *British and Foreign Medical Review* 16: 155–187.

Laycock, T. (1860). *Mind and Brain, or, The Correlations of Consciousness and Organisation: with their Applications to Philosophy, Zoology, Physiology, Mental Pathology, and the Practice of Medicine.* Edinburgh: Sutherland and Knox.

Laycock, T. (1871). Lectures on the clinical observation of diseases of the nervous system. *Medical Times and Gazette* i: 31–34, 91–93, 151–153.

Lefrancois, G. R. (1980). *Psychology.* Belmont, CA: Wadsworth.

Leishman, T. (1890–1891). Case of extensive injury of the left frontal lobe from a wound. *Edinburgh Medical and Surgical Journal* 36: 327–329.

Leny, R. (1793). Remarkable case of a boy, who lost a considerable portion of brain, and who recovered, without detriment to any faculty, mental or corporeal. *Medical Commentaries* 8: 301–316. (Original work published 1792)

Leonardo, R. A. (1943). *History of Surgery.* New York: Froben Press.

Le Page, J. F. (1881). A case of compound fracture of the skull, with laceration of the brain and loss of brain substance. *Lancet* ii: 789.

LeUnes, A. (1974). Contributions to the history of psychology: 20. A review of selected aspects of texts in abnormal psychology. *Psychological Reports* 35: 1319–1326.

Levitt, R. A. (1981). *Physiological Psychology.* New York: Holt, Rinehart, and Winston.

Lewis, N. D., and Landis, C. (1957). Freud's library. *Psychoanalytic Review* 44: 327–354.

Lewis, W. B. (1883). Cerebral localisation in its relationships to psychological medicine. *British Medical Journal* ii: 624–628.

Leys, R. (1990). *From Sympathy to Reflex: Marshall Hall and His Opponents.* New York: Garland Publishing.

Licht, W. (1983). *Working for the Railroad: The Organization of Work in the Nineteenth Century.* Princeton, NJ: Princeton University Press.

Lichterman, B. (1998). Roots and routes of Russian neurosurgery (from surgical neurology towards neurological surgery). *Journal of the History of the Neurosciences* 7: 125–135.

Little, G. T. (1882). *The Descendants of George Little, Who Came to Newbury, Massachusetts, in 1640.* Auburn, ME: Author.

Lloyd, J. H., and Deaver, J. B. (1888). A case of focal epilepsy successfully treated by trephining and excision of the motor centres. *American Journal of the Medical Sciences* 96: 477–487.

Lucas, M. S. (1940). *Elements of Human Physiology.* Philadelphia: Lea and Febiger.

Lund, F. H. (1927). *Psychology: The Science of Mental Activity.* New York: Seiler.

Luria, A. (1966a). *Higher Cortical Functions in Man* (B. Haigh, trans.). London: Tavistock. (Original work published 1962)

Luria, A. (1966b). *Human Brain and Psychological Processes* (B. Haigh, trans.). New York: Harper. (Translation of manuscript)

Luzzatti, C., and Whitaker, H. (1996). Johannes Schenck and Johannes Jakob Wepfer: Clinical and anatomical observations in the prehistory of neurolinguistics and neuropsychology. *Journal of Neurolinguistics* 9: 157–164.

Lyman, G. D. (1925). *The Beginnings of California's Medical History*. San Francisco, CA: n.p. (Original work published 1925)

McBurney, M. D., and Starr, M. A. (1893). A contribution to cerebral surgery. *American Journal of the Medical Sciences* 105: 361–387.

M'carthy, J. (1882–1883). Compound fracture of skull, and abscess of frontal lobes. *Biological Bulletin of the Marine Biological Laboratory, Woods Hole, Mass.* 5: 559–561.

McCaw, J. F. (1919). Gangrene of the temporosphenoidal lobe, right side, of otitic origin—operation and extensive excision of the lobe—with recovery. *Annals of Otology, Rhinology and Laryngology* 28: 823–827.

McCollom, I. N. (1973). Psychological classics: Older journal articles frequently cited today. *American Psychologist* 28: 363–365.

McDougall, W. (1920). *Outline of Psychology*. New York: Scribner's.

Macewen, W. (1879). Tumour of the dura mater—Convulsions—Removal of tumour by trephining—Recovery. *Glasgow Medical Journal* 11: 210–213.

Macewen, W. (1881). Inter-cranial lesions illustrating some points in connexion with the localisation of cerebral affections and the advantages of antiseptic trephining. *Lancet* ii: 541–543, 581–583.

Macewen, W. (1888). An address on the surgery of the brain and spinal cord. *British Medical Journal* ii: 302–309.

MacGillivray, P. H. (1864). On a case of compound fracture of the skull, with laceration of the brain and hernia cerebri. Recovery. *Australian Medical Journal* 9: 163–164.

Mackay, G. (1853). Case of gun-shot wound of the left lung terminating in recovery, and a case of gun-shot wound of the skull, followed by great loss of substance. *Monthly Journal of Medical Science* (Edinburgh) 16: 481–486.

Maclaren, P. W. (1861–1862). Case of punctured wound of the brain—Recovery. *Edinburgh Medical and Surgical Journal* 7: 645–648.

McMahon, F. B., and McMahon, J. W. (1982). *Psychology: The Hybrid Science* (4th ed.). Homewood, IL: Dorsey.

Macmillan, M. B. (1986). A wonderful journey through skull and brains: The travels of Mr. Gage's tamping iron. *Brain and Cognition* 5: 67–107.

Macmillan, M. B. (1990). Freud and Janet on organic and hysterical paralyses: A mystery solved? *International Review of Psychoanalysis* 17: 189–203.

Oxford University Press. (1992). *The Oxford English Dictionary on Compact Disc* (2d ed.). Oxford: Oxford University Press.

Packard, F. R. (1901). *The History of Medicine in the United States.* Philadelphia: Lippincott.

Pagel, W. (1958). Medieval and renaissance contributions to knowledge of the brain and its functions. In F. N. L. Poynter, ed., *The History and Philosophy of Knowledge of the Brain and Its Functions* (pp. 95–114). Oxford: Blackwell Scientific.

Parsons, H. (1884). Bullet-wound of the cerebral hemispheres, with hemiplegia: Complete recovery. *British Medical Journal* ii: 759.

Patten, T. H. (1968). *The Foreman: Forgotten Man of Management.* New York: American Management Association.

Peabody, G. A. (1937). *South American Journals, 1858–1859* (ed. J. C. Phillips). Salem, MA: Peabody Museum.

Peake, S. (1820). Case of fractured skull, with loss of portion of the brain, successfully treated. *Edinburgh Medical and Surgical Journal* 16: 513–516.

Pearce, J. M. S. (1982). The first attempt at removal of brain tumors. In F. C. Rose and W. F. Bynum, eds., *Historical Aspects of the Neurosciences* (pp. 239–242). New York: Raven Press.

Penfield, W. (1958). Hippocratic preamble. In F. N. L. Poynter, ed., *The History and Philosophy of Knowledge of the Brain and Its Functions* (pp. 1–4). Oxford: Blackwell Scientific.

Penfield, W., and Evans, J. (1934). Functional defects produced by cerebral lobectomies. *Research Publications of the Association for Research in Nervous and Mental Disease* 13: 352–377. (Original work published 1932)

Penfield, W., and Evans, J. (1935). The frontal lobe in man: A clinical study of maximum removals. *Brain* 58: 115–133.

Pilkington, G. W., and McKellar, P. (1960). Inhibition as a concept in psychology. *British Journal of Psychology* 51: 194–201.

Pillsbury, W. B. (1911). *The Essentials of Psychology.* New York: Macmillan.

Pitres, A. (1877). *Recherches sur les Lésions du Centre Ovale des Hémisphères Cérébraux Étudiées au Point de vue des Localisations Cérébrales.* Paris: Bureaux du Progrès Médical.

Plotnik, R. (1996). *Introduction to Psychology* (4th ed.). Pacific Grove, CA: Brooks/Cole.

Poor, H. V. (1860). *History of the Railroads and Canals of the United States of America.* New York: Schultz.

Porter, G. H. (1858). Case of gunshot wound. *Dublin Medical Press* 11: 386–387.

Pott, P. (1768). *Observations on the Nature and Consequences of Those Injuries to Which the Head Is Liable from External Violence.* London: Hawes, Clarke, and Collins.

Pott, P. (1790). *The Chirurgical Works of Percivall Pott F.R.S.* (Vols. 1–3). London: Johnson, Robinson, Robinson, Cadell, Murray, Fox, Bew, Hayes, and Lowndes.

Pott, P. (1808). *The Chirurgical Works of Percivall Pott F.R.S.* (Vols. 1–3). London: Johnson, and others.

Power, D. (1932). Some bygone operations in surgery: The first localized cerebral tumour. *British Journal of Surgery* 19: 523–526.

Pressman, J. D. (1998). *Last Resort: Psychosurgery and the Limits of Medicine.* Cambridge: Cambridge University Press.

Prewitt, T. F. (1873). A case of gunshot wound in the head—The patient surviving for eleven months, with the bullet in the brain. *St. Louis Medical and Surgical Journal* 10: 610–612.

Prochaska, G. (1851). *Dissertation on the Functions of the Nervous System* (T. Laycock, trans.). London: Sydenham Society. (Original work published 1784)

Putnam, J. J. (1875). Contribution to the physiology of the cortex cerebrii. *Boston Medical and Surgical Journal* 91: 49–53.

Quain, [?]. (1861). Concussion of the brain, with paralysis of the left arm; persistence of the former; recovery, with impaired intellect. *Lancet* ii: 372–373.

Quain, J. (1848). *Elements of Anatomy* (5th ed., R. Quain and W. Sharpey, eds.). London: Taylor, Watson, and Malberly.

Rasmussen, L. J. (1965–1969). *San Francisco Ship Passenger Lists.* Colma, CA: San Francisco Historic Records and Genealogy Bulletin.

Raymond, J. H. (1905). *Human Physiology* (3d ed.). Philadelphia: Saunders.

Restak, R. M. (1984). *The Brain.* New York: Bantam Books.

Rettger, L. J. (1898). *Studies in Advanced Physiology.* Terre Haute, IN: Inland Publishing.

Review of F. E. Anstie's *Stimulants and Narcotics, Their Mutual Relations.* (1864a). *Lancet, ii,* 121–124.

Review of F. E. Anstie's *Stimulants and Narcotics, Their Mutual Relations.* (1864b). *British Medical Journal, ii,* 627–629.

Review of F. E. Anstie's *Stimulants and Narcotics, Their Mutual Relations.* (1864c). *Medical Times and Gazette, ii,* 661–662.

Review of Guthrie's "On injuries of the head affecting the brain." (1843). *British and Foreign Medical Review* 15: 161–180.

Review of Wm. James "Principles of Psychology." (1890–1891). *American Journal of Psychology* 3: 551–552.

Ribot, Th. (1874). *English Psychology.* New York: Appleton.

Ribot, Th. (1891). *Les Maladies de la Volonté* (7th ed.). Paris: Librarie Baillère. (Hinterberger Collection, Item Number 633)

Ribot, Th. (1894). *The Diseases of the Will* (4th English ed. from 8th French ed., M.-M. Snell, trans.). Chicago: Open Court.

Rice, D. (1849). Remarkable case of recovery from gun-shot wound of the head. *Boston Medical and Surgical Journal* 40: 323–324.

Riese, W. (1958). Descartes's ideas of brain function. In F. N. L. Poynter, ed., *The History and Philosophy of Knowledge of the Brain and Its Functions* (pp. 115–134). Oxford: Blackwell Scientific.

Roberts, G. M. (1957). *The Vital and Cemetery Records of the Town of Enfield, Grafton County, New Hampshire*. N.p.: G. M. Roberts.

Roberts, W. (1838–1839). Novel mode of treating injuries of the brain. *Lancet* i: 655–656.

Robertson, J. W. (1894). Cerebral localization—What is known, what is surmized, and what is its surgical value. *Journal of the American Medical Association* 23: 192–196.

Robertson, J. W. (1896). Brain surgery and operations based on cerebral localization. *American Medico-Surgical Bulletin* 10: 203–206.

Robin, A., and Macdonald, D. (1975). *Lessons of Leucotomy*. London: Henry Kimpton.

Rogers, [?]. (1827). Case of injury to the head. With remarks by Mr. Tyrrell. *Medico-Chirurgical Transactions* 13: 282–292.

Rose, J. (1858). On a case of fracture of the cranium with protrusion of brain. *Lancet* i: 35–36.

Rosenhan, D., and Seligman, M. E. P. (1984). *Abnormal Psychology*. New York: Norton.

Rosenzweig, M. R., and Leiman, A. R. (1982). *Physiological Psychology*. Lexington, MA: Heath.

Royal Medical and Chirurgical Society. (1885). Reports of Societies: Royal Medical and Chirurgical Society, Tuesday May 12th, 1885. *British Medical Journal* i: 988–989.

Ruch, J. C. (1984). *Psychology: The Personal Science*. Belmont, CA: Wadsworth.

Russell, W. R. (1948). Function of frontal lobes. *Lancet* i: 356–360.

Rutland and Burlington Railroad Company. (1850). *Report of the Directors of the Rutland and Burlington Railroad Company at their Annual Meeting*. Burlington, VT: Free Press.

Rylander, G. (1939). *Personality Changes after Operations on the Frontal Lobes: A Clinical Study of 32 Cases*. Copenhagen: Munksgaard.

Saunders, J. B. deC. M., and O'Malley. C. D. (1950). *The Illustrations from the Works of Andreas Vesalius of Brussels*. Cleveland, OH: World. (Dover reprint edition, 1973)

Savage, E. H. (1873). *Police Records and Recollections, or Boston by Daylight and Gaslight for Two Hundred and Forty Years*. Boston: Dale; Montclair, NJ: Patterson Smith reprint, 1971.

Saxon, A. H. (1989). *P. T. Barnum: The Legend and the Man.* New York: Columbia University Press.

Schele de Vere, M. (1872). *Americanisms: The English of the New World.* New York: Scribner.

Schiller, F. (1979). *Paul Broca: Founder of French Anthropology, Explorer of the Brain.* Berkeley and Los Angeles: University of California Press.

Scott, J. N. (1796). Two cases, showing that the anterior part of the brain may sustain considerable injury without fatal consequence. *Annals of Medicine* (Edinburgh) 1: 358–370.

Sdorow, L. (1990). *Psychology.* Dubuque, IA: Brown.

Seccombe, T. (1921–1922). Thomas Laycock. In L. Stephen and S. Lee, eds., *Dictionary of National Biography* (pp. 744–745). Oxford: Oxford University Press.

Sechenov, I. (1935). Physiologische studien über die Hemmungsmechanismen für die Reflexthätigkeit des Rüuckenmarks im Gehirne des Frosches. In I. Sechenov *Selected Works* (pp. 153–176). Moscow: XVth. International Physiological Congress (Amsterdam: Bonset reprint 1968. Original work published 1862)

Sechenov, I. ([1965a?]). Physiology of the nervous system (selected chapters). In G. Gibbons, ed., *I. Sechenov: Selected Physiological and Psychological Works* (S. Belsky, trans., pp. 511–525). Moscow: Foreign Languages Publishing House. (Original work published 1866)

Sechenov, I. (1965b). *Autobiographical Notes* (K. Hanes, trans.). Washington, DC: American Institute of Biological Sciences. (Original work published 1904)

Seguin, E. C. (1868). A statement of the aphasia question, together with a report of fifty cases. *Quarterly Journal of Psychological Medicine* (New York) ii: 74–119.

Sewall, T. (1828). Two cases of injury to the head, accompanied with a loss of brain. *American Journal of the Medical Sciences* 2: 62–63.

Shattuck, L. (1855). *Memorials of the Descendants of William Shattuck* (Vol. 1). Boston: Dutton and Wentworth. (Vol. 2 in 1977 by B. M. Larson).

Sherrington, C. S. (1906). *The Integrative Action of the Nervous System.* New York: Scribner's.

Sherrington, C. S. (1937). Sir David Ferrier. In J. R. H. Weaver, ed., *The Dictionary of National Biography 1922–1930* (pp. 302–304). Oxford: Oxford University Press.

Shipman, A. B. (1848). Cases of injury of the head, with remarks. *Boston Medical and Surgical Journal* 38: 353–380.

Shuck, O. T. (1894). *Official Roll of San Francisco ab initio.* San Francisco: Press of Dempster Brothers.

Shutts, D. (1982). *Lobotomy: Resort to the Knife.* New York: Van Nostrand Reinhold.

Signoret, J. L., Castaigne, P., Lhermitte, F., Abelanet, R., and Lavorel, P. (1984). Rediscovery of Leborgne's brain: Anatomical description with CT scan. *Brain and Language* 22: 303–319.

Singer, C. (1952). *Vesalius on the Human Brain*. London: Oxford University Press.

Singer, S., and Hilgard, H. R. (1978). *The Biology of People*. San Francisco: W. H. Freeman.

Sizer, N. (1882). *Forty Years in Phrenology: Embracing Recollections of History, Anecdote, and Experience*. New York: Fowler and Wells.

Smith, A. (1984). *The Mind*. London: Hodder and Stoughton.

Smith, A. (1985). *The Body*. Harmondsworth, England: Penguin.

Smith, C. U. M. (1970). *The Brain: Towards an Understanding*. London: Faber and Faber.

Smith, P. B. (1892). Revolver wound of the brain; lodgment of the bullet; recovery. *British Medical Journal* ii: 627–629.

Smith, R. (1992). *Inhibition: History and Meaning in the Sciences of Mind and Brain*. Berkeley and Los Angeles: University of California Press.

Smith, R. E. (1993). *Psychology*. Minneapolis-St. Paul, MN: West.

Smith, T. (1879). A case of bullet-wound of the anterior lobes of the brain. *Lancet* i: 622–624.

Smith, W. (1858). Report of a case of fracture of the skull, with severe injury of the brain; recovery. *Lancet* i: 626.

Soury, J. (1892). *Les Fonctions du Cerveau*. Paris: Bureau du Progrés Médical.

Spence, G. W. (1856–1857). Remarkable case of gunshot wound of the face, orbit, and brain. *Edinburgh Medical Journal* 84: 416–418.

Spillane, J. D. (1981). *The Doctrine of the Nerves: Chapters in the History of Neurology*. London: Oxford University Press.

Spurling, R. G. (1929). Lobectomy for left occipital lobe tumour. *Kentucky Medical Journal* 27: 525.

Stainbrook, E. (1948). The use of electricity in psychiatric treatment during the nineteenth century. *Bulletin of the History of Medicine* 22: 156–177.

Standing Committee on Surgery. (1850). Report. *Transactions of the American Medical Association* 3: 345.

Stapleton, M. H. (1858). Case of wound of the head. *Dublin Medical Press* 40: 387.

Starling, E. H. (1897). *Manual of Human Physiology* (3d ed.). London: Churchill.

Starr, M. A. (1884a). Cortical lesions of the brain. A collection and analysis of the American cases of localized cerebral disease. *American Journal of the Medical Sciences* 87: 366–391.

Starr, M. A. (1884b). Cortical lesions of the brain. A collection and analysis of the American cases of localized cerebral disease. *American Journal of the Medical Sciences* 88: 114–141.

Stearns, E. S., Whitcher, W. F., and Parker, E. E. (1908). *Genealogical and Family History of the State of New Hampshire: A Record of the Achievements of Her People in the Making of a Commonwealth and the Founding of a Nation.* New York: Lewis.

Steegmann, A. T. (1962). Dr. Harlow's famous case: The "impossible" accident of Phineas P. Gage. *Surgery* 52: 952–958.

Steno, N. (1950). *Discours de Monsieur Stenon sur l'anatomie du Cerveau* (E. Gotfredsen, ed., and G. Douglas, trans.). Copenhagen: Busck. (Original work published 1669)

Stern, M. B. (1971). *Heads and Headlines: The Phrenological Fowlers.* Norman: University of Oklahoma Press.

Stern, M. B. (1987). *The Selected Letters of Louisa May Alcott.* Boston: Little, Brown.

Stevens, L. A. (1971). *Explorers of the Brain.* New York: Knopf.

Stewart, G. N. (1899). *A Manual of Physiology* (3d ed.). Philadelphia: Saunders.

Stone, J. L. (1999). Transcranial brain injuries caused by metal rods or pipes over the past 150 years. *Journal of the History of the Neurosciences* 8: 227–234.

Stone, J. L. (1991). Paul Broca and the first craniotomy based on cerebral localization. *Journal of Neurosurgery* 75: 154–159.

Stone, J. L., Rifai, M. H. S., and Moody, R. A. (1981). An unusual case of penetrating head injury with excellent recovery. *Surgical Neurology* 15: 369–371.

Stone, W. L. (1901). *Washington County, New York: Its History to the Close of the Nineteenth Century.* New York: New York History Company.

Stookey, B. (1954). A note on the early history of cerebral localization. *Bulletin of the New York Academy of Medicine* 30: 559–578.

Stout, G. F. (1899). *A Manual of Psychology.* New York: Hinds and Noble.

Stuss, D. T. (1996). Frontal lobes. In J. G. Beaumont, P. M. Kennedy, and M. J. C. Rogers, eds., *The Blackwell Dictionary of Neuropsychology* (pp. 346–353). Oxford: Blackwell.

Stuss, D. T., and Benson, D. F. (1983). Emotional concomitants of psychosurgery. In K. H. Heilman and P. Satz, eds., *Neuropsychology of Human Emotion* (pp. 111–140). New York: Guilford.

Suinn, R. M. (1970). *Fundamentals of Behavior Pathology* (2d ed.). New York: Wiley.

Sutton, W. L. (1850–1851). A centre shot. *Boston Medical and Surgical Journal* 43: 241.

Svanevik, M., and Burgett, S. (1992). *Pillars of the Past: A Guide to Cypress Lawn Memorial Park, Colma, California.* San Francisco: Custom and Limited Editions.

Svanevik, M., and Burgett, S. (1995). *City of Souls: San Francisco's Necropolis at Colma.* San Francisco: Custom and Limited Editions.

Swetland, B. S., ed. (1907). *Partial Genealogy of the Swetland Family*. Brocton, NY: Brocton Enterprise Press.

Tavris, C., and Wade, C. (1997). *Psychology in Perspective* (2d ed.). New York: Longman.

Taylor, J. (1920). John Hughlings Jackson. In S. Lee, ed., *The Dictionary of National Biography Supplement 1901–1911* (pp. 302–304). Oxford: Oxford University Press.

Temkin, O. (1953). Remarks on the neurology of Gall and Spurzheim. In E. A. Underwood, ed., *Science, Medicine and History* (Vol. 2, pp. 282–289). London: Oxford University Press. (Reprinted in 1975 in New York by ARNO Press)

Teuber, H.-L. (1964). The riddle of frontal function in man. In J. M. Warren and K. Akert, eds., *The Frontal Granular Cortex and Behavior* (pp. 410–444). New York: McGraw-Hill.

Theodoric. (1955). *The Surgery of Theodoric. ca. A.D. 1267* (E. Campbell and J. Colton, trans.). New York: Appleton-Century-Crofts. (Original work published 1267)

Thomas, F., de Troisvèvre. (1826). *Physiologie des Tempéramens ou Constitutions, Nouvell doctrine applicable à la Médicine pratique*. Paris: Baillère.

Thomas, R. K., and Young, C. D. (1993). A note on the early history of electrical stimulation of the human brain. *Journal of General Psychology* 120: 73–81.

Thompson, Z. (1842). *History of Vermont, Natural, Civil and Statistical*. Burlington, VT: Chauncey Goodrich.

Thornton, J. (1896). *Human Physiology* (2d ed.). London: Longmans, Green.

Tilney, F., and Riley, H. A. (1921). *The Form and Function of the Central Nervous System*. New York: Hoeber.

Todd, R. B., and Bowman, W. (1845). *The Physiological Anatomy and Physiology of Man* (Vols. 1 and 2). London: Parker.

Todd, R. B., and Bowman, W. (1856). *The Physiological Anatomy and Physiology of Man* (Vols. 1 and 2). London: Parker.

Tow, P. M. (1955). *Personality Changes Following Frontal Leucotomy*. London: Oxford University Press.

Treisman, M. (1968). Mind, body, and behavior: Control systems and their disturbances. In P. London and D. Rosenhan, eds., *Foundations of Abnormal Psychology* (pp. 460–518). New York: Holt, Rinehart, and Winston.

Trotter, W. (1934). A landmark in modern neurology. *Lancet* ii: 1207–1210.

Troy Conference Academy. (1838a). *Catalogue of the Corporation, Faculty, and Students for the Fall and Winter Term of 1837–1838*. Rutland, VT: [Troy Conference Academy?].

Troy Conference Academy. (1838b). *Catalogue of the Corporation, Faculty, and Students for the Spring and Summer Term of 1838*. Lansingburgh, VT: [Troy Conference Academy?].

Turner, W. (1866). The convolutions of the human cerebrum topographically considered. *Edinburgh Medical Journal* 11: 1105–1122.

Tyler, K. L., and Tyler, H. R. (1982). A "Yankee Invention": The celebrated American crowbar case. *Neurology* 32: A191.

Urdang, L., Hunsinger, W. W., and LaRoche, N., eds. (1985). *Picturesque Expressions: A Thematic Dictionary*. Detroit, MI: Gale.

Unzer, J. A. (1851). *Principles of Physiology* (T. Laycock, trans.). London: Sydenham Society. (Original work published 1771)

U. S. Bureau of the Census. (1960). *Historical Statistics of the United States. Colonial Times to 1957*. Washington, DC: U.S. Government Printing Office.

U. S. Census Office. (1841). *Sixth Census or Enumeration of the Inhabitants of the United States in 1840*. Washington, DC: Blair and Rives.

U. S. Census Office. (1853). *Seventh Census of the United States: 1850*. Washington, DC: Robert Armstrong.

U. S. Surgeon General's Office. (1865). *Circular No. 6: Reports on the Extent and Nature of the Materials Available for the Preparation of a Medical and Surgical History of the Rebellion*. Philadelphia: SGO/Lippincott.

U. S. Surgeon General's Office. (1870). *The Medical and Surgical History of the War of the Rebellion*. Washington, DC: U.S. Government Printing Office.

U. S. Surgeon General's Office. (1871). *Circular No. 3: A Report of Surgical Cases Treated in the Army of the United States*. Washington, DC: U.S. Government Printing Office.

Valenstein, E. S. (1986). *Great and Desperate Cures: The Rise and Decline of Psychosurgery and Other Radical Treatments for Mental Illness*. New York: Basic Books.

Viets, H. R. (1930). *A Brief History of Medicine in Massachusetts*. Boston: Mifflin.

Vincent, J. D. (1996). Sexuality. In J. G. Beaumont, P. M. Kennedy, and M. J. C. Rogers, eds., *The Blackwell Dictionary of Neuropsychology* (pp. 661–665). Oxford: Blackwell.

Vital Records of Acton, Massachusetts to the Year 1850. (1923). Boston: New England Historic Genealogical Society.

von Chelius, J. M. (1847). *A System of Surgery* (Vols. 1 and 2, J. F. South, trans.). London: Renshaw (translation of 6th German edition of ? 1843).

Vulpian, A. (1866). *Leçons sur le Physiologie Générale et Comparée du Systéme Nerveux*. Paris: Baillière.

Waite, F. C. (1949). *The First Medical College in Vermont: Castleton: 1818–1862*. Montpelier: Vermont Historical Society.

Walke, J. W. (1849). Case of extensive fracture of the os frontis with escape of a portion of the cerebral substance—Recovery. *American Journal of the Medical Sciences* 17: 238.

Walker, A. E. (1951). *A History of Neurological Surgery*. Baltimore: Williams and Wilkins.

Walker, A. E. (1957a). The development of the concept of cerebral localization in the nineteenth century. *Bulletin of the History of Medicine* 31: 99–121.

Walker, A. E. (1957b). Stimulation and ablation: Their role in the history of cerebral physiology. *Journal of Neurophysiology* 20: 435–449.

Walker, A. E. (1959). The dawn of neurosurgery. In *Congress of Neurological Surgeons, Clinical Neurology* Vol. 6, pp. 1–40. Baltimore: Williams and Wilkins.

Wallace, E. R. (1992). Freud and the mind-body problem. In T. Gelfand and J. Kerr, eds., *Freud and the History of Psychoanalysis* (pp. 231–269). Hillsdale, NJ: Analytic Press.

Walsh, A. A. (1976a). The "New Science of the Mind" and Philadelphia physicians in the early 1800's. *Transactions and Studies of the College of Physicians of Philadelphia* 43: 397–415.

Walsh, A. A. (1976b). Phrenology and the Boston medical community in the 1830's. *Bulletin of the History of Medicine* 50: 261–273.

Walsh, K. W. (1978). *Neuropsychology: A Clinical Approach*. Edinburgh: Churchill Livingstone.

Walsh, K. W. (1985). *Understanding Brain Damage: A Primer of Neuropsychological Evaluation*. Edinburgh: Churchill Livingstone.

Walton, E. P. (1846). *Walton's Vermont Register and Farmer's Almanac for 1846*. Montpelier, VT: Walton.

Walton, E. P. (1847). *Walton's Vermont Register and Farmer's Almanac for 1847*. Montpelier, VT: Walton.

Walton, E. P. (1857). *Walton's Vermont Register and Farmer's Almanac for 1857*. Montpelier, VT: Walton.

Walton, E. P. (1858). *Walton's Vermont Register and Farmer's Almanac for 1858*. Montpelier, VT: Walton.

Ware, W. P., and Lockhard, T. C. (1980). *P. T. Barnum Presents Jenny Lind*. Baton Rouge: Louisiana State University Press.

Warner, J. H. (1986). *The Therapeutic Perspective: Medical Practice, Knowledge, and Identity in America, 1820–1885*. Cambridge: Harvard University Press.

Warren, H. C. (1912). *A History of the Association Psychology*. New York: Scribner's.

Warren, H. C. (1920). *Human Psychology*. Boston: Mifflin.

Way, P. (1993). *Common Labour: Workers and the Digging of North American Canals 1780–1860*. Cambridge: Cambridge University Press.

Weber, E. F. W., and Weber, E. H. W. (1966). Experiments by which it is proved that when stimulated with a rotary electro-magnetic apparatus the vagus nerves slow down and, to a considerable extent, interrupt the heart-beat. In J. F. Fulton, ed., *Readings in the History of Physiology* (2d ed., p. 296). Springfield, IL: Thomas. (Original work published 1845)

Weisfeld, G. E. (1997). Discrete emotions theory with specific reference to pride and shame. In N. L. Segal, G. E. Weisfeld, and C. C. Weisfeld, eds., *Uniting Psychology and Biology: Integrative Perspectives on Human Development* (pp. 419–443). Washington, DC: American Psychological Association.

Werner, M. R. (1926). *Barnum*. Garden City, NY: Garden City.

Wharton, J. (1818). A case of fracture of the cranium, attended with a loss of cerebral substance. *American Medical Recorder* (Philadelphia) 1: 11–13.

Wheeler, L. (1952). *History of Cavendish, Vermont*. Proctorsville, VT: Author.

Whitaker, H. (1998). History of neurolinguistics: Neurolinguistics from the Middle Ages to the pre-modern era. In B. Stemmer and H. Whitaker (eds.), *Handbook of Neurolinguistics* (pp. 27–54). San Diego, CA: Academic Press.

Whitaker, H., and Luzzatti, C. (1997, June). *The third ventricle: Memory and memory disorders in the late Middle Ages and Renaissance*. Paper presented to the 2nd Meeting of the International Society for the History of the Neurosciences and the 6th Meeting of the European Club on the History of Neurology, Leiden, Netherlands.

Whitaker, H. A., Stemmer, B., and Joanette, Y. (1996). A psychosurgical chapter in the history of cerebral localization: The six cases of Gottlieb Burckhardt (1891). In C. Code, C.-W. Wallesch, A.-R. Lecours, and Y. Joanette, eds., *Classic Cases in Neuropsychology* (pp. 275–304). London: Erlbaum.

Wiersma, C. A. G. (1961). Inhibitory neurons: A survey of the history of their discovery and of their occurrence. In E. Florey, ed., *Nervous Inhibition* (pp. 1–7). Oxford: Pergamon.

Willett, R. A. (1960). The effects of psychosurgical procedures on behaviour. In H. J. Eysenck, ed., *Handbook of Abnormal Psychology* (pp. 566–610). London: Pitman Medical.

Williams, IV., E. H. (1997). A sketch of Dr. Edward H. Williams. *Root and Branch* 3: 1–8. (Published by the Williams Family Association)

Williams, S. W. (1835). Case of extensive injury of the brain, from the kick of a horse. *Boston Medical and Surgical Journal* 11: 212–214.

Wilson, A. (1879). The old phrenology and the new. *Gentleman's Magazine* 244: 68–85.

Wilson, C. (1969). *The Philosopher's Stone*. London: Barker.

Windsor, W. (1921). *Phrenology the Science of Character*. Big Rapids, MI: Ferris-Windsor.

Wood Jones, F., and Porteus, S. D. (1928). *The Matrix of the Mind*. Honolulu: University Press Association.

Woodill, G., and LeNormand, M.-T. (1991, January). *The concept of aphasia before Freud: A sociology of science approach*. Paper presented to the History of Brain Functions Conference, Ft. Myers, Florida.

Wooldridge, D. E. (1963). *The Machinery of the Brain*. New York: McGraw-Hill.

Woollam, D. H. M. (1958). Concepts of the brain and its functions in classical antiquity. In F. N. L. Poynter, ed., *The History and Philosophy of Knowledge of the Brain and Its Functions* (pp. 5–18). Oxford: Blackwell Scientific.

Woolsey, C. N. (1951, April). *David Ferrier's contributions to cerebral localization*. Paper presented at the Wisconsin Medical History Seminar, Madison.

Wriston, J. W. (1991). *Vermont Inns and Taverns, Pre-Revolution to 1925: An Illustrated and Annotated Checklist*. Rutland, VT: Academy Books.

Wundt, W. (1897). *Outlines of Psychology* (C. H. Judd, trans.). New York: Stechert. (Original work published 1896)

WNET/13 (1984). *The Brain* (Episode 4: Stress and Emotion). New York: WNET/13.

Yakovlev, P. I. (1958). The "Crowbar Skull" and mementoes of "Phrenological Hours." *Harvard Medical Alumni Bulletin*, October: 19–24.

Yerkes, R. M. (1911). *Introduction to Psychology*. New York: Holt.

Young, R. M. (1970). *Mind Brain and Adaptation in the Nineteenth Century*. Oxford: Clarendon.

Zimbardo, P. G., and Ruch, F. L. (1979). *Psychology and Life* (10th ed.). Glenview, IL: Scott, Foresman.

Index

Bridgeman, Benjamin Hatch, 101;
121n. 11
Bridgman, A. M., 365n. 5; 366n. 12
Broadbent, W. H., 203n. 17
Broca, Paul, 201n. 13; 202nn. 15, 16;
226n. 1
 diagnosis and brain surgery (1871),
 205–208
 theory of aphasia and localization, 4,
 189–195
Brooke, [?], 68n. 7
Brooks, N., 304n. 6
Browder, J., 311; 251n. 6; 334n. 8
Brown, B., 65; 68n. 7; 69n. 17
Brown, H., 252n. 9; 334nn. 15, 18,
20; 336n. 30
Brown, J. W., 201n. 13
Browne, W. A. F., 201n. 14
Brown-Sequard, C. E., 193; 203n. 17
Brunton, T. L., 255–256; 276nn. 1, 3
Buell, P. L., and Sizer, N., 32n. 12;
345; 347–348; 366nn. 7, 9
Bull, J. W. D., 251n. 4
Burckhardt, G., 231–233, 249–250;
251n. 2
Burrage, W. L., 120n. 5; 367n. 15

"C.'s" letter about Gage, 40–41
Cabot, S., 68n. 7; 69n. 13
Caldwell, C., 366n. 8
Calkins, M. W., 334n. 9
Callander, R., 269
Campbell, A. W., 373; 379n. 3
Capen, N., 171n. 8
Capon, H. J., 68n. 7
Cardno, J., 172n. 20
Carlson, N. R., 252n. 9; 326; 334n.
16; 335nn. 18, 21; 336n. 34; 337n.
39
Carmichael, [?], 68n. 7; 69nn. 12, 13,
16
Carola, R., Harley, J. P., and Noback,
C. R., 277n. 12
Carpenter, W. B., 146; 170n. 1; 172n.
21; 333n. 2

posterior localization of intellectual
functions, 334n. 6
Carr, M., 31n. 4
Carter, K. C., 68n. 4
Cases
Joe A. (Brickner's patient), 237–239;
251n. 5
Lewis Henry Avery (Noyes's patient),
62–64; 69n. 15
Frau Borel (Burckhardt's patient),
231–232; 251n. 2
Charles Burklin (Prewitt's patient),
220–222; 228n, 15
The forty-year-old farmer (McBurney
and Starr's patient), 206, 215–216;
226n. 1, 227n. 10
The fourteen-year-old girl
(Macewen's patient), 206, 212–213;
226n. 1, 227n. 7
Mr. Henderson (Bennett and
Godlee's patient), 206, 210–211;
226n. 1, 227n. 6
Joel Lenn (Jewett's patient), 66, 113,
435–438, 440
The male lacking decency (Elder and
Miles's patient), 216–217; 227n. 11
K. M., (Milner's case, Hebb and
Penfield's patient), 373–374; 380n.
4
Friedrich August N. (Burckhardt's
patient), 232–233; 251n. 2
Mary Rafferty (Bartholow's patient),
208–210; 226n. 4
Corporal George Washington Stone
(Union Army patient), 220–221;
228n, 14
The thirty-eight-year-old man
(Broca's patient), 205–206, 207–
208; 226n. 1
The young man (Macewen's patient),
206, 208; 226nn. 1, 3
Castaigne, P., Lhermitte, F., Signoret,
J. L., and Abelant, R., 202n. 15
Castiglioni, A., 201n. 14
Castleton Medical College, 365n. 3

See also Bigelow, H. J.; Harlow, J. M.

Gage, Phineas (fiction and semifiction)
Blackington's "The Man with a Hole in His Head," 293–295
The Brain (WNET/13 television series), 284–286
Brooks's "The Man with a Hole in His Head," 290–293
in folklore, popular history and culture, 298
Lamere's "Phineas Gage Had a Headache," 295–296
Madness (Miller's television series), 286–288
Sur les Traces de Phineas Gage (Georget's television film), 288–290
Wilson's *The Philosopher's Stone*, 296–297

Gage, Phineas (physiological damage)
Bigelow's assessment, 42–45
to brain, 82–87
Harlow's assessment, 51–55, 82–83
left lateral ventricle, 80, 83, 84, 142
to skull, 71–82
as standard for brain injuries, 66–67

Gage, Phineas (postaccident behavior and experiences)
additions to Harlow's accounts, 116–119, 319–324
his balance, 319–320
Bigelow's account (1850), 41–47, 390–400, 444–460
descriptions of changes, 372
evidence of drinking problem, 329–330
his fitfulness, irritability, and obstinance, 320–322
Harlow's account (1848), 12, 72–74, 82, 86, 90–94, 168, 371, 383–387, 388–389, 443–460
Harlow's account (1868), 12–13, 41–42, 72–74, 82–83, 86, 90–94, 169, 332, 371, 403–422, 443–460
Harlow's account of postrecovery life, 94–116

immediate postaccident behavior, 90–92
longer-term changes, 94
newspapers (1848, 1849), 11–12, 35–41
newspaper stories about, 298–301
his profanity, 320
relationship with P. T. Barnum, 98–100, 330–331
short-term postrecovery behavior, 92–94
Sizer's account in context of phrenology, 347–351
various elaborations, 322–324

Gage, Phineas (preaccident behavior and experiences)
assumptions about education of, 16–17; 31n. 5
description by Harlow, 13, 318
location of parent's farm, 31n. 5
modified descriptions based on Harlow, 318–319
and psychology, 90
railroad employment, 12–13, 17–23
tamping iron donation, 46–47

Gainotti, G., 334n. 14
Galen, 126, 133, 136; 144n. 9
Gall, Franz Josef, 144n. 16; 170nn. 1, 2, 3, 4, 5; 171nn. 6, 7, 8, 9, 10
answers charge of materialism, 171n. 9
brain's language function, 149
correlation of his faculties with Ferrier's centers, 203n. 19
discovery of brain's faculties, 142–143, 145, 150–151
explanations of human traits and behavior, 147–151, 268
faculties as nonmaterial "essences," 149; 171n. 9
fails to see connection between hemiplegia and aphasia, 201n. 14
first empirical psychologist, 170n. 4
inferences about brain injury effect on language, 149, 188–189, 192